THIRD EDITION

D0521079

DREEBEN-IRIMIA'S INTRODUCTION TO
Physical Therapist Practice

for Physical Therapist Assistants

Christina M. Barrett, PT, MEd

Program Director

Physical Therapist Assistant Program

Lake Area Technical Institute

Watertown, South Dakota

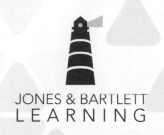

JONES & BARTLETT
LEARNING

World Headquarters
Jones & Bartlett Learning
5 Wall Street
Burlington, MA 01803
978-443-5000
info@jblearning.com
www.jblearning.com

Jones & Bartlett Learning books and products are available through most bookstores and online booksellers. To contact Jones & Bartlett Learning directly, call 800-832-0034, fax 978-443-8000, or visit our website, www.jblearning.com.

Substantial discounts on bulk quantities of Jones & Bartlett Learning publications are available to corporations, professional associations, and other qualified organizations. For details and specific discount information, contact the special sales department at Jones & Bartlett Learning via the above contact information or send an email to specialsales@jblearning.com.

Production Credits

VP, Executive Publisher: David D. Cella
Publisher: Cathy L. Esperti
Associate Acquisitions Editor: Kayla Dos Santos
Associate Director of Production: Julie C. Bolduc
Marketing Manager: Grace Richards
VP, Manufacturing and Inventory Control: Therese Connell

Composition: Cenveo Publisher Services
Cover Design: Scott Moden
Rights & Media Specialist: Jamey O'Quinn
Cover Image: © Knikola/Shutterstock
Printing and Binding: LSC Communications
Cover Printing: LSC Communications

Library of Congress Cataloging-in-Publication Data

Names: Barrett, Christina M., 1967- , author. | Dreeben-Irimia, Olga.
   Introduction to physical therapy for physical therapist assistants.
   Preceded by (work):
Title: Dreeben-Irimia's introduction to physical therapist practice for
   physical therapist assistants / Christina Barrett.
Other Titles: Introduction to physical therapist practice for physical
   therapist assistants
Description: Third edition. | Burlington, MA : Jones & Bartlett Learning,
   2016. | Preceded by Introduction to physical therapy for physical
   therapist assistants / Olga Dreeben-Irimia. 2nd ed. 2011. | Includes
   bibliographical references and index.
Identifiers: LCCN 2015041962 | ISBN 9781449681852 (pbk.)
Subjects: | MESH: Physical Therapy Specialty–methods. | Physical Therapist
   Assistants. | Physical Therapy Modalities.
Classification: LCC RM705 | NLM WB 460 | DDC 615.8/2–dc23
LC record available at http://lccn.loc.gov/2015041962

6048

Printed in the United States of America
20 19 18   10 9 8 7 6 5

To all my past, present, and future students for understanding my crazy awesome love of physical therapy.

Brief Contents

Contents

PART II   Physical Therapist Practice   71

CHAPTER 4   Examination, Evaluation, and Plan of Care 73

CHAPTER 5   Physical Therapy Practice Areas 85

PART IV   Communication   139

CHAPTER 8   Communication Basics. 141

CHAPTER 9   Introduction to Documentation and the Medical Record. . . 155

PART V   Planning for Success   191

CHAPTER 12   Student Learning Success   193

CHAPTER 13   Lifelong Success   203

Preface

I have been given a wonderful opportunity, a privilege really, to revise Olga Dreeben-Irimia's *Introduction to Physical Therapy for Physical Therapist Assistants* textbook. This textbook has been a mainstay of physical therapist assistant (PTA) education and has provided beginning physical therapist assistant students with the basic understanding of the role and profession. I hope that this *Third Edition* lives up to the expectations of the readers and helps them develop an understanding and enthusiasm for the profession.

When students choose to enter physical therapist assistant school, their decision usually revolves around the idea that they enjoy helping people. Service professions are rooted in the intrinsic feelings that helping others gives and the satisfaction of seeing progress in patients' function. The understanding of pathology, development of skills, and assimilation of behaviors are all required to enter the role of a physical therapist assistant. This textbook's goal is to present information in a way that students appreciate all that is necessary to learn to become an effective physical therapist assistant. Knowledge of the basics begins with an introduction to the profession and health care. An overall grasp of what will be learned helps students realize how the components of a physical therapist assistant curriculum connect to prepare them for this role. This will help the students map out a plan for success in both their education and career.

STRUCTURE OF THE TEXT

The textbook is broken into five parts:

- *Part I: The Profession of Physical Therapy* introduces the reader to the profession of physical therapy.
  - *Chapter 1: The Physical Therapist Profession*, a historical overview, describes the progression of the profession in both skills and creation of a unique identity that separates it from other professions. With an appreciation of the history and growth of physical therapist practice, it is easier to understand how the role of the physical therapist assistant can work effectively in a health care team.
  - *Chapter 2: The Physical Therapist Assistant as a Member of the Health Care Team* introduces the reader to each of the members of the health care team and describes what role the physical therapist assistant has in the team. A detailed discussion of the relationship between the physical therapist and physical therapist assistant describes the supervisory and collaborative role the two have in patient care.
  - *Chapter 3: Physical Therapist Clinical Practice* completes the introduction by explaining practice issues to assist the learner in appreciating patient-related components of physical therapist practice and management issues. An understanding of the *Guide to Physical Therapist Practice* helps the student see the broad picture of physical therapy. Practice settings are explained including: acute care, primary care centers, sub acute facilities, outpatient care, rehabilitation hospitals, chronic care facilities, hospice, home health services, school systems, and private practice facilities. An understanding of job applications, resumes, and interviews will allow the PTA student to learn skills and effective behaviors that will be nurtured and developed throughout the professional program coursework.
- *Part II: Physical Therapist Practice* covers physical therapy evaluation and the major physical therapist practice specialties.
  - *Chapter 4: Examination, Evaluation, and Plan of Care* explains the components of the initial

visit with the patient. An understanding of the process and terminology of physical therapy will assist the student in being more effective in treating the patient.

- *Chapter 5: Physical Therapy Practice Areas* explains the specific areas of practice: orthopedic, neurologic, pediatric, geriatric, cardiopulmonary, and integumentary.

- *Part III: Ethical and Legal Issues* includes *Chapter 6: Ethics and Professionalism* and *Chapter 7: Laws and Regulations*. This part explains the ethical, legal, and professional components of providing health care services. An understanding of confidentiality, cultural competence, and laws along with the expectations of conduct for a PTA provides the basis for PTA interaction with the patients.
- *Part IV: Communication* comprises Chapters 8–11 and describes aspects of communication.
  - *Chapter 8: Communication Basics* lays the groundwork for learning the skills for successful verbal and nonverbal communication with patients and with colleagues.
  - *Chapter 9: Introduction to Documentation and the Medical Record* introduces the basics to writing effective documentation and appropriate written communication with a variety of audiences.
  - *Chapter 10: Teaching and Learning* discusses teaching techniques for patient instruction that will help students develop skills that will work in a variety of settings and with a variety of patients.
  - *Chapter 11: Reimbursement and Research* helps students understand reimbursement by a variety of payer sources and allows an understanding of restrictions that may be in place. Research techniques and an understanding of evidence-based practices complete Part IV.
- *Part V: Planning for Success* completes the textbook by describing how the student can be most successful during PTA school (*Chapter 12: Student Learning Success*) and how to develop career success (*Chapter 13: Lifelong Success*).

NEW TO THE *THIRD EDITION*

- The addition *Chapter 6: Ethics and Professionalism* will allow the student to understand the process of dealing with ethical issues and work through the process to make a decision.

- *Part V: Planning for Success* is entirely new, including two chapters to assist students in educational success and career development. The focus is on developing career-ready skills and behaviors and understanding how to develop a plan for lifelong learning and career success.

- Important data updates have been made throughout the text. As the student will learn, health care and physical therapy are constantly being updated with research on effective techniques, changes in health care policy, and new technology advances. These updates bring the book up to speed with the latest *APTA Guide 3.0*.

- APTA documents have been added, including the Vision Statement, Strategic Plan, Minimum Skills of the PTA Graduate at Entry-Level, the Decision-Making Guide, and the Value-Based Behaviors for the PTA.

- Practice issues such as elder abuse, harassment, the development of professional attributes, and good teaching practices are introduced.

KEY FEATURES

Students will find learning tools developed specifically for the development of understanding the concepts presented in the textbook. Each chapter includes the following:

- **Learning Objectives** are new to this edition and have been included to focus the reader's learning on the core concepts.
- **Discussion Questions** push the reader's learning further with questions that assess and stretch the knowledge gained throughout the chapter.
- **Learning Opportunities** replace lab activities from the previous edition and present additional activities for readers to deepen their understanding.

- **Key Terms** are listed at the start of each chapter and defined in the new **end-of-book glossary** to provide readers with a quick guide to important terminology.

INSTRUCTOR RESOURCES

Instructors also have access to numerous resources including the following:

- **Clinical Scenarios** present real-world examples of the concepts introduced in the text and include questions that instructors can utilize to assess students' application of those concepts.

- **Slides with Lecture Outlines** for each chapter include slide decks that instructors can use as a starting point for teaching the content in their course. These slides now include additional notes for the instructor and additional images.

- **Test Banks** have been extensively revised from the previous edition and new questions added.

- **Practice Activities** have been supplied as suggested questions for students to use to study the material.

Note from Olga Dreeben-Irimia

My wonderful journey writing and publishing a new edition of *Introduction to Physical Therapy for Physical Therapist Assistants* is coming to an end. Although I feel a little sad for not being able to continue this trip of enhancing information and knowledge in the profession, I am happy to pass the torch to a new author, Professor Barrett.

Good luck to all of you in your new and exciting quest to become a physical therapist assistant!

Olga Dreeben-Irimia, PhD, (R)PT

About the Author

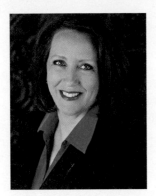

Christina M. Barrett is the Physical Therapist Assistant Program Director at Lake Area Technical Institute in Watertown, South Dakota. She received her Bachelor's degree in Physical Therapy from the University of North Dakota and a Masters of Education degree from the University of Phoenix. In her 20 years in academia, she has taught the fundamental theories and skills of physical therapy in all areas of practice to hundreds of students. She continues to work in clinical practice spending time in a variety of practice settings for Big Stone Therapies, Inc. She has been a proud member of the American Physical Therapy Association since 1989. She has had opportunities to work in leadership as both Delegate and President of the South Dakota chapter, and currently serves as membership chair. This membership has allowed her to work closely with her peers in promoting the continued development of the physical therapy profession.

Reviewers

Frank J. Bates, PT, DPT, MBA
Director and Assistant Professor
Physical Therapist Assistant Program
University of Indianapolis
Indianapolis, Indiana

Paula W. Duffy, PT
Instructor
Physical Therapist Assistant Program
Bishop State Community College
Mobile, Alabama

Julie Feeny, PTMS
Program Director
Physical Therapist Assistant Program
Illinois Central College
East Peoria, Illinois

Renae H. Gorman, PT, DPT, MTC, OCS, ACCE
Assistant Professor
Springfield Technical Community College
Springfield, Massachusetts

Charlene S. Jensen, PT, DPT
Program Director
Physical Therapist Assistant Program
Riverside College of Health Careers
Newport News, Virginia

Kelly McGovern, PT, DPT
Academic Coordinator of Clinical Education,
Instructor
Physical Therapist Assistant Program
Lackawanna College
Hawley, Pennsylvania

Kimberly Salyers, PTA, MA Ed
Physical Therapist Assistant Program
Coordinator
Physical Therapist Assistant Program
Florida Gateway College
Lake City, Florida

Debbie Van Dover, PT, MEd
Program Director
Physical Therapist Assistant Program
Mt. Hood Community College
Gresham, Oregon

Bruce Wassung, PTA, MSPH, PhD (cand)
Chair
Physical Therapist Assistant Program
Terra State Community College
Fremont, Ohio

PART I

The Profession of Physical Therapy

This part is divided into three chapters:

- CHAPTER 1: The Physical Therapist Profession
- CHAPTER 2: The Physical Therapist Assistant as a Member of the Health Care Team
- CHAPTER 3: Physical Therapist Clinical Practice

In these three chapters, we will discuss the history of rehabilitation treatments including therapeutic exercises, and the organization, history, values, and culture of the profession of physical therapy. We will also explore the differences in role, function, and supervisory relationship of the physical therapist (PT), the physical therapist assistant (PTA), and other health care practitioners and ancillary personnel.

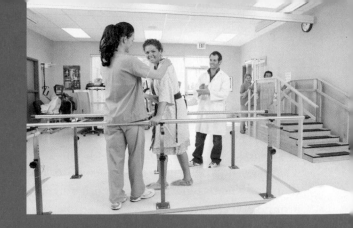

CHAPTER 1

The Physical Therapist Profession

OBJECTIVES

After studying this chapter, the reader will be able to:

1. Discuss the history of rehabilitation treatments (including therapeutic exercises) from ancient times through the 1900s.
2. Describe the history of the physical therapy profession and its five cycles of growth and development.
3. Identify the values and culture of the physical therapy profession.
4. Describe the APTA's mission and its goals in regard to PTs and PTAs.
5. Explain the organizational structure of the APTA.
6. Discuss the benefits of belonging to a professional organization.
7. Name the other organizations involved in the physical therapy profession.

KEY TERMS

American Physical Therapy Association (APTA)
Commission on Accreditation in Physical Therapy Education (CAPTE)

disability
functional limitations

History of Rehabilitation Treatments Including Therapeutic Exercises

It may be difficult to believe that some types of treatments utilized in physical therapy today, such as therapeutic massage, hydrotherapy (water therapy), and therapeutic exercises, were used in antiquity—around 3000 BC by the Chinese and around 400 BC by the Greeks and Romans. Therapeutic exercise and massage with aromatic oils were probably the first therapeutic modalities applied by the Greeks and Romans in a purposeful way to cure health problems. Written and pictorial records from the ancient civilizations of China, Japan, India, Greece, and Rome also contain descriptions and depictions of massage and exercise. Researchers have found evidence that the application of heat, cold, water, exercise, massage, and sunlight was often used to abate physical afflictions even during prehistoric times.

ANCIENT CHINA, INDIA, AND GREECE

Writings about therapeutic exercises came from the Taoist priests in China and originated sometime before 1000 BC. These writings describe a type of exercise called Cong Fu that was able to relieve pain and other symptoms. Later, around 500 BC in ancient Greece, Herodicus, a Greek physician, wrote about an elaborate system of exercises called *Ars Gymnastica*[1] or *The Art of Gymnastics*. In ancient Greece around 400 BC, Hippocrates, who is considered the father of medicine, recognized the value of muscle strengthening using exercises (**FIGURE 1-1**). Hippocrates[1] was the first physician in his time to recommend therapeutic exercises to his patients because he understood the principle of muscle, ligament, and bone atrophy (wasting) due to inactivity. In regard to rehabilitation treatments, Hippocrates wrote about the utility of friction after ligament tears and dislocations, and recommended abdominal kneading massage and chest clapping massage to improve digestion and relieve colds. Hippocrates was the first to

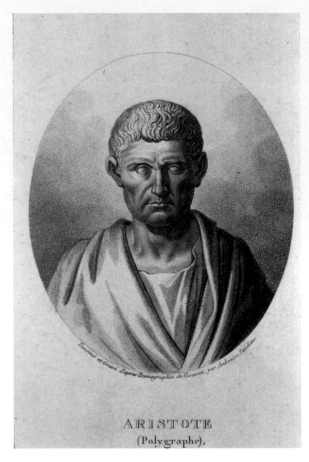

FIGURE 1-2 Aristotle.
© National Library of Medicine

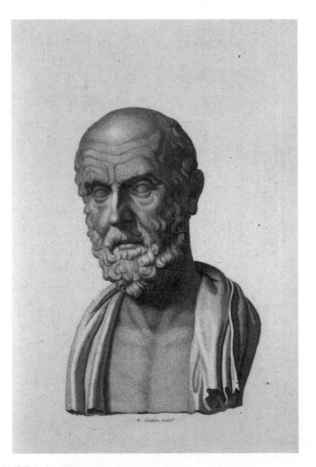

FIGURE 1-1 Hippocrates.
© National Library of Medicine

use electrical stimulation, applying torpedo-fish poultices for headaches. The torpedo fish has an electrical charge of approximately 80 volts to stun its prey. Also in the area of treatments, the Greek philosopher Aristotle[1] recommended rubbing massage using oil and water as a remedy for tiredness (**FIGURE 1-2**).

Around 180 BC, the ancient Romans[1] adopted a form of therapeutic exercises that they called *gymnastics*. The Roman gladiators and athletes used gymnastics in the Roman arenas and in popular exhibitions of athletics. Later, in the second century AD, Galen,[1] the renowned physician of ancient Rome, believed that moderate exercises strengthened the body, increased body temperature, allowed the pores of the skin to open, and improved a person's spiritual well-being (**FIGURE 1-3**). Galen[1] was also an authority on trauma surgery and musculoskeletal injuries. His extensive writings, advanced for his era, describe from a kinetic principle the roles of anatomy and physiology in human movement.

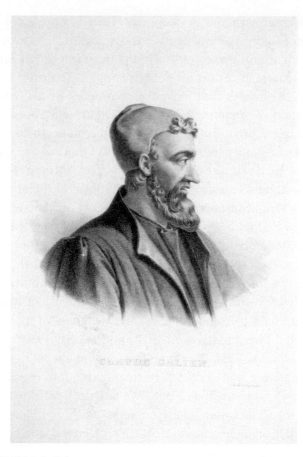

FIGURE 1-3 Galen.
© National Library of Medicine

EUROPE AND AMERICA FROM THE 1500S TO THE 1900S

In Europe around the 1400s, after the Middle Ages, therapeutic exercises[2] were introduced in schools as physical education courses. During the 1500s, the first printed book on exercise, entitled *Libro del Exercicio* and written by Christobal Mendez of Jaen,[2] was published in Spain. During the 1600s and 1700s, more books were written about exercises. These works promoted moderate exercises, stating that exercises give the body agility and vigor and also have the ability to cleanse the muscles and ligaments of waste.[2]

In the United States, massage, hydrotherapy, and exercises were first introduced around the year 1700. These rehabilitation treatments were based on ideas originating mostly in England. They were further developed in the 1800s and early 1900s.

In Europe in 1723, Nicolas Andry,[3] a professor at the Medical Faculty in Paris, was the first scientist to relate the movements created by exercises to the musculoskeletal system. Andry is considered to be the "grandfather"[3] of orthopedics.

During the 1800s, Per Henrik Ling,[4] a Swedish poet, fencing master, playwright, and educator, contributed to the growth of physical exercise by initiating the gymnastic movement. These gymnastic techniques, similar to Chinese manipulative therapy, were adopted in the 1800s by Dr. Johan Georg Mezger of Holland[4] (a Dutch practitioner). Dr. Mezger gave these types of manipulative therapy French names such as "effleurage," "petrissage," and "tapotement." These techniques (describing some of Ling's movements) became known as the *Swedish massage*.

Around the 1860s, George H. Taylor, an American physician[5] from Vermont who was the medical director of the Remedial Hygienic Institute in New York, introduced Ling's Swedish gymnastics for the first time in America. Swedish gymnastics became very popular in American public schools and had a significant impact upon physical education classes. Ling's exercises, consisting of passive and active movements, were also used to treat chronic disease conditions. In addition, Ling's medical gymnastics contributed to the development of Swedish massage as a therapeutic activity. Although Ling's system of exercise was effective, it required the continuous personal attention of a gymnast. In 1864, Gustav Zander,[6] a Swedish physician, invented different exercise machines that offered assistance and resistance to the patient.

Later, at the beginning of the 1900s, with the advent of World War I (1917), "reconstruction aides" (who began physical therapy in the United States) used Zander's machines as well as Ling's Swedish movement for the rehabilitation of disabled soldiers. In those early times, physical therapy was performed in various specialized rooms; one of the rooms was for "mechanotherapy" and contained Zander's exercise machines. Zander's apparatus seemed to work very well during the war.

At the beginning of the 1920s, after the passage of the Rehabilitation Bill in New Jersey, orthopedic surgeons[7] became enthusiastic about the future of rehabilitation and of "reconstruction aides or teachers of vocational and educational forms of work that are therapeutic in purpose."[7(p.39)] An article written in February 1920 in the *Journal of the Medical Society of New Jersey* described modern developments in rehabilitation, especially for "industrially injured"[7(p.43)] individuals. It was considered that "the sooner an industrially injured man gets safely back to work" the better it would be for his morale and physical well-being. In the 1920s, this required the injured worker to receive "active, voluntary joint-motion and muscle exercises."[7(p.44)] It is interesting that in the 1920s, orthopedic surgeons believed that these forms of rehabilitation using active exercises were to be provided by a "reconstruction aide," who was described as a combination of "the school teacher"[7(p.46)] and "the professional nurse."[7(p.46)]

In the 1860s, electrical stimulation was first introduced in the United States as a therapeutic modality, having originated in Europe and been used in France, England, and Germany. In the 1890s, the American Electro-Therapeutic Association was formed. Members included interested U.S. practitioners who promoted specialized training in electrotherapy, electrotherapeutic research, and the use of reliable electrotherapeutic equipment. Also in the 1890s, Nikola Tesla[8] introduced diathermy as an electrotherapeutic modality; however, it was not until the 1900s that diathermy's beneficial role as a deep heating agent for joints and the circulatory system was discovered.

In England around the beginning of the 1950s, a neurophysiologist (physician) named Herman Kabat[9] utilized newly discovered neurological concepts of stretch reflex, flexion reflex, and tonic neck reflex to develop neurological exercises called "proprioceptive facilitation." Around 1968, Margaret Knott and Dorothy Voss expanded[9] proprioceptive neuromuscular facilitation (PNF) as a form of physical therapy intervention for patients with paralysis. As is done today, the PNF method was recommended and utilized for patients who had paralysis produced by stroke, cerebral palsy, or another neurological dysfunction. Additionally, regarding neurological exercises and rehabilitation, toward the end of the 1800s, H.S. Frenkel[10] of Switzerland was able to improve an ataxic (unstable) gait resulting from nerve cell destruction by repetitive attempts at supervised ambulation. Frenkel did not rely on equipment, but instead marked the floor for successive placement of the feet in walking (as we do today using Frenkel's exercises). Frenkel advocated walking in groups of three to six patients with similar degrees of ataxia for long walking paths, insisting on repetitions.

In the United States during the 1900s, the area of therapeutic exercises was built up by physicians, physical therapists (PTs), surgeons, psychologists, and other scientists. All therapeutic exercises developed in the early 1900s greatly influenced the growth of physical therapy interventions. Robert Lovett's[11] concept was an example of such growth and development. Lovett, a professor of orthopedic surgery at Harvard, discovered in 1916 that muscle training exercises were the most important early therapeutic measures for polio treatment. Ten years later in 1926, Lovett's idea was put into practice by his senior assistant, Wilhelmine G. Wright. Wright[12] developed the training technique of ambulation with crutches (using the upper extremity muscles) for patients who had paraplegia or paralysis caused by polio. She also introduced the manual muscle testing procedure in physical therapy. In 1928, Wright authored the book[12] *Muscle Function* (which she started with Dr. Lovett), in which she described the systematic method of manual muscle testing using palpation, gravity, external manual resistance, and the arc of active movement. Wright believed in the importance of muscle testing on polio patients and the use of stronger muscles to compensate for the weakness of muscles affected by polio. Between 1917 and the early 1950s, several PTs and rehabilitation clinicians[12] made changes to Wright's method of muscle testing, taking into consideration variables such as a patient's fatigue, body position, and incoordination. These clinicians included Florence Kendall, Signe Brunnstrom, Marjorie Dennen, and Catherine Worthingham.

Another example of the developments made to combat the devastating effects of paralysis caused by the polio epidemic was Charles Leroy Lowman's[13] method of "hydrogymnastics." In California in 1924, he converted a lily pond into two treatment pools for the treatment of spasticity and paralysis caused by cerebral palsy. In the 1920s at Warm Springs, Georgia, Carl Hubbard[13] (an American engineer) installed the first metal tank (known today as the Hubbard tank) in a hospital for hydrogymnastics use. In 1928, U.S. President Franklin D. Roosevelt,[13] who had polio, used the hydrogymnastics therapy at Warm Springs Institute for rehabilitation. During the late 1920s, Roosevelt developed the institute known today as the Georgia Warm Springs Foundation, which has become an international polio treatment facility.

In the area of exercise for vascular disease, in 1924 Leo Buerger (a urologist) and Arthur W. Allen (a surgeon) created the Buerger-Allen exercises[14] for arterial insufficiency in the legs. The exercises used the effects of gravity and posture and applied those to the vascular musculature and blood circulation. Additionally, during the 1900s physicians began to treat back pain more efficiently. This was due to the use of x-rays to visualize and identify bone abnormalities and the dysfunction of curvature of the spine. An example of exercise development for back pain was Joel E. Goldthwait's discovery that the reasons for backaches were faulty posture[15] and habits. As a result, in 1934, Goldthwait and his colleagues wrote the book *Essentials of Body Mechanics*. In regard to back pain and exercises, in 1953, Paul C. Williams proposed a series of postural exercises, known today as the Williams exercises. These helped to strengthen the spine flexors and extensors and relieve back pain. Still in regard to exercises, around 1934, Ernest A. Codman, a Boston surgeon, introduced shoulder exercises known as Codman pendulum exercises. He pointed out that a diseased supraspinatus muscle could relax if the shoulder is abducted in the stooping position, allowing the arm to be under the influence of gravity. In the 1920s and 1930s, additional developments in the area of exercise were attributed to surgeons' findings that exercises could be helpful after surgery and that customary bed rest should be eliminated.

In 1938, Daniel J. Leithauser,[16] who performed appendectomies, was amazed to see that one of his patients who did not follow the usual bed rest routines was able to rapidly return to daily activities. Leithauser[16] prescribed early rising and physical activity for all postoperative appendectomies and abdominal surgeries. By 1947, there were many "convalescent centers," in the United States where patients were prescribed "convalescent exercises" or "reconditioning exercises" to counteract the deconditioning effect and the abuse of rest. In these centers, patients performed exercises in groups according to the **disability**. There were ankle classes, shoulder classes, or wheelchair basketball for patients who had paraplegia. Special centers were also created for major disabilities; for example, the centers for patients with amputations required PTs to exercise the amputated extremity early and through maximum range of motion to prepare it for the prosthesis.

In 1945, much of the greatest stimuli to the development of exercises came from an Alabama physician, Thomas DeLorme. Following his own knee surgery, DeLorme[17] found that he could rapidly restore his quadricep muscles to full strength by increasing the resistance applied to the exercising muscles. DeLorme's method first introduced the technique of progressive resistive exercise (PRE),[17] which is still used today.

During the second half of the 1900s, the area of therapeutic exercises in the United States was advanced tremendously by the arrival of isokinetic and biofeedback exercises. For example, in 1967, the Cybex I Dynamometer was introduced based on Helen Hislop and James Perrine's concept of isokinetic exercise. Hislop and Perrine found that muscular performance can be reduced to the physical parameters of force, work, power, and endurance, and that specificity of exercise should be determined by an exercise system designed to control each training need. Another type of exercise called biofeedback was also introduced in the second half of the 1900s as a result of advances in scientific behavioral psychology and clinical electromyography. Furthermore, Williams's back-flexion exercises were complemented in the 1950s and 1960s by Robin McKenzie's back-extension exercises that relieved pressure posteriorly on the spinal disk. Swiss ball exercises,[18] developed by physiotherapists in Switzerland in the 1960s, found their way to the United States in the 1970s and became popular in physical therapy rehabilitation in the 1980s.

History of the Physical Therapy Profession

The creation of the physical therapy profession centered around two major events in U.S. history: the poliomyelitis epidemics and the negative effects of World War I and World War II. The profession can be compared with a living entity, changing from an undeveloped, young occupation in its formative years (1914 to 1920) to a firm, growing establishment in its development years (1920 to 1940). As a mature profession, during its fundamental accomplishment years (1940 to 1970), physical therapy was able to achieve significant organizational, executive, and educational skills. In the mastery years (1970 to 1996), the profession acquired greater control, proficiency, and respect within the health care arena, growing largely in the areas of education, licensure, specialization, research, and direct access. From 1996 to 2005, in its adaptation years, physical therapy had to adapt, review, and make changes in its objectives and goals due to political, social, and economic changes in the United States. Additionally, the profession went through rapid educational expansion and research growth, and significant developmental and scientific goals were achieved. From 2006 to the present, in its vision and scientific pursuit years, physical therapy has been emerging as a vigorous participant in U.S. health care reform, having large responsibilities in the areas of research, education, and sociopolitical transformations.

FORMATIVE YEARS: 1914 TO 1920

Division of Special Hospitals and Physical Reconstruction

In the United States, physical therapy had its beginnings between 1914 and 1919, in a time known as the Reconstruction Era. Prior to the "Great War" (World War I), most Americans regarded disability as irreversible, requiring little or no medical intervention. The war changed this concept of irreversibility because of the large number of young U.S. men returning home as disabled veterans. As mentioned prior, physical therapy was created because of World War I and the poliomyelitis epidemics. These two devastating events in U.S. history brought a great degree of disease and disability to U.S. society. The first major outbreak of poliomyelitis occurred in New York State in 1916.[19] The methods of treatment at that time[19] were bed rest, isolation, and splinting and casting of the person's legs. Unfortunately, these forms of healing increased the individual's weakness in the legs and back, and as a result, the person required some form of exercise and physiotherapy.

Prior to and during World War I, support for people with disabilities had been growing gradually.[19] For example, the Medical Department of the U.S. Army had two divisions that influenced the growth of physical rehabilitation in the United States, the Division of Orthopedic Surgery and the Division of Physical Reconstruction. The newly created Division of Physical Reconstruction was needed to apply physiotherapy treatments such as massage and mechanical hydrotherapy to wounded soldiers. The Division of Physical Reconstruction drew its "training corps" personnel from schools of allied health therapies and physical training.[19] The Division of Physical Reconstruction had three sections:[19] surgery (including general, orthopedic, and head surgery) and neuropsychiatry, education, and physiotherapy (including gymnasiums and equipment).

In April 1917, the United States entered World War I. The U.S. Congress authorized the military draft and passed legislation to rehabilitate all servicemen permanently disabled from war-related injuries. In August 1917, the Surgeon General of the United States, William Gorgas, authorized the creation of the Division of Special Hospitals and Physical Reconstruction.[20] The role of the division was to give soldiers who were disabled "reconstruction therapy." The people involved in the reconstruction therapy

were newly trained physical reconstruction aides. They consisted of a handful of physicians called orthopedists and 1,200 young women called reconstruction aides. These people were the physical therapy and occupational therapy pioneers[20] who treated the injured soldiers from World War I. The division included two different groups of reconstruction aides. One group who assisted physicians was to become today's PTs. They provided exercise programs, massage, hydrotherapy, and other forms of therapeutic modalities including patient education. The other group of reconstruction aides was to become today's occupational therapists. They provided training in the vocational skills that would help wounded soldiers return to work.

These forms of rehabilitation enabled soldiers to return either to combat or to their civilian prewar lives.[20] The division had almost a dozen small facilities set up in Europe and more extensive centers and hospitals in New York Harbor; Lakewood, New Jersey; Tacoma Park, Maryland (a suburb of Washington, D.C.); Fort McPherson, Georgia; and San Francisco, California. Each hospital had a physical therapy unit containing a gymnasium, a whirlpool room, a massage room, a pack room, and other rooms for mechanotherapy[20] and "electricity" (electrotherapy). The mechanotherapy room was an exercise room equipped with various apparatuses such as pulley-and-weight systems, trolleys, and ball-bearing wheels.

From its creation, the division recruited unmarried women between the ages of 25 and 40 to be trained as reconstruction aides. Applicants who had certificates showing practical and theoretical training in any of the treatments performed such as hydrotherapy, electrotherapy, mechanotherapy, or massage received priority and were accepted first. Nevertheless, they still were given additional preparation in all other necessary treatments.

First Physical Therapists: Marguerite Sanderson and Mary McMillan

The first reconstruction aides who made big contributions to the physical therapy profession during the Reconstruction Era were Marguerite Sanderson and Mary McMillan. Marguerite Sanderson was a physiotherapist who graduated from the Boston Normal School of Gymnastics and used to work with Dr. Joel Goldthwait, an orthopedic surgeon who later became the chairman of the War Reconstruction Committee of the American Orthopedic Association. Because of her prior physiotherapy experience, in 1917, Dr. Goldthwait appointed Sanderson as the first

Supervisor of Reconstruction Aides. Her role was to recruit and arrange for training of reconstruction aides and also send them to Europe to help the wounded soldiers. In 1922, Sanderson married and withdrew from active participation in the school.

The training program for the reconstruction aides took place at Walter Reed General Hospital. The program at Walter Reed was assigned to a reconstruction aide named Mary Livingston McMillan (**FIGURE 1-4**). Mary McMillan was a mature, educated woman who was born in the United States from Scottish ancestry. When she was 5 years old, her mother and sister died of consumption (tuberculosis). Mary was sent to live with relatives in Liverpool, England. Although acquiring a higher education was unusual at that time for a young woman, as an avid and eager learner Mary received a college degree in physical education and a postgraduate degree in her

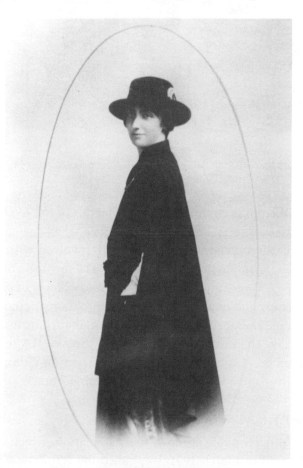

FIGURE 1-4 Mary McMillan, one of the founders and the first president of the American Physical Therapy Association (WWI Era/1918/1919).

chosen career, the science of physical therapy. McMillan's physical therapy degree included topics such as corrective exercises, massage, electrotherapy, aftercare of fractures, dynamics of scoliosis, psychology, neurology, and neuroanatomy.[20] In 1910, McMillan took her first professional position in Liverpool, England, working with Sir Robert Jones, nephew and professional heir of the great orthopedist Hugh Owen Thomas. Jones, an orthopedic physician, was renowned for using the Thomas splint (invented by his famous uncle) and performing progressive massage and orthopedic manipulations (invented by the French orthopedist Lucas-Championniere and British surgeon James B. Mennell). Lucas-Championniere and Mennell were pioneers of the principle that following an injury, early movement can enhance healing and prevent disability.

In 1916, McMillan returned home to her family in Massachusetts. Because of her education and experience, she was hired immediately at the Children's Hospital in Portland, Maine, where for 2 years she was director of massage and medical gymnastics, treating children with scoliosis, congenital hip dislocations, and other childhood orthopedic bone and joint abnormalities.[20] In 1918, at the recommendation of Sir Robert Jones, Elliott Bracket, a Boston orthopedist and one of the organizers of the army's Reconstruction Program, asked McMillan to consider service with the U.S. Army. In February 1918, McMillan was sworn in as a member of the U.S. Army Medical Corps. As a reconstruction aide she was assigned to Walter Reed General Hospital in Tacoma Park, Maryland. Shortly after, in June 1918, due to her experience and education in England, McMillan was asked to go to Reed College in Portland, Oregon, to train reconstruction aide applicants in the practical, hands-on segment of the War Emergency Training Program. With her contribution, Reed College's physical therapy curriculum became the standard by which other emergency war training programs were measured. In January 1919, McMillan was awarded the position of Chief Reconstruction Aide[20] in the department of physiotherapy at Walter Reed General Hospital.

Between 1919 and 1920, the number of physical therapy reconstruction aides was reduced primarily because of a major postwar decrease in military hospitals (at home and overseas). The number of hospitals shrank from 748 to 49. Despite this cutback, the army's commitment to maintain physical therapy as an important part of its medical services was established (**FIGURE 1-5**). In 1920, McMillan resigned her duties in the army because she felt her work

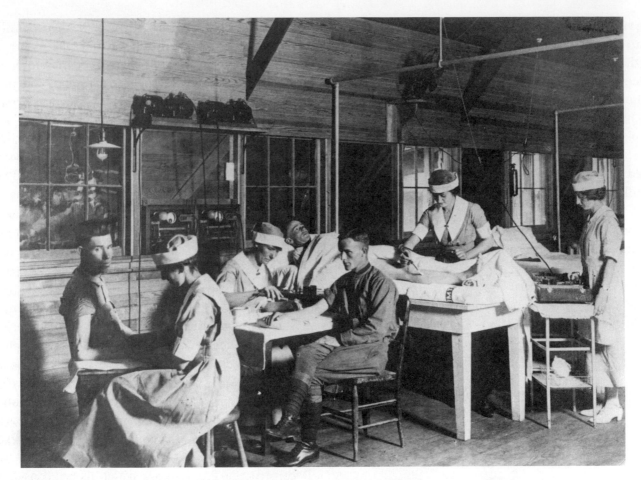

FIGURE 1-5 Reconstruction aides treat soldiers at Fort Sam Houston, Texas, in 1919 (WWI Era).

Reproduced from Murphy W: *Healing the Generations: A History of Physical Therapy and the American Physical Therapy Association*. Alexandria, American Physical Therapy Association, 1995; Commemorative Photographs; APTA—75 Years of Healing the Generations, with permission of the American Physical Therapy Association. This material is copyrighted, and any further reproduction or distribution is prohibited.

was essentially completed. She returned to civilian life in Boston as a staff therapist in an orthopedic office. In 1921, McMillan published her book, *Massage and Therapeutic Exercise.*

DEVELOPMENT YEARS: 1920 TO 1940

The Development of Professional Organization

During her work as a reconstruction aide, Mary McMillan was convinced that physical therapy had a vital future role in America's health care. Before resigning her duties in the army, McMillan wanted to maintain a nucleus of trained people who were capable of carrying out such a role. She contacted 800 former reconstruction aides and civilian therapists and received 120 enthusiastic responses. On January 15, 1921, at Keene's Chop House, an eatery in Manhattan, New York,[20] McMillan and 30 former reconstruction aides organized themselves into the first association of PTs. The organization was called the American Women's Physical Therapeutics Association (AWPTA).

McMillan was elected president. The role of the AWPTA was to establish and maintain professional and scientific standards for individuals who were involved with the profession of physical therapeutics.[19] The members of the AWPTA[19] were graduates of recognized schools of physiotherapy and of physical education programs trained in massage, therapeutic exercises, electrotherapy, and hydrotherapy. The executive committee of the AWPTA represented geographically diverse reconstruction aides; the first year there were 274 members coming from 32 states.

The P.T. Review *and Constitution*

The official publication of the Association, which first appeared in March 1921, was called the *P.T. Review.*[20] It was published quarterly and included the Association's constitution and bylaws, professional interest articles, and even a column called "S.O.S." for job classified advertisements. Also in 1921, the first textbook written by a physiotherapist (Mary McMillan) was published.

The first edition of the *P.T. Review* reported the full text of the constitution and bylaws of the Association. The basic reasons for the Association's existence, as described in its constitution,[20] were to have professional and scientific standards for its members, to increase competency among members by encouraging advanced studies, to promulgate medical literature and articles of professional interest, to make available efficiently trained members, and to sustain professional socialization.[20] The Association's bylaws specified three categories of membership in the Association: charter members, who were the reconstruction aides in physiotherapy; active members, who were graduates of recognized schools of physiotherapy or physical education; and honorary members, who were graduates of medical schools.

American Physiotherapy Association

At its first conference in Boston in 1922, the Association changed its name to the American Physiotherapy Association because although its members were all women, they recognized that men also practiced physiotherapy. At that time, there were a few male reconstruction aides who provided physiotherapy services during World War I.

In 1922, new schools of physiotherapy were opened at Harvard Medical School and in New York City. The graduates of these schools were called physiotherapists. By 1923 the membership in the Association had risen appreciably, and McMillan stepped down as president, giving way to a new president, one of the former reconstruction aides, Inga Lohne.[20]

In 1926, the Committee on Education and Publicity was formed to draft the minimum standard curriculum for schools offering a complete course in physical therapy. The committee's report, which was published in 1928,[20] was recommending a 9-month course with 33 hours of physical therapy–related instruction per week for a total of 1,200 hours. The entrance requirement was graduation from a recognized school of physical education or nursing. In 1930, there were 11 schools[20] that met or exceeded the minimum standards set by the committee. By 1934, there were 14 approved physiotherapy schools[20] including higher standard educational institutions such as Harvard Medical School in Boston, Massachusetts; Stanford University Hospital in Stanford, California; and the College of William and Mary in Williamsburg, Virginia.

In the early years, the American Physiotherapy Association tried to stay side by side with the medical profession.

During the 1920s and 1930s, physical therapy physicians became organized[21] in order to belong to the American Medical Association (AMA). The AMA recognized their efforts and educated other physicians about the value of physical therapy in rehabilitating World War I veterans. As a result, in 1925, a group of physical therapy physicians founded[21] the American College of Physical Therapy (ACPT). Later that year, the ACPT joined the AMA and changed its name to the American Congress of Physical Therapy. Physical therapy physicians decided to call themselves "physiatrists." Although their name was not officially changed until 1946, the physiatrists established the American Registry of Physical Therapy Technicians to separate the physiotherapists from the medical profession.

In 1930, the American Physiotherapy Association was incorporated and decided to work with the AMA to create standards of education for physiotherapists, to encourage the regulation of physical therapy practice by law, and to cooperate with, or under the direction of, the medical profession to provide a central registry for physiotherapists.[22] Consequently, by the 1930s, due to pressure from the AMA, registered physiotherapists were called technicians and settled to work under the referral of physical therapy physicians. It seems, however, that members of the AMA were concerned that the public might consider physiotherapists to be physicians, because their designation as physiotherapists ended in "ists," the same as radiologists, orthopedists, and so on. The AMA wanted no confusion in regard to medical school education of physiatrists as compared to physiotherapists. Finally, in the 1940s, the name physiotherapists changed to physical therapists.

Poliomyelitis and the Great Depression

By the 1930s, members of the American Physiotherapy Association were confronted with two calamities[20] in U.S. life—the growing severity of poliomyelitis and its resulting infantile paralysis (which began in the summer of 1916) and the Great Depression of 1929 (**FIGURE 1-6**). The poliomyelitis epidemic started in 1916 and continued into the 1930s and 1940s. As an example of the high incidence and magnitude of this disease, between May and November 1934, approximately 2,500 cases of poliomyelitis were treated at just one hospital,[19] the Los Angeles County General Hospital. The fact that the President of the United States, Franklin Delano Roosevelt, was treated for poliomyelitis by physiotherapists generated large public recognition of the physical therapy profession. At that time, physical

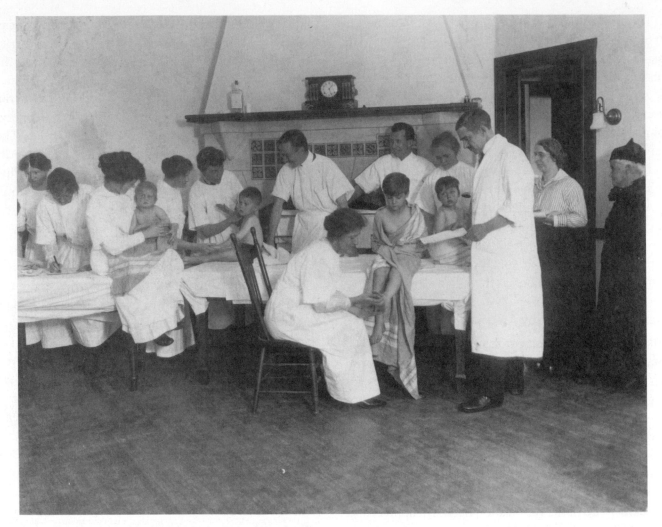

FIGURE 1-6 PTs and physicians work together to treat children at a New York poliomyelitis clinic in 1916 (WWI Era).

therapy for poliomyelitis consisted of hydrotherapy, exercises, massage, heat and light modalities, and assistive and adaptive equipment.[19] For home care, especially in rural areas, the physiotherapists provided "homemade" braces and splints.

In 1929, the Depression closed many hospitals and private medical practices, substantially reducing the number of physical therapy services.

Because the country was looking for a cure for poliomyelitis, in 1937, the National Foundation for Infantile Paralysis was founded. The foundation, using federal funding and money from charitable organizations such as the March of Dimes, opened new facilities and lent equipment to families and hospitals for polio aftercare. The National Foundation for Infantile Paralysis also financially contributed to the development of physical therapy education and

the growth of physical therapy schools. PTs who had no work during the Great Depression were able to pick and choose positions. They were needed to work in diagnostic clinics, outpatient centers, orthopedic hospitals, convalescent homes, schools for children with disabilities, and restorative services.

In 1937, although the physiotherapists were still dominated by their technician mindsets, their plans for the future were progressive, and included unity, research, and provision of educational standards. For example, the aims of the American Physiotherapy Association in 1937 were:[19]

- To form a nationwide organization that would establish and maintain professional and scientific standards for its members
- To promote the science of physical therapy

- To aid in the establishment of educational standards and scientific research in physical therapy
- To cooperate with, and to work only under the prescription of, members of the medical profession
- To provide available information to those interested in physical therapy
- To unite several chapters
- To create a central registry (available for the medical profession) that will make physiotherapists the only "trained assistants"[19(p.6)] in physical therapy

FUNDAMENTAL ACCOMPLISHMENT YEARS: 1940 TO 1970

The Professional and Educational Developments of Physical Therapy

During World War II, the American Physiotherapy Association continued to grow under its experienced president, Catherine Worthingham.[20] She was the first PT to hold a doctoral degree in anatomy and served as president of the Association from 1940 to 1945. The governance of the American Physiotherapy Association changed substantially to accommodate increased growth and responsibilities and a more national approach. In the summer of 1941, six months before the bombing of Pearl Harbor, the first War Emergency Training Course of World War II was initiated at Walter Reed General Hospital. Emma Vogel[20] directed the Walter Reed General Hospital program to train PTs (**FIGURE 1-7**). The course at Walter Reed consisted of 6 months of concentrated didactic instruction followed by 6 months of supervised practice at a military hospital.

The physiotherapists graduating from the Emergency Training Course were no longer called reconstruction aides but instead were physiotherapy aides. In 1943, the U.S. Congress passed a bill stating that graduates of the Emergency Training Course should be called physical therapists. Inadvertently, with the change of their titles, PTs started to have increased recognition and wideranging responsibilities. These new tasks were related to the treatment of wounded veterans including rehabilitation for amputations, burns, cold injuries, wounds, fractures, and nerve and spinal cord injuries. Additionally, immediately after the war, the U.S. government allocated $1 million for the enhancement of prosthetic services. This gave PTs the opportunity to participate in the teaching and training programs of the 25-year-old Artificial Limb Program at the University of California at Berkeley,

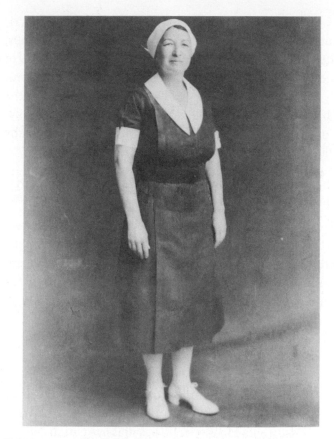

FIGURE 1-7 Emma Vogel directed the Walter Reed General Hospital program for PTs. After the outbreak of World War II, Vogel was deployed to direct the War Emergency Training courses at 10 Army hospitals (Post WWI through WWII Era).

Reproduced from Murphy W: *Healing the Generations: A History of Physical Therapy and the American Physical Therapy Association.* Alexandria, American Physical Therapy Association, 1995; Commemorative Photographs; APTA—75 Years of Healing the Generations, with permission of the American Physical Therapy Association. This material is copyrighted, and any further reproduction or distribution is prohibited.

New York University, and the University of California at Los Angeles. Furthermore, in 1946, because of the passing of the Hill-Burton Act and founding of a nationwide hospital-building program, PTs increased their hospital-based[19] practice. The work of PTs expanded even more in the 1950s with the outbreak of the Korean War.

In 1944, the American Physiotherapy Association membership voted for a separate internal legislative branch called the House of Delegates.[20] The House of Delegates had the same legislative powers as it does today—to amend or repeal the bylaws of the Association. In 1946, physical therapy physicians practicing physical medicine officially changed their specialty name to physiatrist. In the same year, the American Physiotherapy Association changed its name to its current one, the **American Physical Therapy Association (APTA)**. By 1959, membership in the APTA had increased to 8,028 PTs.

In 1947, the length of physical therapy schools' curricula increased from 9 months to 12 months. By the 1950s, there were 31 accredited schools in the United States, 19 of them offering 4-year integrated bachelor degree programs. By 1959, most of the states had licensure laws adopting the Physical Therapy Practice Act. In 1951, the Joint Commission on Accreditation of Hospitals was formed, raising the standards for institutional staffing and health care.

The Polio Vaccine and the Journal of the American Physical Therapy Association

Because new cases of polio were seen every year, PTs were called upon from all over the country to help either part-time or full-time as volunteers dealing with polio epidemics. In 1952, there were 58,000 cases of poliomyelitis in the United States. Between 1948 and 1960 nearly 1,000 PTs participated in the polio volunteer program. In 1954, 63 PTs were dispatched to 44 states to help with clinical studies of the polio vaccine developed by Jonas Salk. After successful clinical trial inoculations of 650,000 children, the Salk vaccine was determined to be safe and was approved for commercial production in 1955 by the Food and Drug Administration. Finally, in 1955, a massive national vaccination program started using the Salk vaccine. As a result, poliomyelitis cases were virtually eradicated.

Jessie Wright, PT, MD, was one of the PTs who helped with polio clinical studies by evaluating patients' strength. In 1954, Wright and her staff introduced the abridged muscle grading system. Wright, who specialized in physical medicine and rehabilitation at the University of Pittsburgh, Pennsylvania, was a visionary in regard to helping patients achieve function. Wright believed that "the first goal of physical therapy was to relax tight muscles"[11(p.77)] allowing complete range of motion in the joints and as a result giving the patient "functional use of residual power, helpful body mechanics and assistive devices."[11(p.78)]

The role of the PT in the 1950s expanded[19] from a technical position to that of a professional practitioner. Private practices expanded and, in 1957, the Physical Therapy Fund was established to foster scientific, literary, and educational programs.[20] PTs' licensure started in 1913 in Pennsylvania and in 1926 in New York; it expanded during the 1950s and by 1959,[20] 45 states and the territory of Hawaii offered licensure.

In 1964, the APTA formed a committee on research in order to improve the development of scientific inquiry. In regard to dissemination of information (including scientific discovery) among the members of the physical therapy profession, just 2 years earlier (1962), the APTA changed the name of the official journal, the *P.T. Review* to the *Journal of the American Physical Therapy Association*. In 1963 the journal modified its format and expanded its content with the help of its editor, Helen Hislop.[20] In 1964, the journal changed its name to the *Journal of Physical Therapy*. Later, the name was changed to *Physical Therapy*.

The Beginning of Physical Therapy Assistants

In the 1960s the U.S. population was changing, primarily because of the doubling of the number of elderly, but also because people were becoming more health conscious. As with other health professions, physical therapy was expanding rapidly with a high demand for physical therapy services. In addition, the change in physical therapy insurance reimbursement (through diagnostic related groups introduced by Medicare) and the enactment in 1965 and 1966 of Medicare and Medicaid programs created an even greater demand for PTs. As a result, in 1967 the APTA adopted a policy statement that set the foundation for the creation of the physical therapy assistant and the establishment of educational programs for the training of physical therapy assistants. The policy statement adopted by the House of Delegates recommended the following:[20]

- The APTA had to establish the standards for physical therapy assistant education programs.
- A supervisory relationship existed between the PT and the physical therapy assistant.
- The functions of assistants were to be identified.
- Mandatory licensure or registration was encouraged.
- Membership in the APTA was to be established for the assistants.

By 1969, the occupational title changed from physical therapy assistant to physical therapist assistant (PTA). Also, training programs were to be called physical therapist assistant programs. At that time there were already two colleges in the country that enrolled students in their programs: Miami Dade Community College in Miami, Florida, and St. Mary's Campus of the College of St. Catherine in Minneapolis, Minnesota.

MASTERY YEARS: 1970 TO 1996

The Societal Developments of Physical Therapy

In 1969, the first 15 PTAs graduated with associate degrees from Miami Dade College and College of St. Catherine. By

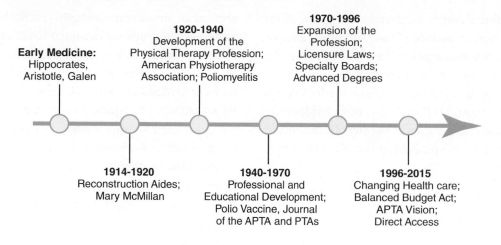

FIGURE 1-8 Timeline.

1970 there were nine PTA education programs, mostly due to federal financial assistance to junior colleges. In the same year, the APTA offered temporary affiliate membership to PTAs. By 1973, eligible PTAs were admitted as affiliate members in the national association, having the right to speak and make motions, to hold committee appointments, and to chapter representation in the House of Delegates. In 1983, PTAs formed the Affiliate Special Interest Group, and in 1989 the House of Delegates approved the creation of the Affiliate Assembly, which gave PTAs a formal voice in the Association. The first president of the Affiliate Assembly was Cheryl Carpenter-Davis, PTA, MEd.

The Expansion of the Physical Therapy Profession

During the 1970s and 1980s, the physical therapy profession continued to grow and expand. Because of the establishment of the Occupational Safety and Health Administration (OSHA) by the Department of Labor, physical therapy practices related to prevention, work management, and job injuries and compensation also developed. This contributed to PTs' advancement of practice from hospital-based to private. In 1972, Congress added physical therapy services to the Social Security Act as services that were to be reimbursed[20] when they were furnished by an individual PT in his or her office or in the patient's home. In 1975, the Individuals with Disabilities Education Act (IDEA) was passed. This helped physical therapy expand into treatment of children with disabilities in public schools.

In 1971, the AMA dissolved the American Registry, and by 1976, all states had physical therapy licensure laws in place. In 1981 and 1982, the House of Delegates adopted

the policy that PT practice that was independent of practitioner referral was ethical[19] (as long as it was legal in that specific state). This separated PTs from the physician's control, giving them the right to practice without a physician's referral.

During the early 1970s, the APTA formed sections for state licensure and regulations, sports physical therapy, pediatrics, clinical electrophysiology, and orthopedics. The state licensure and regulations section later became the health policy, legislation, and regulation section. In 1976, the first combined sections meeting took place in Washington, D.C. In 1977, the APTA, through the Commission on Accreditation in Physical Therapy Education, became the sole accrediting agency for all educational programs for PTs and PTAs in the United States, Canada, and Europe.

In 1978, the American Board of Physical Therapy Specialties was created by the APTA to allow members a mechanism to receive certification and recognition as a clinical specialist in a certain specialty area. During the late 1970s, the sections on obstetrics and gynecology (now called women's health) and on geriatrics were created. By 1985, the American Board for Physical Therapy Specialties—Certified Cardiopulmonary Specialists was formed, giving cardiopulmonary specialist certifications. Shortly, other specialty certifications followed such as orthopedic, pediatric, electrophysiology, neurology, and sports. In 1983, the APTA purchased its first four-story building in Alexandria, Virginia.

In 1990, the Americans with Disabilities Act assured the involvement of PTs as consultants to guarantee every individual with disabilities rightful access to all aspects of life. Many major changes occurred during the 1990s; managed care, point of service plans, and other alternative organizational structures such as health economics resources also impacted physical therapy delivery. Nevertheless, physical therapy practice developed in the areas of work conditioning, women's health, and work hardening.[19]

During the last two decades of the twentieth century, the following major developments occurred in the physical therapy profession:

- In 1980, the House of Delegates established its goal to raise the minimum entry-level education in physical therapy to a postbaccalaureate degree.
- During the early 1980s, the sections on veterans' affairs, hand rehabilitation, and oncology were established.
- In 1986, the *PT Bulletin* was initiated. In the same year, setting goals and objectives became part of the APTA's annual self-review process.
- In 1989, the House of Delegates approved the formation of the Affiliate Assembly, composed entirely of PTA members. In this way, PTAs had a formal avenue to come together and discuss issues that directly concerned them.
- By 1988, direct access was legal in 20 states, providing patients and clients the ability to seek direct physical therapy services without first seeing a physician.
- The academic preparation of PTs changed from a bachelor's degree to postbaccalaureate degrees. By January 1994, 55 percent of physical therapy education programs were at the master's level.
- In 1995, the American Board of Physical Therapy Specialties inaugurated nationwide electronic testing and the APTA celebrated the 75th anniversary of the association and the physical therapy profession.
- Also in 1995, the APTA hosted the 12th World Confederation for Physical Therapy Congress in Washington, D.C. The Congress had record-breaking crowds.[19]
- In 1995, the APTA received representation on the AMA Coding Panel, facilitating a better development of PT practice codes.

ADAPTATION YEARS: 1996 TO 2005

The Balanced Budget Act

In August 1997, President Clinton signed the Balanced Budget Act (BBA) to eliminate the Medicare deficit. The Balanced Budget Act, which took effect in January 1999,

applied an annual cap of $1,500 (for both physical therapy and speech therapy services) per beneficiary for all outpatient rehabilitation services. As an effect of the Balanced Budget Act and its resultant reduction in rehabilitation services to Medicare patients, many new graduate PTs and PTAs could not find jobs. Also, some experienced PTs and PTAs suffered an appreciable decrease in income and in the number of working hours. Due to pressure from the Association, its members, patients, and the general public, in November 1999 President Clinton signed the Refinement Act, which suspended the $1,500 cap for 2 years in all rehabilitation settings starting on January 3, 2000. Nonetheless, the Balanced Budget Act was detrimental to the treatment of many Medicare patients and also created a hardship for PTs and PTAs for at least 3 years. An APTA survey[23] in October 2000, found that as a result of the Balanced Budget Act, PTAs were hurt the most, with an unemployment rate of 6.5 percent. The PTs also reported that their hours of employment had been involuntarily reduced. In March 2001, the same survey discovered that the unemployment rate among PTAs had improved, going down to 4.2 percent. PTs also reported an improvement, with the reduction in working hours only 10.8 percent. The reduction in the number of working hours for PTAs was even greater than the PTs, at 24.5 percent in October 2000; in March 2001 it went down to 19.8 percent.

During 2005, the effects of the Balanced Budget Act of 1997 were still influencing the future of rehabilitation services. On February 17, 2005, the APTA stated in a news release that "Senior citizens across the country are looking to the 109th Congress to keep much needed rehabilitation services available under Medicare."[24] Rehabilitation providers and patients urged Congress to pass the Medicare Access to Rehabilitation Services Act of 2005 to eliminate the threat that seniors and individuals with disabilities would have to pay out of pocket for rehabilitation or to alter the course of their rehabilitation care. This Act was considered significant to repeal the cap that was originally instituted through the Balanced Budget Act (BBA) of 1997. From 1997 to the beginning of 2005, Congress enforced a moratorium three times that delayed implementation of the cap. On December 31, 2005, the moratorium expired. As a result, on January 1, 2006, the Medicare cap was reimplemented by the Centers for Medicare and Medicaid Services (CMS). From January 1, 2006 to December 31, 2006, the dollar amount of the therapy cap was $1,740 for physical therapy and speech language pathology combined and $1,740 for occupational therapy.

The APTA has been working diligently during each Congressional session to reduce the drastic impact the BBA has had on patient care. Although the therapy cap went into effect in 2006, because of the pressure from the APTA, clinicians, and consumer groups, Congress authorized Medicare to allow exceptions for beneficiaries who needed additional rehabilitation services based on diagnosis and clinicians' evaluations and judgments. Consequently, Congress acted to extend these exceptions through December 31, 2009. On January 1, 2010, without Congressional action, authorization for exceptions to the therapy caps expired. The APTA states on its website that "on March 23rd, 2010, President Obama signed H.R. 3590, the Patient Protection and Affordable Care Act, making it law." This Act includes a health care reform package that extended the therapy cap exception process until December 31, 2010. For details of the Act and more information, visit the APTA's website at: www.apta.org.

APTA Events

In 1999, two significant events affected the APTA: the suspension of the $1,500 Medicare cap and the publication of the *Normative Model of Physical Therapist Assistant Education: Version 1999,* which guides PTA education programs. In 2000, the Association adopted the new "Evaluative Criteria for the Accreditation of Education for Physical Therapist Assistants," launched *PT Bulletin* online, and published the *Normative Model for Physical Therapist Professional Education: Version 2000.* In 2001, the Association introduced the second edition of the *Guide to Physical Therapist Practice* and worked hard to maintain PTs' rights in certain states to perform manipulations and provide orthotics and prosthetics within the scope of physical therapy practice. The Association launched Hooked on Evidence on the Web in 2002 to help clinicians review the research literature and utilize the information to enhance their clinical decision making and practice. In January 2002, all physical therapy educational programs changed to the master's level. In the same year, Pennsylvania became the 35th state to achieve direct access, and the APTA released the *Interactive Guide to Physical Therapist Practice.* In 2003, the Association built support in Congress for the Medicare Patient Access to Physical Therapists Act to allow

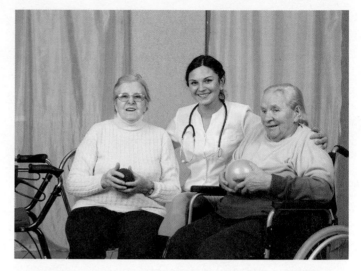

© GBZero/Shutterstock

licensed PTs to evaluate and treat Medicare patients without a physician's referral.

VISION AND APPLICATION OF SCIENTIFIC PURSUIT YEARS: 2006 TO TODAY

From 2006 to today, the roles of PTs have become more dependent on the application of the scientific method in clinical practice and finding new evidence-based approaches for disease prevention and health promotion. PTAs were delegated with important responsibilities as the only individuals permitted to assist PTs in selected interventions (under the direction and supervision of PTs).

The American Physical Therapy Association's Vision

The House of Delegates updated the vision statement in 2013. The new vision for the APTA is "Transforming society by optimizing movement to improve the human experience."[25]

The previous vision statement was created in 2000 and guided the Association for 13 years. The guiding principles were critical for directing the profession to its current vision statement.[26]

Vision 2020 states: "By 2020, physical therapy will be provided by physical therapists who are doctors of physical therapy, recognized by consumers and other health care professionals as the practitioners of choice to whom consumers have direct access for the diagnosis of, interventions for, and prevention of impairments, **functional limitations**, and disabilities related to movement, function, and health."

APTA Vision Statement for Physical Therapy 2020 includes the following:[26]

- Physical therapy will be provided by PTs who are doctors of physical therapy and who may be board-certified specialists.
- Consumers will have direct access to PTs in all environments for patient/client management, prevention, and wellness services.
- PTs will be practitioners of choice in patients/clients' health networks and will hold all privileges of autonomous practice.
- PTs may be assisted by PTAs who are educated and licensed to provide PT–directed and supervised components of interventions.
- Guided by integrity, lifelong learning, and a commitment to comprehensive and accessible health programs for all people, PTs and PTAs will render evidence-based services throughout the continuum of care and improve quality of life for society.
- PTs and PTAs will provide culturally sensitive care distinguished by trust, respect, and an appreciation for individual differences.
- While fully availing themselves of new technologies, as well as basic and clinical research, PTs will continue to provide direct patient/client care.
- PTs and PTAs will maintain active responsibility for the growth of the physical therapy profession and the health of the people it serves.

The terminology used in the vision sentence/statement relates to the following:[26]

- *Autonomous physical therapy practice environments* include all physical therapy practice settings where PTs accept the responsibility to practice autonomously and collaboratively to provide best practice to the patient/client. Such PT practices are characterized by independent, self-determined, professional judgments and actions.
- *Direct access* means that throughout his or her lifetime, every consumer has the legal right to directly access a PT for the diagnosis of, interventions for, and prevention of impairments, functional limitations, and disabilities related to movement, function, and health.

- The *Doctor of Physical Therapy (DPT)* is a clinical doctorate degree (entry level) that reflects the growth in the body of knowledge and expected responsibilities that a professional PT must master to provide best practice to the consumer. All PTs and PTAs are obligated to engage in the continual acquisition of knowledge, skills, and abilities to advance the science of physical therapy and its role in the delivery of health care.
- *Practitioner of choice* means PTs who personify the elements of the Vision 2020 and are recognized among consumers and other health care professionals as the preferred providers for the diagnosis of, interventions for, and prevention of impairments, functional limitations, and disabilities related to movement, function, and health.
- *Evidence-based practice* means access to, and application and integration of evidence to guide clinical decision making to provide best practice for the patient/client. Evidence-based practice includes the integration of best available research, clinical expertise, and patient/client values and circumstances related to patient/client management, practice management, and health care policy decision making. Plans for evidence-based practice include enhancing patient/client management and reducing unwarranted variation in the provision of physical therapy services.
- *Professionalism* means that PTs and PTAs consistently demonstrate core values by aspiring to and wisely applying principles of altruism, excellence, caring, ethics, respect, communication, and accountability, and by working together with other professionals to achieve optimal health and wellness in individuals and communities.

BEYOND VISION 2020

The APTA vision statement adopted in 2013 includes new guiding principles:[25]

- Identity. The physical therapy profession will be recognized as the experts in movement systems in practice, education, and research.
- Quality. The physical therapy profession will identify, adopt and utilize evidence-based principles in practice, education, and research.
- Collaboration. The physical therapy profession will identify and value interprofessional collaboration in order to provide integrated services for society and consumers.

- Innovation. The physical therapy profession will develop inventive practices in research, education, and practice to lead health care.
- Consumer-centricity. The physical therapy profession will value patient needs as core to all interactions and will create a culture that values the cultures of all people.
- Access/Equity. The physical therapy profession will identify and develop creative avenues to reach all people in need of physical therapy care and education.
- Advocacy. The physical therapy profession will be an advocate for consumers in research, education, and practice.

Achieving Direct Access

Direct access means the ability of the public to directly access a PT's services such as physical therapy evaluation, examination, and intervention. Direct access eliminates the patient's need to visit his or her physician to ask for a physician's referral. Licensed PTs are qualified to provide physical therapy services without referrals from physicians. Direct access decreases the cost of health care and does not promote overutilization. The APTA assigned direct access to PTs as a high priority in the Association's federal government affairs activities. In 2005, the Medicare Patient Access to Physical Therapists Act was introduced in the House of Representatives, and its companion bill in the Senate. The Act and the bill recognized the ability of licensed PTs to evaluate, diagnose, and treat Medicare beneficiaries requiring outpatient physical therapy services under Part B of the Medicare program, without a physician referral. In 2014, all 50 states and the District of Columbia passed legislation that allows PTs to evaluate and treat patients without a physician's referral.[27]

PTA Caucus

In June 2005, the National Assembly of Physical Therapist Assistants was dissolved and the Physical Therapist Assistant (PTA) Caucus was formed. The National Assembly of PTAs was formed in 1998 as the Affiliate Assembly. The PTA Caucus's purpose was to more fully integrate PTA members into the APTA's governance structure and increase PTAs' influence in the Association.[28] The PTA Caucus represents the PTAs' interests, needs, and issues in the APTA governance.[28] The caucus includes a chief delegate and four delegates representing five regions.[28] Additionally, there are 51 PTA Caucus members representing 51 chapters.[28] Each PTA Caucus representative is elected or selected by his or her state chapter. The PTA Caucus also elects one chief delegate and four delegates (representing five regions) to the APTA's House of Delegates. The PTA Caucus representatives work with their chapter delegates and provide input to the delegates to the House of Delegates (HOD) and the advisory panel of PTAs. Each delegate has the ability to speak, debate, and make and second motions providing representation in the HOD for a particular region of the country.

Membership in the American Physical Therapy Association

The APTA is the national organization that represents the profession of physical therapy. Membership in the Association is voluntary. Active members of the Association are PTs, PTAs (also called affiliate members), and PT and PTA students. Other Association members are retired members, honorary members (people who are not PTs or PTAs but who made remarkable contributions to the Association or the health of the public), and Fellow members (called Catherine Worthingham Fellows of the American Physical Therapy Association). The Fellow member is an active member for 15 years who has made notable contributions to the profession. As of 2013, the APTA membership consisted of approximately 88,000 PTs, PTAs, and student members. The APTA includes 51 chapters operating in the United States and its territories. Each chapter offers a variety of events, professional development activities, and other opportunities for members' interaction.

The requirement for membership in the APTA is to be a graduate of an accredited PT or PTA program or to be enrolled in an accredited PT or PTA program. PT or PTA students are welcome as student members of the Association.

The Association describes the following 12 specific benefits for student members:[29]

How Will APTA Membership Jump-Start Your Career?

1. Enjoy significant members-only savings on APTA's products, services, and conferences.

2. Explore new topics and research you won't find in the classroom through podcasts, newsletters, and more.

3. Get solid advice from people who have been in your shoes through APTA's mentoring programs.

4. Find the right job—studies have shown that when they have the option, employers prefer to hire APTA members.

5. Become involved in professional issues and debates by participating in the Student Assembly and student special-interest groups.

6. Stay current through *Guide to Physical Therapist Practice,* podcasts, ArticleSearch, *PT in Motion, PTJ Online, Student Assembly Pulse,* and other publications.

7. Connect with students, educators, and clinicians now and build lifelong contacts and friendships you can rely on for years.

8. Explore APTA's 18 special-interest sections now and know exactly where your interests lie when you embark on your new career.

9. Build leadership skills and make a difference—take on active volunteer roles in the Student Assembly and your state chapter.

10. Protect your future with APTA-endorsed plans and programs for professional liability, education loans, and more.

11. Save 50% upon graduating when you convert to PT or PTA membership—APTA's graduation gift to you.

12. Do your part to ensure the best possible future for the profession. APTA is the voice of physical therapy, actively representing the profession on Capitol Hill, in state legislatures, and with regulators.

The American Physical Therapy Association. Membership & Leadership. Membership Benefits for Students. Reprinted from http://www.apta.org, with permission of the American Physical Therapy Association. Copyright (c) 2015 American Physical Therapy Association. APTA is not responsible for the translation from English.

As of 2013, most members of the APTA were females, with an average age of 44.1 years.[30] Members averaged 18.4 years working as a PT, with the majority of members practicing for more than 31 years.

As of 2013, the APTA's demographic profiles[31] for PTA members indicate that most of the PTAs were female (79 percent). In regard to age, in 2013, the highest percentage (16.4 percent) were between 45 and 49 years old, the second highest (15.7 percent) were between 35 and 39, and the lowest percentage (0.1 percent) were over 65 years of age.[31] In 2013, 82.3 percent of all PTA members were working full-time, and 14.4 percent were working part-time.[31] In regard to education, in 2013, 60.2 percent of PTAs had associate degrees, 32.5 percent had baccalaureate degrees, 6.1 percent had master's degrees, and 0.5 percent had doctorate degrees (not DPTs or tDPTs).[31]

THE APTA'S MISSION

The APTA is the principal membership organization that stands for and promotes the profession of physical therapy. Its purpose is to "improve the health and quality of life of individuals in society by advancing physical therapist practice."[25]

The 2013 Strategic Plan identified four major goals for the APTA.[25]

1. "APTA will better enable physical therapists to consistently use best practice to improve the quality of life of their patients and clients."[25] The major push for this goal has been the development of the Physical Therapy Outcomes Registry. It will be a location for data that will lead researchers, educators, and practitioners to better outcomes for our patients. In addition, the sections began the process of creating clinical practice guidelines to support practice decisions.

2. "APTA will be the recognized leader in supporting physical therapists in the delivery of patient- and client-centered care across the lifespan."[25] As leaders and experts in the movement system, the APTA has developed an annual physical therapy exam to be used with patients to identify the health of a person's movement system. In addition, this goal is pushing for more interdisciplinary work for the betterment of patients and society. This goal has created specific tools to assist with health throughout the lifespan by developing education such as FitAfter 50, Fittest Cities for Baby Boomers, and Painless Parenting 101.

3. "APTA will empower physical therapists to demonstrate and promote high standards of professional and intellectual excellence."[25] In a continued effort to create experts in movement systems, the APTA created Residency/Fellowship Physical Therapist Centralized Application Services to allow applicants to fill out one application form when applying to multiple programs. In addition, the continuation of the American Board of Physical Therapist Specialists shows growth in numbers. The APTA Learning Center has enhanced its offerings to allow for up-to-date learning on a variety of topics.

4. "APTA will be the recognized leader in setting the standards for physical therapy service delivery and establishing and promoting the value of physical therapist practice to all stakeholders."[25]

The APTA is known as a strong voice in Washington, D.C. politics for physical therapy services and patient advocacy. In addition, the APTA has worked for payment reform and insurance provider education.

APTA COMPONENTS

The components of the APTA are chapters, sections, and assemblies. The Association has 51 chapters including chapters in the 50 states and the District of Columbia. Membership in a chapter is automatic. Members must belong to the chapter of the state in which they live, work, or attend school (or of an adjacent state if more active participation is possible). Chapters are significant for governance at the state level and for contributing to a national integration of members in the Association. The APTA has 18 sections. They are organized at the national level, providing an opportunity for members with similar areas of interest to meet, discuss issues, and encourage the interests of the respective sections. The sections usually have an annual combined sections meeting in February.

The Association has two assemblies: the PTA Caucus and the Student Assembly. The assemblies are composed of members from the same category and provide means for members to communicate and contribute at the national level to their future governance. One of the important positions expressed in 2004 by the National Assembly for the Physical Therapist Assistants was that the PTA is the only educated individual whom the PT may direct and supervise for providing selected interventions in the delivery of physical therapy services. The PTA Caucus is benefiting from and also reinforcing the PTA role in the APTA. A 2014 meeting identified the need for the APTA to develop a membership value plan specifically for the PTA member.[32]

THE HOUSE OF DELEGATES AND THE BOARD OF DIRECTORS

The House of Delegates (HOD) is the highest policy-making body of the APTA. It is composed of delegates from all chapters, sections, and assemblies, as well as the members of the board of directors. The HOD is composed of chapter voting delegates; section, assembly, and PTA Caucus nonvoting delegates; and consultants. The number

of voting chapter delegates is determined each year based on membership numbers as of June 30. The annual session of the APTA is the meeting of the HOD. It usually takes place every year at the Association's NEXT Conference and Exposition in June.

The role of the board of directors is to carry out the mandates and policies established by the HOD and to communicate issues to internal and external personnel, committees, and agencies. The board of directors of the APTA is composed of 15 members—6 officers and 9 directors. Members of the board assume office at the close of the HOD at which they were elected. A complete term for a board member is 3 years. Only active members of the APTA in good standing for at least 5 years can serve on the board of directors. No member is allowed to serve more than three complete consecutive terms on the board or more than two complete consecutive terms in the same office. The board meets at least once a year, and the executive committee meets at least twice a year.

The six officers of the APTA are the president, vice president, secretary, treasurer, speaker of the HOD, and vice speaker of the HOD. The president of the APTA presides at all meetings of the board of directors and the executive committee and serves as the official spokesperson of the Association. The president is also an ex officio member of all committees appointed by the board of directors except the ethics and judicial committee. The vice president of the APTA assumes the duties of the president in the absence or incapacitation of the president. In the event of vacancy in the office of president, the vice president will be the president for the unexpired portion of the term. In this situation, the office of the vice president will be vacant. The secretary of the APTA is responsible for keeping the minutes of the proceedings of the HOD, the board of directors, and the executive committee; for making a report in writing to the HOD at each annual session and to the board of directors on request; and for preparing a summary of the proceedings of the HOD for publication. The treasurer of the APTA is responsible for reporting in writing on the financial status of the Association to the HOD and to the board of directors on request. The treasurer also serves as the chair of the finance and audit committee. The speaker of the HOD presides at sessions of the HOD, serves as an officer of the HOD, and is an ex officio member of the reference committee. The vice speaker of the HOD serves as an officer of the HOD and assumes the duties of the speaker of the HOD in the absence or incapacitation of the speaker. In the event of a vacancy in the office of the speaker of the HOD, the vice speaker succeeds to the office of the speaker for the unexpired term. In this situation, the office of the vice speaker will be vacant.

APTA'S HEADQUARTERS

The Association's headquarters are in Alexandria, Virginia. The Association's personnel are available online at www.apta.org and at the toll-free number (800) 999-2782. The address of the Association is 1111 North Fairfax Street, Alexandria, VA, 22314-1488.

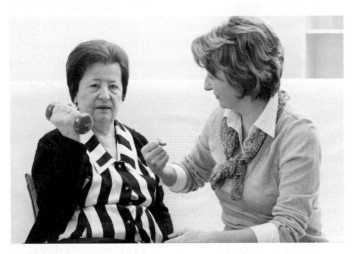

© Baki/Shutterstock

Other Organizations Involved with Physical Therapy

COMMISSION ON ACCREDITATION IN PHYSICAL THERAPY EDUCATION

The **Commission on Accreditation in Physical Therapy Education (CAPTE)** grants specialized accreditation status to qualified entry-level education programs for PTs and PTAs. The commission is a national accrediting agency recognized by the U.S. Department of Education and the Council for Higher Education Accreditation. The APTA and CAPTE work together to ensure that persons entering educational programs for PTs and PTAs receive formal preparation related to current requirements for professional practice. CAPTE accredits professional (entry-level) programs in the United States for the PT at the master's and doctoral degree levels and programs

for the PTA at the associate degree level. CAPTE also accredits two PT education programs in Canada and one in Scotland.

CAPTE states that its mission is "to serve the public by establishing and applying standards that assure quality and continuous improvement in the entry-level preparation of PTs and PTAs, and that reflect the evolving nature of education, research, and practice."[33] CAPTE consists of three panels: the Physical Therapist Review Panel, Physical Therapist Assistant Review Panel, and Central Panel. Appointment to CAPTE is done through the APTA staff members, who provide the APTA board of directors with a list of all individuals[33] qualified for open positions who consent to serve. CAPTE reviews the list and makes recommendations of those individuals who best meet CAPTE's needs. The board of directors considers the recommendations of CAPTE and makes final decisions[33] for appointments to CAPTE. The term of appointment is 4 years.

AMERICAN BOARD OF PHYSICAL THERAPY SPECIALTIES

The American Board of Physical Therapy Specialties (ABPTS) is the governing body for certification and recertification of clinical specialists by coordinating and supervising the specialist certification process. The ABPTS is composed of 11 individuals:[34] eight individuals appointed by the ABPTS for 4-year terms, one member of the APTA board of directors (BOD) appointed by the APTA BOD for a 1-year term, one consumer representative appointed by the BOD for a 2-year term, and one tests and measurement expert appointed by the ABPTS for a 2-year term.

The specialist certification program was established in 1978 by the APTA to provide formal recognition for PTs with advanced clinical knowledge, experience, and skills in a special area of practice, and to assist consumers and the health care community in identifying these PTs. The APTA describes specialization as a process by which a PT increases his or her professional education and practice and develops greater knowledge and skills related to a particular area of practice. Specialist recertification is a process by which a PT verifies current competence as an advanced practitioner in a specialty area by increasing his or her education and professional growth.

The Specialty Council on Cardiopulmonary Physical Therapy was the first to complete the process, and the cardiopulmonary specialist certification examination was first administered in 1985. Since then, seven additional specialty areas were established: clinical electrophysiology, geriatrics, neurology, orthopedics, pediatrics, sports, and women's health physical therapy.

The purposes of APTA's Clinical Specialization Program are as follows:[34]

- To contribute to the identification and development of appropriate areas of specialty practice in physical therapy.
- To promote the highest possible level of care for individuals seeking physical therapy services in each specialty area.
- To promote the development of the science and the art underlying each specialty area of practice.
- To provide a reliable and valid method for certification and recertification of individuals who have attained an advanced level of knowledge and skill in each specialty area.
- To help the consumers, the health care community, and others in identifying certified clinical specialists in each specialty area.
- To serve as a resource in specialty practice for APTA, the physical therapy profession, and the health care community.

FEDERATION OF STATE BOARDS OF PHYSICAL THERAPY

The Federation of State Boards of Physical Therapy (FSBPT) develops and administers the National Physical Therapy Examination (NPTE)[35] for both PTs and PTAs in 53 jurisdictions: the 50 states, the District of Columbia, Puerto Rico, and the Virgin Islands. The purpose of the FSBPT is to protect the public by providing leadership and service that encourage competent and safe physical therapy practice.[35] The exams assess the basic entry-level competence for first-time licensure or registration as a PT or PTA within the 53 jurisdictions. FSBPT's vision[35] is that the organization will achieve a high level of public protection through a strong foundation of laws and regulatory standards in physical therapy, effective tools and systems to assess entry-level and continuing competence, and public and professional awareness of resources for public protection.

For PT and PTA graduates who are candidates to sit for the NPTE, the federation offers a Candidate Handbook that includes all the necessary information about the exam and exam administration. The handbook can be viewed or downloaded online at www.fsbpt.org. The federation has been working with the state boards within its jurisdiction toward licensure uniformity supporting one passing score on the NPTE. This uniformity in scores assists PTs and PTAs to work across states.

In 2004, the FSBPT developed for purchase an online Practice Exam and Assessment Tool (PEAT) to help PT and PTA candidates prepare for the NPTE. The online PEAT allows the candidates to take a timed, multiple-choice exam similar to the NPTE and receive feedback on it. When receiving feedback, the candidates have access to the correct answer rationale and the references used for each question. PTA candidates can purchase a PTA PEAT that has two different 200-question exams.

APTA'S POSITION IN REGARD TO LICENSURE

In regard to licensure, the APTA requires that all PTs and PTAs should be licensed or otherwise regulated in all U.S. jurisdictions. State regulation of PTs and PTAs should require at a minimum graduation from an accredited physical therapy education program (or in the case of an internationally educated PT, an equivalent education) and passing an entry-level competency exam; should provide title protection; and should allow for disciplinary action. In addition, PTs' licensure should include a defined scope of practice. Relative to temporary jurisdictional licensure, the APTA supports the elimination of temporary jurisdictional licensure of PTs or temporary credentialing of PTAs for previously non-U.S.-licensed or non-U.S.-credentialed applicants in all jurisdictions.[32]

POLITICAL ACTION COMMITTEE

The physical therapy political action committee (PT-PAC) of the APTA is a vital aspect of the Association's success on Capitol Hill in Washington, D.C. The PT-PAC ensures that future legislative actions on Capitol Hill are helpful to physical therapy practice. PT and PTA members make donations to the political action committee. The PT-PAC committee uses membership donations to influence legislative and policy issues through lobbying efforts directed toward policy decision makers. The purpose of the PT-PAC is "to further the legislative aims of APTA."[36] The tasks of the PT-PAC are:[36]

- To raise funds to contribute to campaigns of candidates for national and state office with attention to PTs as candidates for public office.
- To encourage and facilitate APTA member participation in the political process.

PHYSICAL THERAPY EDUCATION

In regard to PT and PTA education, as of June 11, 2014, there were:[37]

- 224 DPT (Doctor of Physical Therapy) accredited PT education programs
- 1 MS/MPT accredited PT education program (which is changing to DPT)
- 29 developing DPT PT education programs
- 327 PTA accredited PTA education programs
- 47 developing PTA education programs

Outside of the United States there were three PT accredited programs, two in Canada and one in Scotland.

Discussion Questions

1. List the values of the APTA.
2. A second-year student member of the APTA is developing a presentation to incoming students. What should the student highlight as the purpose and value of becoming a member of the APTA?
3. After reviewing the APTA vision statement and goals, list contributions that PTAs can make to the APTA and profession.
4. Utilizing the APTA webpage, locate the *Information for Prospective Students*. Identify the role and benefits of being a PTA.

Learning Opportunities

1. Go online at www.apta.org and research information about the APTA.
2. Create a brochure identifying the vision, mission, and function of the APTA and the benefits of belonging to the APTA.
3. Participate in a district or chapter/subchapter meeting of the APTA.

CHAPTER 2

The Physical Therapist Assistant as a Member of the Health Care Team

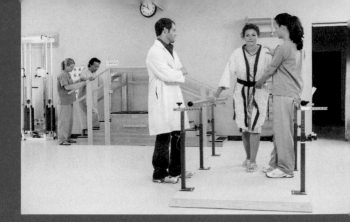

OBJECTIVES

After studying this chapter, the reader will be able to:

1. Discuss the supervisory role of the physical therapist on the health care team.
2. Describe the differences in role, function, and supervisory relationships of the physical therapist, physical therapist assistant, and other health care personnel.
3. List the events taking place in the collaborative path between physical therapist and physical therapist assistant.
4. Compare and contrast the types of health care teams.
5. Identify the members of the rehabilitation team and their responsibilities.

KEY TERMS

direct personal supervision
general supervision
interdisciplinary team
intradisciplinary team

multidisciplinary team
physical therapist assistant (PTA)
plan of care (POC)

Direction and Supervision of the Physical Therapist Assistant

The American Physical Therapy Association (APTA) defines a **physical therapist assistant (PTA)** as "a technically educated health care provider who assists the PT in the provision of physical therapy."[33] The Association considers a PTA to be the only individual who assists the PT in the delivery of selected physical therapy interventions. A PTA is also a graduate of a PTA education program accredited by the Commission on Accreditation in Physical Therapy Education (CAPTE).

LEVELS OF SUPERVISION

Per the APTA, a PTA delivering selected physical therapy interventions must be under a level of supervision called **general supervision**. This means the PT is not required to be physically present on-site for direction and supervision of the PTA, but must be available by telecommunications at all times. Some states, however, require that the PTA deliver selected physical therapy interventions only under the **direct personal supervision** of the PT. Direct personal supervision means the PT must be physically present and immediately available on-site at all times to direct and supervise tasks related to patient and client management. The direction and supervision is continuous throughout the time these tasks are performed.

In all physical therapy practice settings, the PTA's performance must be safe and legal. His or her performance also depends on many variables, including the type of clinical practice, the environmental surroundings of the practice, the type of communication between the PT and the PTA, the experience of the PTA, the patient/client's needs, the type of PTA supervision offered in emergency events, the PT's expectations for the patient/client, the necessary modification(s) to the **plan of care (POC)**, and the accessibility of the PT.

THE ROLE OF THE PTA IN A CLINICAL SETTING

The practice of physical therapy is conducted by the PT. The PT remains the only individual responsible for the physical therapy services when the PTA is involved with provision of selected interventions (treatments). The PT must provide direction and supervision of PTAs and other personnel for the provision of quality physical therapy services. Many considerations are involved to assure quality in physical therapy clinical settings. These considerations can have direct consequences in clinical practice, and may include the PT and PTA's education, experience, and responsibilities, along with the organizational structure in which the physical therapy services are provided. The PT is directly responsible for the actions of the PTA regarding patient/client management.[33]

APTA MINIMUM REQUIRED SKILLS OF PTA GRADUATES AT ENTRY LEVEL[38]

This document was developed by a committee to develop a list of required skills for a new graduate PTA. This list includes skills considered essential for any PTA graduate include musculoskeletal, neurological, cardiovascular pulmonary, and integumentary systems. The terms used in this list are based on the *Guide to Physical Therapist Practice* and an asterisk (*) denotes a skill identified on the PTA (NPTE) Test Content Outline.

PTA Skill Category	Description of Minimum Skills for PTA

Plan of Care Review
 	
• **Review of physical therapy documents**
 	
• **Review of medical record**
 	
• **Identification of pertinent information**
 	
• **Identification of indications, contraindications, precautions, safety considerations, and expected outcomes**
 	
• **Access to related literature**
 	
• **Match patient goals to selected interventions**
 	
• **Identification of role in patient care**
 	
• **Identification of items to be communicated to the physical therapist**
	1. Read all physical therapy documentation, including initial examination and plan of care.
	  A. Note indications, contraindications, precautions and safety considerations for the patient.
	  B. Note goals and expected outcomes.
	  C. Seek clarification from physical therapist, as needed.
	
	2. Review information in the medical record at each visit, including:
	  A. Monitor medical record for changes in medical status and/or medical procedures.
	  B. Collect data on patient's current condition, compare results to previously collected data and safety parameters established by the physical therapist, and determine if the safety parameters have been met.
	  C. Seek clarification from appropriate health professions' staff for unfamiliar or ambiguous information.
	
	3. Identify when the directed interventions are either beyond the scope of work or personal scope of work of the PTA.
	
	4. Communicate to the physical therapist when there are significant changes in the patient's medical status, physician referral, or when the criticality and complexity of the patient is beyond the knowledge, skills, and abilities of the PTA.
	
	5. Explain the rationale for selected interventions to achieve patient goals as identified in the plan of care.

APTA MINIMUM REQUIRED SKILLS OF PTA GRADUATES AT ENTRY LEVEL

PTA Skill Category	Description of Minimum Skills for PTA

Provision of Procedural Interventions
 	
· **Compliance with policies, procedures, ethical standards, etc.**
 	
· **Risk management strategies**
 	
· **Protection of patient privacy, rights, and dignity**
 	
· **Competent provision of interventions, including:**
 	
  · **Therapeutic exercise**
 	
  · **Functional training**
 	
  · **Manual therapy techniques**
 	
  · **Application and adjustment of devices and equipment***
 	
  · **Airway clearance techniques**
 	
  · **Integumentary repair and protection techniques**
 	
  · **Electrotherapeutic modalities***
 	
  · **Physical agents and mechanical modalities***
 	
· **Assessment of patient response**
 	
· **Clinical problem solving**
 	
· **Ability to modify techniques**
	1. Provide interventions compliant with federal and state licensing requirements, APTA standards documents (e.g. *Guide for Conduct for the PTA, Code of Ethics*), and facility policies and procedures.
	
	2. Assure safety of patient and self throughout patient care.
	  A. Identify the need for and take action when safety of patient or self may be at risk or has been compromised.
	  B. Utilize risk management strategies (e.g. universal precautions, body mechanics).
	
	3. Assure patient privacy, rights, and dignity.
	  A. Follow HIPAA requirements and observe Patient Bill of Rights.
	  B. Position/drape to protect patient modesty.
	
	4. Provide competent provision of physical therapy interventions, including:
	
	Therapeutic exercise
	  A. Aerobic Capacity/Endurance Conditioning or Reconditioning
	    1. Increase workload over time
	    2. Movement efficiency and energy conservation training
	    3. Walking/wheelchair propulsion programs
	  B. Balance, coordination, and agility training
	    1. Developmental activities training
	    2. Neuromuscular education or reeducation
	    3. Postural awareness training
	    4. Standardized, programmatic, complementary exercise approaches (protocols)
	    5. Task-Specific Performance Training (e.g. transfer training, mobility exercises, functional reaching)
	  C. Body mechanics and postural stabilization
	    1. Body mechanics training
	    2. Postural stabilization activities
	    3. Postural awareness training
	  D. Flexibility exercises
	    1. Range of motion
	    2. Stretching (e.g. passive, active, mechanical)
	  E. Gait and locomotion training
	    1. Developmental activities training
	    2. Gait training (with and without devices)
	    3. Standardized, programmatic, complementary exercise approaches
	    4. Wheelchair propulsion and safety
	  F. Neuromotor development training
	    1. Developmental activities training
	    2. Movement pattern training
	    3. Neuromuscular education or reeducation
	  G. Relaxation
	    1. Breathing strategies (with respect to delivery of an intervention)
	    2. Relaxation techniques (with respect to delivery of an intervention)

(continues)

APTA MINIMUM REQUIRED SKILLS OF PTA GRADUATES AT ENTRY LEVEL

PTA Skill Category	Description of Minimum Skills for PTA

	H. Strength, power, and endurance training for head, neck, limb, trunk, and ventilatory muscles
	    1. Active assistive, active, and resistive exercises, including concentric, dynamic/isotonic, eccentric, isometric, diaphragmatic breathing, and low-level plyometrics (e.g. kicking a ball, throwing a ball)
	
	Functional training in self-care and home management
	A. Activities of daily living (ADL) training
	    1. Bed mobility and transfer training
	    2. Activity-specific performance training
	B. Device and equipment use and training
	    1. Assistive and adaptive device or equipment training during ADL
	C. Injury prevention or reduction
	    1. Injury prevention education during self-care and home management
	    2. Injury prevention or reduction with use of devices and equipment
	    3. Safety awareness training during self-care and home management
	
	Manual therapy techniques
	A. Therapeutic massage
	B. Soft tissue mobilization
	C. Passive range of motion
	
	Application and adjustment of devices and equipment
	A. Adaptive devices
	    1. Hospital beds
	    2. Raised toilet seats
	B. Assistive devices
	    1. Canes
	    2. Crutches
	    3. Long-handled reachers
	    4. Walkers
	    5. Wheelchairs
	C. Orthotic and prosthetic devices
	    1. Braces
	D. Protective devices
	    1. Braces
	E. Supportive devices, such as:
	    1. Compression garments
	    2. Elastic wraps
	    3. Soft neck collars
	    4. Slings
	    5. Supplemental oxygen
	
	Breathing strategies/oxygenation
	    1. Identify patient in respiratory distress
	    2. Reposition patient to improve respiratory function

APTA MINIMUM REQUIRED SKILLS OF PTA GRADUATES AT ENTRY LEVEL

PTA Skill Category	Description of Minimum Skills for PTA
	3. Instruct patient in a variety of breathing techniques (pursed lip breathing, paced breathing, etc.)
	4. Administration of prescribed oxygen during interventions
	Integumentary protection
	1. Recognize interruptions in integumentary integrity
	2. Repositioning
	3. Patient education
	4. Edema management
	Electrotherapeutic modalities, such as:
	1. Electrotherapeutic delivery of medications
	2. Electrical muscle stimulation
	3. Electrical stimulation for tissue repair
	4. Functional electrical stimulation
	5. High-voltage pulsed current
	6. Neuromuscular electrical stimulation
	7. Transcutaneous electrical nerve stimulation
	Physical agents
	1. Cryotherapy (e.g. cold pack, ice massage, vapocoolant spray, hydrotherapy)
	2. Ultrasound
	3. Thermotherapy (e.g. dry heat, hot packs, paraffin baths, hydrotherapy)
	Mechanical modalities
	1. Compression therapies
	2. Mechanical motion devices
	3. Traction devices
	5. Determine patient's response to the intervention:
	A. Interview patient and accurately interpret verbal and nonverbal responses.
	B. Identify secondary effects or complications caused by the intervention.
	C. Determine outcome of intervention (positive or negative), including data collection and functional measures.
	6. Use clinical problem solving skills in patient care.
	A. Determine if patient is safe and comfortable with the intervention, and, if not, determine appropriate modifications.
	B. Compare results of intervention to previously collected data and determine if there is progress toward the expectations established by the PT or if the expectations have been met.
	C. Determine if modifications to the interventions are needed to improve patient response.
	7. Modify interventions to improve patient response.
	A. Determine modifications that can be made to the intervention within the plan of care.
	B. Communicate with physical therapist when modifications are outside scope of work or personal scope of work of PTA.
	C. Select and implement modification.
	D. Determine patient outcomes from the modification.

(continues)

APTA MINIMUM REQUIRED SKILLS OF PTA GRADUATES AT ENTRY LEVEL

PTA Skill Category	Description of Minimum Skills for PTA
Patient Instruction · **Application of principles of learning** · **Use of variety of teaching strategies** · **Methods to enhance compliance** · **Clarity in instructions** · **Assessment of patient response**	1. Apply principles of learning using a variety of teaching strategies during patient instruction. 2. Provide clear instructions (e.g. verbal, visual). 3. Apply methods to enhance compliance (e.g. handouts, reporting forms). 4. Determine patient response/understanding of instruction.

Patient Progression
 	
· **Competent patient progression**
 	
· **Communication of pertinent information**
 	
· **Relationship of psychosocial factors to progress**
 	
· **Clinical problem solving**
	1. Implement competent patient progression.
	  A. Identify the need to progress via data collection.
	  B. Determine what progression can be made within the plan of care.
	  C. Identify possible progressions that will continue to advance patient response.
	  D. Select and implement the progression of the intervention.
	  E. Determine outcomes of the intervention.
	2. Communicate pertinent information.
	  A. Identify changes in patient response due to intervention.
	  B. Describe adjustments to intervention within plan of care.
	  C. Describe response to change in intervention.
	3. Recognize when other variables (psychological, social, cultural, etc.) appear to be affecting the patient's progression with the intervention.
	4. Determine if patient is progressing toward goals in plan of care. If no, determine if modifications made to the intervention are required to improve patient response.

Data Collection
 	
· **Competent data collection**
 	
· **Interview skills**
 	
· **Accurate and timely**
 	
· **Clinical problem solving**
 	
· **Ability to modify techniques**
 	
· **Documentation and communication**
	1. Provide accurate, reproducible, safe, valid, and timely collection and documentation of data to measure the patient's medical status and/or progress within the intervention as indicated in the following categories:
	
	Anthropometric characteristics
	  1. Measure body dimensions (e.g. height, weight, girth, limb length).
	
	Arousal, attention, and cognition
	  1. Determine level of orientation to situation, time, place, and person.
	  2. Determine patient's ability to process commands.
	  3. Determine level of arousal (lethargic, alert, agitated).
	  4. Test patient's recall ability (e.g. short-term and long-term memory).
	
	Assistive and adaptive devices
	  1. Measure for assistive or adaptive devices and equipment.
	  2. Determine components, alignments and fit of device and equipment.
	  3. Determine patient's safety while using the device.
	  4. Monitor patient's response to the use of the device.
	  5. Check patient or caregiver's ability to care for device and equipment (maintenance, adjustment, cleaning).
	
	Body mechanics
	  1. Determine patient's ability to use proper body mechanics during functional activity.
	
	Environmental barriers, self-care, and home management
	  1. Identify potential safety barriers.
	  2. Identify potential environmental barriers.

APTA MINIMUM REQUIRED SKILLS OF PTA GRADUATES AT ENTRY LEVEL

PTA Skill Category	Description of Minimum Skills for PTA
	3. Identify potential physical barriers.
	4. Determine ability to perform bed mobility and transfers safely in the context of self-care home management.
	Gait, locomotion, and balance
	1. Determine patient's safety while engaged in gait, locomotion, balance, and mobility.
	2. Measure patient's progress with gait, locomotion, balance, and mobility, including use of standard tests.
	3. Describe gait deviations and their effect on gait and locomotion.
	Integumentary integrity
	1. Identify activities, positioning, and postures that may produce or relieve trauma to the skin.
	2. Identify devices and equipment that may produce or relieve trauma to the skin.
	3. Observe and describe skin characteristics (e.g. blistering, continuity of skin color, dermatitis, hair growth, mobility, nail growth, sensation, temperature, texture, and turgor).
	4. Observe and describe changes in skin integrity, such as presence of wound, blister, incision, hematoma, etc.
	5. Test for skin sensation and describe absent or altered sensation.
	Muscle function
	1. Perform manual muscle testing.
	2. Observe the presence or absence of muscle mass.
	3. Describe changes in muscle tone.
	Neuromotor function
	1. Identify the presence or absence of developmental reflexes, associated reactions, or abnormal tone.
	2. Identify performance of gross and fine motor skills.
	Orthotic and prosthetic devices and equipment
	1. Check components, ensure alignment and fit of orthotic devices, braces, and/or splints.
	2. Determine effectiveness of components (Is it working or not?), alignment, and fit of orthotic devices, braces, and splints during functional activities.
	3. Determine patient/caregiver's ability to don/doff orthotic, device, brace, and/or splint.
	4. Determine patient/caregiver's ability to care for orthotic device, brace, and/or splint (e.g. maintenance, adjustments, and cleaning).
	Pain
	1. Define location and intensity of pain.
	Posture
	1. Determine postural alignment and position (static and dynamic, symmetry, deviation from midline).
	Range of motion
	1. Perform tests of joint active and passive movement, muscle length, soft tissue extensibility, tone and flexibility (goniometry, tape measure).
	2. Describe functional range of motion.

(continues)

APTA MINIMUM REQUIRED SKILLS OF PTA GRADUATES AT ENTRY LEVEL

PTA Skill Category	Description of Minimum Skills for PTA

	Sensory response
	  1. Perform tests of superficial sensation (coarse touch, light touch, cold, heat, pain, pressure, and/or vibration).
	  2. Check peripheral nerve integrity (sensation, strength).
	Vital signs
	  1. Monitor and determine cardiovascular function (e.g. peripheral pulses, blood pressure, heart rate).
	  2. Monitor and determine physiological responses to position change (e.g. orthostatic hypotension, skin color, blood pressure, and heart rate).
	  3. Monitor and determine respiratory status (e.g. pulse oximetry, rate, and rhythm, pattern).
	2. Provide timely communication to the physical therapist regarding findings of data collection techniques.
	3. Recognize when intervention should not be provided or should be modified due to change in patient status.

Documentation • **Select relevant information** • **Accuracy** • **Ability to adapt**	1. Document in writing/electronically patient care using language that is accurate, complete, legible, timely, and consistent with institutional, legal, and billing requirements. 2. Use appropriate grammar, syntax, and punctuation in communication. 3. Use appropriate terminology and institutionally approved abbreviations. 4. Use an organized and logical framework to document care. 5. Identify and communicate with the physical therapist when further documentation is required.
Safety, CPR, and Emergency Procedures • **Safety** • **Initiate emergency response system** • **CPR**	1. Ensure safety of self and others in the provision of care in all situations. 2. Initiate and/or participate in emergency life support procedures (simulated or actual). 3. Initiate and/or participate in emergency response system (simulated or actual). 4. Maintain competency in CPR. 5. Prepare and maintain a safe working environment for performing interventions (e.g., clear walkways, equipment checks, etc.).
Health Care Literature	1. Reads and understands the health care literature.
Education • **Colleagues** • **Aides, volunteers, peers, coworkers** • **Students** • **Community**	1. Instruct other members of the health care team, using established techniques, programs, and instructional materials, commensurate with the learning characteristics of the audience. 2. Educate colleagues and other health care professionals about the role, responsibilities, and academic preparation and scope of work of the PTA.
Resource Management • **Human** • **Fiscal** • **Systems**	1. Follow legal and ethical requirements for direction and supervision of other support personnel. 2. Select appropriate nonpatient care activities to be directed to support personnel. 3. Identify and eliminate obstacles to completing patient related duties. 4. Demonstrate efficient time management. 5. Provide accurate and timely information for billing and reimbursement purposes. 6. Adhere to legal/ethical requirements, including billing. 7. Maintain and use physical therapy equipment effectively.

APTA MINIMUM REQUIRED SKILLS OF PTA GRADUATES AT ENTRY LEVEL

PTA Skill Category	Description of Minimum Skills for PTA
Behavioral Expectations • **Accountability** • **Altruism** • **Compassion and caring** • **Cultural competence** • **Duty** • **Integrity** • **Social responsibility**	Accountability 1. Adhere to federal and state legal practice standards and institutional regulations related to patient care and fiscal management. 2. Act in a manner consistent with the *Standards of Ethical Conduct for the Physical Therapist Assistant* and *Guide for Conduct of the Physical Therapist Assistant*. 3. Change behavior in response to understanding the consequences (positive and negative) of the physical therapist assistant's actions. Altruism 1. Place the patient/client's needs above the physical therapist assistant's self-interests. Compassion and caring 1. Exhibit compassion, caring, and empathy in providing services to patients; promote active involvement of the patient in his or her care. Cultural competence 1. Identify, respect, and act with consideration for the patient's differences, values, preferences, and expressed needs in all physical therapy activities. Duty 1. Describe and respect the physical therapists' and other team members' expertise, background, knowledge, and values. 2. Demonstrate reliability in meeting normal job responsibilities (e.g. attendance, punctuality, following direction). 3. Preserve the safety, security, privacy, and confidentiality of individuals. 4. Recognize and report when signs of abuse/neglect are present. 5. Actively promote physical therapy. Integrity 1. Demonstrate integrity in all interactions. 2. Maintain professional relationships with all persons. Social responsibility 1. Analyze work performance and behaviors and seek assistance for improvement as needed.
Communication	Interpersonal communication 1. Develop rapport with patients/clients and others to promote confidence. 2. Actively listen and display sensitivity to the needs of others. 3. Ask questions in a manner that elicits needed responses. 4. Modify communication to meet the needs of the audience, demonstrating respect for the knowledge and experience of others. 5. Demonstrate congruence between verbal and nonverbal messages. 6. Recognize when communication with the physical therapist is indicated. 7. Initiate and complete verbal and written communication with the physical therapist in a timely manner. 8. Ensure ongoing communication with the physical therapist for optimal patient care. 9. Recognize role and participate appropriately in communicating patient status and progress within the health care team.

(continues)

APTA MINIMUM REQUIRED SKILLS OF PTA GRADUATES AT ENTRY LEVEL

PTA Skill Category	Description of Minimum Skills for PTA
	Conflict management/negotiation 1. Recognize potential for conflict. 2. Implement strategies to prevent and/or resolve conflict. 3. Seek resources to resolve conflict when necessary.
Promotion of Health, Wellness, and Prevention	1. Demonstrate health-promoting behaviors. 2. Recognize opportunities to educate the public or patients about issues of health, wellness, and prevention (e.g. benefits of exercise, prevention of falls, etc.) and communicate opportunity to the physical therapist. 3. Educate the public or patients about issues of health, wellness, and prevention (e.g. benefits of exercise, prevention of falls, etc.). 4. Recognize patient indicators of willingness to change health behaviors and communicate to the physical therapist.
Career Development	1. Engage in self-assessment. 2. Identify individual learning needs to enhance role in the profession. 3. Identify and obtain resources to increase knowledge and skill. 4. Engage in learning activities (e.g. clinical experience, mentoring, skill development). 5. Incorporate new knowledge and skill into clinical performance.

American Physical Therapy Association. Minimum Required Skills of Physical Therapist Assistant Graduate at Entry-Level. Reprinted from http://www.apta.org, with permission of the American Physical Therapy Association. Copyright (c) 2015 American Physical Therapy Association. APTA is not responsible for the translation from English.

The PTA cannot evaluate, develop, or change the POC or the treatment plan, and cannot write a discharge plan or a summary.[39] Furthermore, the APTA has a position that the PTA cannot perform joint mobilization techniques and sharp debridement wound therapy because it requires evaluative skills during the application of the intervention. Some PTs choose to allow PTAs who have the appropriate knowledge and skills to perform these interventions. And while it is not mandated as a minimum skill of PTA graduates, many PTA programs teach the basics of joint mobilization with the understanding that some clinical practice sites expect PTAs to perform these interventions. States' physical therapy practice acts differ in regard to the PTA's responsibilities and may prohibit or allow different skills, including joint mobilization.

THE PHYSICAL THERAPIST'S RESPONSIBILITIES IN THE CLINICAL SETTING

The PT integrates the five elements of patient/client management to optimize patient/client outcome(s). These five elements are examination, evaluation, diagnosis, prognosis, and intervention. The PT's POC may involve having the PTA assist with selected interventions. The PT is responsible for directing and supervising the PTA consistent with the APTA's House of Delegates positions (Direction and Supervision of the Physical Therapist Assistant[39]). All selected interventions are directed and supervised by the PT. Also, there should be ongoing communication regarding the patient/client's care between the PT and the PTA.

Regardless of the setting in which the services are provided, while supervising the PTA, the APTA has established that the PT has the following responsibilities:[39]

- Referral interpretation
- Initial examination, evaluation, diagnosis, and prognosis
- Development or modification of a POC based on the initial examination and reexamination; the POC includes the physical therapy goals and outcomes.
- Determination of when the expertise and decision-making capability of the PT requires the PT to personally administer physical therapy interventions and when it may be appropriate to utilize the PTA. A PT must determine the most appropriate use of the PTA in order to provide safe, effective, and efficient physical therapy services.
- Reexamination of the patient/client considering the patient/client's goals and revision of the POC

- Establishment of the discharge plan and documentation of discharge summary/status
- Oversight of all documentation for physical therapy services rendered to each patient/client

Ultimately, the PT remains responsible for the physical therapy services provided when the PT's POC involves the PTA assisting with selected interventions. When determining the appropriate extent of assistance from the PTA, the PT must consider the following:[39]

- The PTA's education, training, experience, and skill level
- Patient/client stability, criticality, acuity, and complexity
- The predictability of the consequences
- The type of setting in which physical therapy services are provided
- Liability and risk management concerns
- Federal and state statutes
- The mission of physical therapy services for that specific clinical setting
- The needed frequency of reexamination

The APTA's recommendations for ongoing communication between the supervising PT and the PTA in off-site settings may include the following actions:[39]

- The supervising PT must be accessible by telecommunications to the PTA at all times while the PTA is treating patients/clients. This requirement is dependent on the jurisdiction of the clinical site. Some jurisdictions require general supervision whereas others require direct, on-site supervision.
- There must be regularly scheduled and documented conferences between the supervising PT and the PTA regarding patients/clients. The frequency of these conferences must be determined by the needs of the patient/client and the needs of the PTA. In those situations in which a PTA is involved in the care of a patient/client, a supervisory visit by the PT will be made for the following reasons:
  - Upon the PTA's request for a patient's reexamination
  - When a change in the POC is needed
  - Prior to any planned discharge

- In response to a change in the patient/client's medical status
- At least once a month, or at a higher frequency when established by the supervising PT, in accordance with the needs of the patient/client

A supervisory visit should include the following: an on-site reexamination of the patient/client, an on-site review of the POC with appropriate revision or termination, and an evaluation of need and recommendation for use of outside resources.

THE COLLABORATION PATH BETWEEN THE PHYSICAL THERAPIST AND THE PHYSICAL THERAPIST ASSISTANT

There is a collaborative path between the PT and the PTA that allows appropriate communication and patient care. This collaborative path includes the following steps:

1. The PT performs the initial examination of the patient/client. During the examination, the PTA helps the PT by gathering specific data that the PT requested. The PTA accepts the delegated tasks within the limits of his or her capabilities and also considering legal, jurisdictional, and ethical circumstances and principles. Although the PTA cannot perform the initial examination and evaluation, he or she may take notes and help gather some data as requested by the PT. Taking notes should not compromise the decision-making process of the PT, the integrity of the evaluation, or the establishment of the POC.
2. The PT performs the initial evaluation of the patient/client by comprehensively assessing all the results of the initial examination. The PT assesses the examination data to make a judgment about the data value. This is called evaluating. The PTA is not involved in this process. The PTA does not interpret the results of the initial examination.
3. The PT establishes a diagnosis by organizing the examination data into defined clusters, syndromes, or categories to be able to determine the prognosis, including the POC. The PTA is not involved in this process.
4. The PT determines the patient/client's prognosis (level of optimal improvement) that may be obtained

through specific interventions; the PT also decides the necessary amount of time, frequency, and types of interventions required to reach the patient/client's optimal level. The PTA is not involved in this process.

5. The PT establishes the goals/outcomes to be accomplished by the POC and the plan for interventions. The PT creates a POC to use various physical therapy procedures and techniques to produce changes in the patient/client's condition.

6. The PT performs the patient/client's interventions, delegating selected patient/client interventions to the PTA.

7. The PTA performs the selected patient/client interventions as directed by the PT. There is established, ongoing communication between the PT and the PTA.

8. The PTA may perform data collection during the course of the patient/client's interventions to record patient/client's progress or lack of progress since the initial examination and evaluation. The PTA may ask the PT for a reexamination. The PTA's utilization and understanding of problem solving is an integral part of patient care. The APTA has developed a Decision Making Algorithm that can assist the PTA in developing this skill. The Algorithm can be located in Appendix E.

9. The PT performs the reexamination and establishes new patient/client outcomes and POC.

10. The PT performs patient/client's new interventions. The PT delegates to the PTA selected new patient/client interventions.

11. The PTA performs new patient/client interventions as directed by the PT. There is again established, ongoing communication between the PT and the PTA.

12. The PT performs the discharge examination and evaluation of the patient/client when the outcomes are met. Just as with the initial examination, the PTA can gather examination data that can be utilized by the PT in the discharge evaluation.

The preferred collaborative relationship between the PT and the PTA is characterized by trust, mutual respect, and value and appreciation for individual and cultural differences. In this relationship, the PTA's role is to offer suggestions, provide feedback, carry out agreed-upon delegated activities, and freely express concerns to the PT about clinical issues or other difficulties. The PT and the PTA modify communication to effectively treat patients,

collaborate as team members, ensure a continuum of care in all settings, and educate patients, families, caregivers, other health care providers, and payers. The mechanisms for effective communication and feedback between the PT and the PTA relating to patient/client care include:

- Discussion of the goals and expectations for the patient
- Frequent and open communication
- Information on response to patient care
- Recommendations for discharge planning
- Discussion of modifications of a POC established by the PT
- Recommendations from other disciplines
- Considerations of precautions, contraindications, or other special problems included in the interventions

The PT is the administrator and supervisor of the clinical services and the PTA can assist with delegated clinical services or administrative tasks.

DIFFERENCES IN SUPERVISION REQUIREMENTS FOR PHYSICAL THERAPIST ASSISTANTS

PTs are licensed providers in all states and PTAs are licensed providers in the majority of states. In regard to supervision, the PTs and PTAs are governed by their state's specific physical therapy practice act. Some states have more stringent standards of supervision than other states. In all situations, the PTs and PTAs must comply with their state practice act. The state-specific practice act dictates the number of assistive personnel (including PTAs) that the PT can supervise. For example, in Arizona one PT can supervise three PTAs, whereas in Kansas he or she can supervise four and in Iowa only two. The majority of states limit the number of personnel a PT can supervise.

In addition, there are supervision requirements for PTAs that relate to the type of insurance that reimburses physical therapy services, such as Medicare, and the types of setting, such as outpatient or inpatient departments, home health agencies, private facilities, and others. For example, in certain settings (reimbursed by Medicare) such as home health agencies (HHA), physical therapy services can be performed safely and effectively under the "general" supervision of a PT. This type of supervision means the PT need not always be present on the premises when the PTA is delivering physical therapy services. However, this Medicare rule for HHAs may be superseded by a specific state physical therapy practice act.

Another example of Medicare supervision for PTAs is the "direct" form of supervision, which takes place in the office of a PT in private practice (PTPP). This means that the supervising PT (who owns his or her physical therapy practice) must always be physically present in the office suite at the time physical therapy services are provided by PTAs (and other PTs). For more information, PTAs must consult the Medicare supervision requirements (at www.apta.org) and their state practice act.

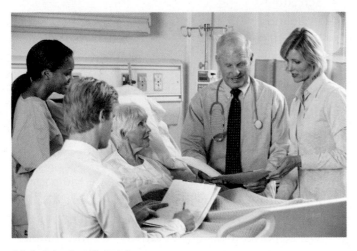

© Monkey Business Images/Shutterstock

The Health Care Team and the Rehabilitation Team

As health care professionals and providers, PTs and PTAs always work together with other professionals and providers. Typically, this collaborative effort between disciplines involves the health care team and the rehabilitation team.

HEALTH CARE TEAM

The health care team is a group of equally important individuals with a common interest: collaborating to develop common goals and building trusting relationships to achieve these goals. Members of the health care team are the patient/client, family member(s), caregiver(s), various health care professionals involved in the patient/client's care, and insurance companies. The patient/client, the patient/client's family, and the caregiver(s) are extremely important in the team. To work effectively as a team, the members of the health care team must be committed to the goals of the team and of the patient. They must address all the patient's medical needs. Team members must communicate

effectively with each other, sharing a common language of care, respect, dedication, and teamwork. All members must also show leadership skills to be able to effectively work together and help the patient/client placed in their care.

There are three types of health care teams: intradisciplinary, multidisciplinary, and interdisciplinary. **Intradisciplinary team** members work together within the same discipline. Other disciplines are not involved. An example of such a team is the PT and the PTA working in a home health care physical therapy practice when other services are not necessary. Although the members collaborate effectively, this team is not the most efficient type because only one discipline is involved. This means the patient/client has only one type of care.

In a **multidisciplinary team**, members work separately and independently in their different disciplines. They do not meet or try to collaborate with each other. The members' allegiance is mostly geared toward their particular discipline. Sometimes, competition between members may develop. An example of such a team may be different medical specialties trying to evaluate a patient for a specific pathology having very little communication with each other. The lack of communication and cooperation between the members of the multidisciplinary team may cause problems for the patient/client. For example, the patient/client's final diagnosis may be controversial because some members of the team have a competitive approach and limited consultation. This is not the most effective team approach; however, its success depends on the members of the team.

Contrary to the first two teams, the **interdisciplinary team** members work together within all disciplines to set goals relevant to a patient/client's individual case. All the members collaborate in decision making; however, the evaluations and interventions are done independently. An example of such an interdisciplinary team would be health care members working together in a skilled nursing facility (SNF). In such a facility, members from different disciplines meet, exchange information, and try to understand each other's discipline in order to help the patients. The outcomes and the goals are team-directed, and not bound to a specific discipline. This team is the most efficient and most successful in regard to a patient's outcomes.

REHABILITATION TEAM

The rehabilitation team may include the PT, the PTA, the occupational therapist, the certified occupational therapist assistant, the SLP, the certified orthotist and prosthetist, the kinesiologist, the primary care physician (a medical doctor such as a physiatrist and/or a doctor of osteopathy or other specialty/physician who is concurrently treating the patient), the physician assistant, the registered nurse, the social worker, and the certified athletic trainer. It may also include the physical therapy aide, the physical therapy volunteer, the PT or the PTA student, and the home health aide.

Physical Therapy Director

The rehabilitation team also includes the physical therapy director (who may also be called the physical therapy manager or physical therapy supervisor). The physical therapy director may be an experienced PT or PTA (with knowledge and experience beyond entry level) who manages and supervises a physical therapy department. He or she is in charge of the functions of the department, the responsibilities of all members of the department, and the relationships of all personnel in the department.

The physical therapy director has to make sure that the department's policies and procedures are applied efficiently and that goals and strategic planning are set for the department. The director also has clinical knowledge and skills plus abilities in administration, education, leadership, and other areas. He or she has the responsibility to:

- Motivate subordinates
- Communicate effectively with supervisors
- Impartially evaluate staff and give feedback
- Educate all employees
- Interview new personnel and help their development of skills
- Delegate tasks to appropriate staff

Physical Therapist

As a member of the rehabilitation team, the PT clinician is a skilled health care professional with a postbaccalaureate degree (doctorate—Doctor in Physical Therapy). The APTA considers attainment of a postbaccalaureate as the minimum professional education qualification for PTs who graduated from a CAPTE-accredited program after 2003.

As of 2014, almost all PT postbaccalaureate degrees were from Doctor of Physical Therapy (DPT) programs.[37] As per the APTA, the DPT is a postbaccalaureate degree conferred upon successful completion of a doctoral-level

professional (entry-level) or postprofessional education program. The transition to the regulatory designation of "DPT" was adopted by the 2014 House of Delegates. This transition will require changes in the practice acts of all states by the year 2025.[32] After graduation, and following successful performance on the National Physical Therapy Examination, every PT is licensed (or registered) by each state or jurisdiction where he or she practices. As a member of the rehabilitation team, the PT is responsible for the patient/client's:

- Screening
- Evaluation
- Diagnosis
- Prognosis
- Intervention
- Education
- Prevention of injury and disease
- Coordination of care
- Referral to other providers

The PT also must prevent or decrease the patient/client's impairments, functional limitations, and disabilities and achieve cost-effective clinical outcomes.

The responsibilities of PTs are various and complex. They provide services that help restore function, improve mobility, relieve pain, and prevent or limit permanent physical disabilities of patients suffering from injuries or disease. They restore, maintain, and promote overall fitness and health. During their daily practice, PTs examine patients' medical histories and then test and measure the patients' strength, range of motion, balance and coordination, posture, muscle performance, respiration, and motor function. They also determine patients' abilities to be independent and reintegrate into the community or workplace after injury or illness. Furthermore, PTs develop treatment plans describing a treatment strategy, its purpose, and its anticipated outcome. For example, in regard to treatments, PTs encourage patients to use their own muscles to increase their flexibility and range of motion before finally advancing to other exercises that improve strength, balance, coordination, and endurance.

The PT's treatment goal is to improve the individual's functions at work and at home. During interventions, PTs also may use electrical stimulation, hot packs or cold compresses, and ultrasound to relieve pain and reduce swelling. They may use traction or deep-tissue massage or other myofascial release (as a form of manual therapy) to alleviate soreness and tenderness of the muscles.

PTs also educate patients, clients, families of patients/clients, and caregivers on how to:

- Use assistive and adaptive devices, such as crutches, prostheses, and wheelchairs
- Perform home exercise programs
- Help facilitate patient independence at home, work, and/or play
- Prevent disease, and promote wellness and healthy behaviors

As treatment continues, PTs document the patient's progress, conduct periodic examinations, and modify treatments as necessary. PTs are also teachers in colleges and universities and perform research contributing to evidence-based physical therapy practice.

According to the U.S. Department of Labor, Bureau of Statistics, "employment of physical therapists is expected to grow by 36 percent from 2012 to 2022, much faster than the average for all occupations."[39] Over the long run, the demand for PTs should continue to rise as the increase in the number of individuals with disabilities or limited function spurs demand for therapy services. The growing elderly population is particularly vulnerable to chronic and debilitating conditions that require therapeutic services. Also, the baby boomer generation is entering the prime age for heart attacks and strokes, increasing the demand for cardiac and physical rehabilitation. Young people will need physical therapy as technological advances save the lives of a larger proportion of newborns with severe birth defects. Future medical developments also should permit a higher percentage of trauma victims to survive, creating additional demand for rehabilitative care. Employment growth in the physical therapy field may also result from advances in medical technology that would permit the treatment of more disabling conditions. In addition, widespread interest in health promotion should increase demand for physical therapy services. A growing number of employers are using PTs to evaluate worksites, develop exercise programs, and teach safe work habits to employees in the hope of reducing injuries.

Physical Therapist Assistant

The PTA is a technically educated health care provider who assists the PT in the provision of physical therapy. The PTA is a graduate of a PTA educational program accredited by CAPTE earning an associate degree from a technical or community college, college, or university. Following successful

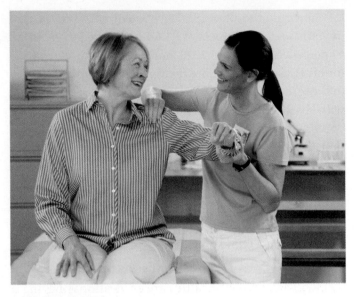

© wavebreakmedia/Shutterstock

performance on the National Physical Therapy Examination (NPTE), administered by the Federation of State Boards of Physical Therapy (FSBPT), every PTA is licensed by each state or jurisdiction where he or she practices.

The PTA is an important member of the rehabilitation team. As discussed earlier, the PT is directly responsible for the actions of the PTA related to patient/client management. The PTA may perform selected physical therapy interventions under the direction and at least general supervision of the PT. The PT can determine the most appropriate use of the PTA to provide delivery of services in a safe, effective, and efficient manner.

PTAs perform a variety of tasks. These treatment procedures, performed under the direction and supervision of PTs, include the following:

- Therapeutic exercises
- Therapeutic massages
- Therapeutic modalities such as electrical stimulation, paraffin baths, hot and cold packs, traction, and ultrasound
- Patient/caregiver/family education

PTAs also record the patient's responses to treatment, and report the outcome of each treatment to the PT.

In addition to clinical practice, PTAs may work in PTA educational programs. They act as program directors, instructors and clinical instructors. They provide students with an appropriate role model of the PT–PTA relationship.

According to the U.S. Department of Labor, Bureau of Statistics, employment of PTAs is expected to grow "by 41 percent from 2012 to 2022, much faster than the average for all occupations."[40] The reasons for growth are similar to those for PTs: the increase in the number of individuals with disabilities or limited function, the growing elderly population vulnerable to chronic and debilitating conditions that require therapeutic services, and the large baby boomer generation in need of rehabilitation. In addition, future medical developments would also create demand for physical therapy services.

Occupational Therapist

The licensed (or registered) **occupational therapist** (OTR/L) is a skilled health care professional having a doctorate or master's degree. All states, Puerto Rico, and the District of Columbia regulate the practice of occupational therapy; however, specific eligibility requirements for licensure vary by state. To obtain a license, applicants must graduate from an accredited educational program and pass a national certification examination. The occupational therapists who pass the exam are awarded the title occupational therapist registered (OTR) or occupational therapist licensed (OTL).

Occupational therapists (OTs) help people improve their ability to perform tasks in their daily living and working environments. They work with individuals who have conditions that are mentally, physically, developmentally, or emotionally disabling. They also help these individuals to develop, recover, or maintain daily living and work skills. OTs help patients and clients not only to improve their basic motor functions and reasoning abilities, but also to compensate for permanent loss of function. OTs' areas of expertise include the following:

- Patient education and training in activities of daily living (ADLs)
- Development and fabrication of orthoses (splints)
- Training, recommendation, and selection of adaptive equipment (such as a long-arm shoehorn)
- Therapeutic activities for a patient/client's functional, cognitive, or perceptual abilities
- Consultation in adaptation of the environment for a physically challenged patient/client

OTs also use computer programs to help patients/clients improve decision-making, abstract-reasoning, problem-solving, and perceptual skills, as well as memory, sequencing, and coordination. All of these skills are important for independent living. OTs instruct those with permanent disabilities, such as spinal cord injuries, cerebral palsy, or muscular dystrophy, in the use of adaptive equipment, including wheelchairs, splints, and aids for eating and dressing. They also design or make special equipment needed at home or at work. Some OTs treat individuals whose ability to function in a work environment has been impaired. These practitioners arrange employment, evaluate the work environment, plan work activities, and assess the client's progress. OTs also may collaborate with the client and the employer to modify the work environment so that the client's work can be successfully completed.

OTs may work exclusively with individuals in a particular age group or with particular disabilities. In schools, for example, they evaluate children's abilities, recommend and provide therapy, modify classroom equipment, and help children participate as fully as possible in school programs and activities. OTs in mental health settings treat individuals who are mentally ill, mentally retarded, or emotionally disturbed. OTs also may work with individuals who are dealing with alcoholism, drug abuse, depression, eating disorders, or stress-related disorders. Assessing and recording a client's activities and progress is an important part of an OT's job. Accurate records are essential for evaluating patients and clients, for billing, and for reporting to physicians and other health care providers. In addition, OTs are specializing in new practices such as driver rehabilitation and fall-prevention training for the elderly.

According to the U.S. Department of Labor, Bureau of Statistics, the largest number of OTs' jobs have been in acute hospitals, rehabilitation centers, and orthopedic settings.[40] Other major employers are offices of other health practitioners (which include offices of OTs), public and private educational services, and nursing care facilities. Some OTs are employed by home health care services, outpatient care centers, offices of physicians, individual and family services, community care facilities for the elderly, and government agencies. A small number of OTs are self-employed in private practice.

Similar to physical therapy, "employment of occupational therapists is expected to increase by 29 percent between 2012 and 2022, much faster than the average for all occupations."[40] The baby boomer generation's movement into middle age and the growth in the population

75 years or older will increase the demand for occupational therapy services. Hospitals will continue to employ a large number of OTs to provide therapy services to acutely ill inpatients. Hospitals also will need OTs to staff their outpatient rehabilitation programs. Employment growth in schools will result from the expansion of the school-age population and extended services for disabled students. OTs will be needed to help children with disabilities prepare to enter special education programs.

Occupational Therapy Assistant

Occupational therapy assistants generally must complete an associate degree or a certificate program from an accredited community college or technical school. Occupational therapy assistants are regulated in most states and must pass a national certification examination after they graduate. Those who pass the test are awarded the title of certified occupational therapy assistant (COTA). The COTA's duties do not include patient evaluation and establishment or revision of a POC. The COTA's areas of practice are in a patient/client's functional deficits of dressing, grooming, personal hygiene, and housekeeping.

The supervisory relationship of the OTR/L and the COTA follow similar guidelines to the supervisory relationship between the PT and the PTA. Occupational therapy assistants work under the direction of occupational therapists to provide rehabilitative services to persons with mental, physical, emotional, or developmental impairments. The ultimate goal is to improve patients/clients' quality of life and ability to perform daily activities. For example, occupational therapy assistants help injured workers reenter the labor force by teaching them how to compensate for lost motor skills; COTAs also help individuals with learning disabilities increase their independence. Occupational therapy assistants help patients/clients with rehabilitative activities and exercises outlined in a treatment plan developed in collaboration with an occupational therapist. Activities range from teaching the proper method of moving from a bed into a wheelchair to the best way to stretch and limber the muscles of the hand. Occupational therapy assistants monitor an individual's activities to make sure they are performed correctly and to provide encouragement. They also record their patient/client's progress for the occupational therapist. In addition, occupational therapy assistants document the billing of the client's health insurance provider.

According to the U.S. Department of Labor, Bureau of Statistics, occupational therapy assistants work in hospitals, offices of other health practitioners (which includes offices of occupational therapists), and nursing care facilities.[40] Some occupational therapy assistants work in community care facilities for the elderly, home health care services, individual and family services, and state government agencies. As per the U.S. Department of Labor, "from 2012 to 2022, employment of occupational therapist assistants is expected to grow by 41 percent, much faster than the average for all occupations."[40] The demand for occupational therapy assistants will continue to rise, due to growth in the number of individuals with disabilities or limited function. Job growth will result from an aging population, which will need more occupational therapy services. Third-party payers, concerned with rising health care costs, are expected to encourage occupational therapists to delegate more hands-on therapy work to occupational therapy assistants.

Speech-Language Pathologist

The speech-language pathologist (SLP) or speech therapist is a skilled health care professional who has a master's degree in speech pathology (including 9 months to 1 year of clinical experience). The SLP needs to pass a national examination to obtain the certification of clinical competence to practice speech and language pathology. The national examination on speech-language pathology is offered through the Praxis Series of the Educational Testing Service (ETS).

Medicaid, Medicare, and private health insurers generally require a SLP practitioner to be licensed to qualify for reimbursement. All states regulate SLPs through licensure or registration. SLPs can also acquire the Certificate of Clinical Competence in Speech-Language Pathology (CCC-SLP) offered by the American Speech-Language-Hearing Association. To earn a CCC, a person must have a graduate degree and 375 hours of supervised clinical experience, complete a 36-week postgraduate clinical fellowship, and pass the Praxis Series examination in speech-language pathology administered by the ETS.

SLPs assess, diagnose, treat, and help to prevent speech, language, cognitive, communication, voice, swallowing, fluency, and other related disorders. The SLP's general area of practice is to restore or improve communication of patients with language and speech impairments. In the rehabilitation team, the SLP works closely with the

PT, PTA, OTR/L, and COTA to correct a patient's swallowing and cognitive deficits. SLPs work with people who cannot make speech sounds, or cannot make them clearly; those with speech rhythm and fluency problems, such as stuttering; people with voice quality problems, such as inappropriate pitch or harsh voice; those with problems understanding and producing language; those who wish to improve their communication skills by modifying an accent; those with cognitive communication impairments, such as attention, memory, and problem-solving disorders; and those with hearing loss who use hearing aids or cochlear implants in order to develop auditory skills and improve communication. SLPs use written and oral tests, as well as special instruments, to diagnose the nature and extent of impairment and to record and analyze speech, language, and swallowing irregularities.

SLPs develop an individualized POC tailored to each patient's needs. For individuals with little or no speech capability, SLPs may select augmentative or alternative communication methods, including automated devices and sign language, and teach their use. They teach these individuals how to make sounds, improve their voices, or increase their language skills to communicate more effectively. SLPs help patients develop, or recover, reliable communication skills so patients can fulfill their educational, vocational, and social roles.

Most SLPs provide direct clinical services to individuals with communication or swallowing disorders. In speech and language clinics, they may independently develop and carry out treatment programs. SLPs in schools develop individual or group programs, counsel parents, and may assist teachers with classroom activities. SLPs keep records on the initial evaluation, progress, and discharge of clients. This helps pinpoint problems, tracks client progress, and justifies the cost of treatment when applying for reimbursement. They counsel individuals and their families concerning communication disorders and how to cope with the stress and misunderstanding that often accompany them. They also work with family members to recognize and change behavior patterns that impede communication and treatment and show them communication-enhancing techniques to use at home. Some SLPs conduct research on how people communicate. Others design and develop equipment or techniques for diagnosing and treating speech problems.

According to the U.S. Department of Labor, Bureau of Statistics, SLPs work in educational services, including preschools, elementary and secondary schools, and colleges and universities.[40] Others work in hospitals; the offices of other health practitioners, including SLPs; nursing care facilities; home health care services; individual and family services; outpatient care centers; child day care services; or other facilities. A few SLPs are self-employed in private practice. They contract to provide services in schools, offices of physicians, hospitals, or nursing care facilities, or work as consultants to industry. As per the U.S. Department of Labor office, "the employment of speech-language pathologists is expected to grow by 19 percent from 2012 to 2022, faster than the average for all occupations."[40] The reasons for this growth may be the members of the baby boomer generation having problems associated with speech, language, swallowing, and hearing impairments, and the high survival rate of premature infants and trauma and stroke victims, whose speech or language may need assessment and possible treatment. Many states now require that all newborns be screened for hearing loss and receive appropriate early intervention services. Employment of SLPs in educational services will increase along with growth in elementary and secondary school enrollments, including enrollment of special education students.

Orthotist and Prosthetist

Both orthotists and prosthetists are important members of the rehabilitation team. They work closely with orthopedic surgeons, physicians from many disciplines, and physical and occupational therapy practitioners. As per the U.S. Department of Labor, "orthotists and prosthetists can fit and prepare orthopedic braces and prosthetic devices for patients/clients who have disabilities of limbs or spine" (including partial or total absence of the limb).[40] In regard to educational requirements, orthotists and prosthetists must complete an accredited bachelor degree program and 1 year of residency in prosthetics and orthotics. Certification as orthotists or prosthetists is available through the American Board for Certification in Orthotics and Prosthetics. The certified orthotist designs, fabricates, and fits patients with orthoses prescribed by the physician. The orthoses can be braces, splints, cervical collars, and corsets. The certified prosthetist designs, fabricates, and fits prostheses for patients with partial or total loss of limb(s). Both prosthetists and orthotists are responsible for making any modifications and alignments of the prosthetic limbs and orthotic braces, evaluating the patients' progress, keeping accurate records on each patient, and teaching the patients how to care for their prosthetic or orthotic devices. Prosthetists and orthotists work in private practice laboratories, hospitals, or government agencies.

Kinesiologist

Kinesiologists are individuals who complete a bachelor or master degree in the study of human movement who try to improve the efficiency and performance of the human body in sports, at work, and during ADLs. Kinesiologists work closely with PTs and PTAs to help patients/clients in specific areas of exercise, biomechanics, psychomotor skills, and the workplace environment. In regard to exercise kinesiology, the kinesiologist will work with the PT to assess and monitor a patient/client's response to exercises. Based on data analysis (from an assessment such as the patient/client's ambulation on a treadmill in cardiac rehabilitation), the PT may ask the kinesiologist to create an exercise program individually designed for the patient. Biomechanics kinesiologists can also collaborate with PTs and prosthetists to improve and maximize prosthetic devices during patient/client ambulation (walking) with a prosthetic limb. A psychomotor kinesiologist will cooperate with physical therapy in the area of neurological impairments that cause motor learning impairments to patients/clients. A kinesiologist in the workplace environment performs workplace and ergonomic analysis together with physical therapy for enhancement of patients/clients' body mechanics and positioning. Some kinesiologists may also coach or train amateur/professional athletes. Others with doctoral degrees (PhD) may teach or be involved in research activities at different universities.

Primary Care Physician

The primary care physician (PCP) is a medical doctor (MD) or an osteopathic doctor (DO). The PCP provides primary care services and manages routine health care needs. Although both MDs and DOs may use all accepted methods of treatment, including drugs and surgery, DOs place special emphasis on the body's musculoskeletal system, preventive medicine, and holistic patient care. DOs are more likely than MDs to be primary care specialists, although they can be found in all specialties. About half of DOs practice general or family medicine, general internal medicine, or general pediatrics. The PCP acts as the "gatekeeper" for patients covered under managed health care systems (such as an HMO), authorizing referrals to other specialties or services including physical therapy.

In general, physicians diagnose illnesses and prescribe and administer treatment for people suffering from injury or disease. They examine patients, obtain medical histories, and order, perform, and interpret diagnostic tests. They counsel patients on diet, hygiene, and preventive health care.

It takes many years of education and training to become an MD: 4 years of undergraduate school, 4 years of medical school, and between a range of 3 to 8 years of internship and residency, depending on the specialty selected. A few medical schools offer combined undergraduate and medical school programs that last 6 years rather than the customary 8 years. The minimum educational requirement for entry into a medical school is 3 years of college; most applicants, however, have at least a bachelor degree, and many have advanced degrees. Acceptance to medical school is highly competitive. Applicants must submit transcripts, scores from the Medical College Admission Test, and letters of recommendation. Schools also consider applicants' character, personality, leadership qualities, and participation in extracurricular activities. Most schools require an interview with members of the admissions committee. Following medical school, almost all MDs enter a residency. Residency is a graduate medical education in a specialty that takes the form of paid on-the-job training, usually in a hospital. Most DOs serve a 12-month rotating internship after graduation and before entering a residency, which may last 2 to 6 years, being also dependent on the selected specialization.

All states, the District of Columbia, and U.S. territories license physicians. To be licensed, physicians must graduate from an accredited medical school, pass a licensing examination, and complete 1 to 7 years of graduate medical education. Although physicians licensed in one state usually can get a license to practice in another without further examination, some states limit reciprocity. Graduates of foreign medical schools generally can qualify for licensure after passing an examination and completing a U.S. residency. MDs and DOs seeking board certification in a specialty may spend up to 7 years in residency training, depending on the specialty. A final examination immediately after residency or after 1 or 2 years of practice also is necessary for certification by the American Board of Medical Specialists or the American Osteopathic Association. There are 24 specialty boards, ranging from allergy and immunology to urology.

In the rehabilitation team, there are five distinct physicians' specialties that PTs and PTAs may interact with the most: family and general practitioners, physiatrists, orthopedic surgeons, neurologists, and pediatricians. Family and general practitioners are often the first point of contact for people seeking health care, acting as the traditional family doctor. They assess and treat a wide range of conditions, ailments, and injuries, from sinus and respiratory infections to broken bones and scrapes. Family and general practitioners typically have a patient base of regular, long-term visitors. Patients with more serious conditions are referred to specialists or other health care facilities for more intensive care.

The physiatrist is a physician specializing in physical medicine and rehabilitation. Physiatrists treat a wide range of problems from sore shoulders to spinal cord injuries. They see patients in all age groups and treat problems that touch upon all the major systems in the body. These specialists focus on restoring function to people. They care for patients with acute and chronic pain and musculoskeletal problems such as back and neck pain, tendonitis, pinched nerves, and fibromyalgia. They also treat people who have experienced catastrophic events resulting in paraplegia, quadriplegia, or traumatic brain injury, and individuals who have had strokes, orthopedic injuries, or neurologic disorders such as multiple sclerosis, polio, or amyotrophic lateral sclerosis (ALS). Physiatrists practice in rehabilitation centers, hospitals, and private offices. They often have broad practices, but some concentrate on one area such as pediatrics, sports medicine, geriatric medicine, brain injury, or many other special interests.

Orthopedic surgeons are highly trained physicians who diagnose, treat, give medical advice, and perform surgery on people with bone and joint disorders including nerve impingement conditions of the spine and hip and knee injuries. They not only have a wide expertise in treating back and neck injuries, but also are often called upon to perform spinal surgeries, such as the removal of a disk. Orthopedic surgeons have one of the longest training periods of all doctors.

Neurologists are physicians skilled in the diagnosis and treatment of diseases of the nervous system including the brain. These doctors do not perform surgery; however, neurologists often help determine whether a patient is a surgical candidate. They are known to employ a wide variety of diagnostic tests such as nerve conduction studies,

and are often called upon to make cognitive assessments and offer medical advice.

Providing care from birth to early adulthood, pediatricians are concerned with the health of infants, children, and teenagers. They specialize in the diagnosis and treatment of a variety of ailments specific to young people and track their patients' growth to adulthood. Most of the work of pediatricians involves treating day-to-day illnesses that are common to children such as minor injuries, infectious diseases, and immunizations. Some pediatricians specialize in serious medical conditions and pediatric surgery, treating autoimmune disorders or serious chronic ailments.

Physician Assistant

The physician assistant (PA) is a skilled health care professional with a baccalaureate degree or a postbaccalaureate degree from an accredited program. Most applicants to PA schools already have a baccalaureate degree. The PA is required to have 1 year of direct patient contact and to pass a national certification examination. All states and the District of Columbia have legislation governing the qualifications or practice of PAs. All jurisdictions require PAs to pass the Physician Assistants National Certifying Examination, administered by the National Commission on Certification of Physician Assistants (NCCPA) and is open to graduates of accredited PA education programs. Only those successfully completing the examination may use the credential "Physician Assistant—Certified."

The PA's responsibilities include therapeutic, preventive, and health maintenance services in settings where physicians practice. The PA works under the supervision and direction of a physician; however, PAs may be the principal care providers in rural or inner city clinics where a physician may be present for only one or two days per week. In such instances, the PA must discuss each patient's case with the supervising physician and other medical professionals as necessary. Similar to physicians, PAs may also evaluate and treat patients in hospitals and nursing homes. Nevertheless, they always must report back to and confer with the physician.

In most states, the PA is allowed to prescribe medications and to refer patients to medical and rehabilitation services including physical therapy. PAs are formally trained to provide diagnostic, therapeutic, and preventive health care services, as delegated by a physician. Working as members of the health care team, they take medical histories, examine and treat patients, order and interpret laboratory tests and x-rays, make diagnoses, and prescribe medications. They also treat minor injuries by suturing, splinting, and casting. PAs record progress notes, instruct and counsel patients, and order or carry out therapy.

PAs also may have managerial duties. Some order medical and laboratory supplies and equipment and may supervise technicians and assistants. The duties of PAs are determined by the supervising physician and by state law. Many PAs work in primary care specialties, such as general internal medicine, pediatrics, and family medicine. Other specialty areas include general and thoracic surgery, emergency medicine, orthopedics, and geriatrics. PAs specializing in surgery provide preoperative and postoperative care and may work as first or second assistants during major surgery. In regard to opportunities for work, it is projected that "employment of PAs will grow by 38 percent from 2012 to 2022."[40]

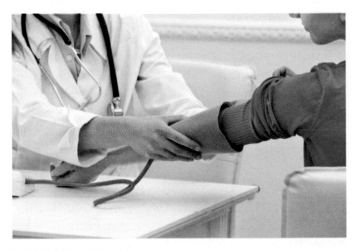

© Monkey Business Images/Shutterstock

Registered Nurse

The registered nurse (RN) is a skilled health care professional who has graduated from an accredited program and is licensed by a state board after successful completion of a licensure examination. In all states and the District of Columbia, nursing students must graduate from an approved nursing program and pass a national licensing examination in order to obtain a nursing license. Nurses may be licensed in more than one state, either by examination, by the endorsement of a license issued by another state, or through a multistate licensing agreement. All states require periodic renewal of licenses, which may involve continuing education.

There are three major educational paths to registered nursing: a bachelor of science degree in nursing (BSN), an associate degree in nursing (ADN), and a diploma program. Most of the nursing educational programs offer degrees at the bachelor level that take about 4 years to complete. ADN programs, offered by community and junior colleges, take about 2 to 3 years to complete. Diploma programs, administered in hospitals, last about 3 years. Only a small and declining number of programs offer diplomas. Generally, licensed nursing graduates of any of the three types of educational programs qualify for entry-level positions as staff nurses. Registered nurses work to promote health, prevent disease, and help patients cope with illness. They are also advocates and health educators for patients, families, and communities. When providing direct patient care, they observe, assess, and record symptoms, reactions, and progress in patients; assist physicians during surgeries, treatments, and examinations; administer medications; and assist in convalescence and rehabilitation. RNs also develop and manage nursing care plans, instruct patients and their families in proper care, and help individuals and groups take steps to improve or maintain their health.

Although state laws govern the tasks that RNs may perform, it is usually the work setting that determines their daily job duties. There are several types of nurses: hospital nurses, office nurses, nursing care facility nurses, home health nurses, public health nurses, occupational health nurses (also called industrial nurses), head nurses (or nurse supervisors), nurse practitioners, clinical nurse specialists, certified registered nurse anesthetists, and certified nurse-midwives. Hospital nurses form the largest group of nurses. Most are staff nurses, who provide bedside nursing care and carry out medical regimens. Office nurses care for outpatients in physicians' offices, clinics, ambulatory surgical centers, and emergency medical centers. They prepare patients for, and assist with, examinations; administer injections and medications; dress wounds and incisions; assist with minor surgery; and maintain records. Some also perform routine laboratory and office work.

Nursing care facility nurses manage care for residents with conditions ranging from a fracture to Alzheimer's disease. Although they often spend much of their time on administrative and supervisory tasks, nursing care facility nurses also assess residents' health, develop treatment plans, supervise licensed practical nurses and nursing aides, and perform invasive procedures, such as starting intravenous fluids. They also work in specialty-care departments, such as long-term rehabilitation units for patients with strokes and head injuries.

Home health nurses provide nursing services to patients at home. Home health nurses assess patients' home environments and instruct patients and their families in various areas of health related to their condition. Home health nurses care for a broad range of patients, such as those recovering from illnesses and accidents, cancer, and childbirth. They must be able to work independently and may supervise home health aides.

Public health nurses work in government and private agencies, including clinics, schools, retirement communities, and other community settings. They focus on populations, working with individuals, groups, and families to improve the overall health of communities. They also work with communities to help plan and implement programs.

Occupational health nurses, also called industrial nurses, provide nursing care at worksites to employees, customers, and others with injuries and illnesses. They give emergency care, prepare accident reports, and arrange for further care if necessary. They also offer health counseling, conduct health examinations and inoculations, and assess work environments to identify potential or actual health problems.

Head nurses or nurse supervisors direct nursing activities, primarily in hospitals. They plan work schedules and assign duties to nurses and aides, provide or arrange for training, and visit patients to observe nurses and to ensure that the patients receive proper care. They also may ensure that records are maintained and equipment and supplies are ordered.

At the advanced level, nurse practitioners provide basic, primary health care. They diagnose and treat common acute illnesses and injuries. Nurse practitioners also can prescribe medications. However, certification and licensing requirements vary by state. Other advanced practice nurses include clinical nurse specialists, certified registered nurse anesthetists, and certified nurse-midwives. Advanced practice nurses must meet educational and clinical practice requirements beyond the basic nursing education and licensing required of all RNs.

In the rehabilitation team, the RN is the primary liaison between the patient and the physician. The RN communicates to the physician changes in the patient's social and medical status, makes patient referrals (under the physician's direction) to other services, educates the patient and patient's family, and performs functional training such

as ambulation or transfers with patients (after instruction from the PT or PTA). The RN also supervises other levels of nursing care such as the licensed practical nurses (LPNs), certified nursing assistants (CNAs), and home health aides.

It is projected that in general, between 2012 and 2022, the occupation of registered nurse is expected to offer over half a million jobs.[40] More new jobs are expected to be created for RNs than for any other occupation in the health care field. Thousands of job openings will result from the need to replace experienced nurses who leave the occupation, especially as the median age of the registered nurse population continues to rise. Faster-than-average growth will be driven by technological advances in patient care, which permit a greater number of medical problems to be treated, and an increasing emphasis on preventive care.[40] In addition, the number of older people, who are much more likely than younger people to need nursing care, is projected to grow rapidly. Employers in many parts of the country are reporting difficulty in attracting and retaining an adequate number of RNs, due primarily to an aging RN workforce and insufficient nursing school enrollments. Imbalances between the supply of and demand for qualified workers should spur efforts to attract and retain qualified RNs.

According to the U.S. Department of Labor, Bureau of Statistics, job opportunities for RNs are expected to be very good.[40] The U.S. Department of Labor indicates that "employment of registered nurses is expected to grow by 19 percent from 2012 to 2022."[40]

Social Worker

In general, a social worker needs a bachelor degree in social work (BSW) to qualify for a job. Although a bachelor degree is sufficient for entry into the field, a master's degree in social work (MSW) or a related field has become the standard for many positions. An MSW is typically required for positions in health care settings and for clinical work. Some social work jobs in public and private agencies also may require an advanced degree, such as a master's degree in social services policy or administration.

All states and the District of Columbia have licensing, certification, or registration requirements regarding social work practice and the use of professional titles. Although standards for licensing vary by state, a growing number of states are placing greater emphasis on communications skills, professional ethics, and sensitivity to cultural diversity issues. Additionally, the National Association of Social Workers (NASW) offers voluntary credentials. Social workers with an MSW may be eligible for the Academy of Certified Social Workers (ACSW), the Qualified Clinical Social Worker (QCSW) credential, or the Diplomat in Clinical Social Work (DCSW) based on their professional experience. Credentials are particularly important for social workers in private practice. Some health insurance providers require social workers to have credentials in order to be reimbursed for services.

Social workers help people function optimally in their environment, deal with their relationships, and solve personal and family problems. Social workers often see clients who face a life-threatening disease or a social problem, such as inadequate housing, unemployment, serious illness, disability, or substance abuse. Social workers also assist families that have serious domestic conflicts, including those involving child or spousal abuse. Social workers often provide social services in health-related settings that are governed by managed care organizations. To contain costs, these organizations are emphasizing short-term intervention, ambulatory and community-based care, and greater decentralization of services.

Most social workers specialize. Although some conduct research or are involved in planning or policy development, most social workers prefer an area of practice in which they interact with clients. There are three classifications of social workers: child, family, and school social workers; medical and public social workers; and mental health and substance abuse social workers.

Child, family, and school social workers provide social services and assistance to improve the social and psychological functioning of children and their families and to maximize the family well-being and academic functioning of children. They also advise teachers on how to cope with problem students. Some child, family, and school social workers may specialize in services for senior citizens. Child, family, and school social workers typically work in individual and family services agencies, schools, or state or local governments.

Medical and public health social workers provide persons, families, or vulnerable populations with the psychosocial support needed to cope with chronic, acute, or terminal illnesses, such as Alzheimer's disease, cancer, or AIDS. They also advise family caregivers, counsel patients, and help plan for patients' needs after discharge

by arranging for at-home services ranging from Meals on Wheels to oxygen equipment. Medical and public health social workers may work for hospitals, nursing, and personal care facilities, individual and family services agencies, or local governments.

Mental health and substance abuse social workers assess and treat individuals with mental illness or substance abuse problems, including abuse of alcohol, tobacco, or other drugs. Such services include individual and group therapy, outreach, crisis intervention, social rehabilitation, and training in skills of everyday living. Mental health and substance abuse social workers are likely to work in hospitals, substance abuse treatment centers, individual and family services agencies, or local governments. These social workers may be known as clinical social workers.

According to the U.S. Department of Labor, Bureau of Statistics, social workers usually spend most of their time in an office or residential facility, but also may travel locally to visit clients, meet with service providers, or attend meetings.[40] To tend to patient care or client needs, many hospitals and long-term care facilities are employing social workers on teams with a broad mix of occupations, including clinical specialists, registered nurses, physical/occupational therapists, PTAs, COTAs, and health aides. Competition for social worker jobs is stronger in cities, where demand for services often is highest and training programs for social workers are prevalent. However, opportunities should be good in rural areas, which often find it difficult to attract and retain qualified staff. Job prospects may be best for those social workers with a background in gerontology and substance abuse treatment.

As per the U.S. Department of Labor, "employment of social workers is expected to increase by 19 percent during the 2012 to 2022 decade, which is faster than the average for all occupations."[40] The growth of social worker jobs will be in home health care services, nursing homes, long-term care facilities, hospices, assisted living communities, and senior communities. This projection is based on the expanding elderly population. Also, the employment of substance abuse social workers will grow rapidly over the 2012 to 2022 projection period. Substance abusers are increasingly being placed into treatment programs instead of being sentenced to prison. As this trend grows, demand will increase for treatment programs and social workers to assist abusers on the road to recovery.

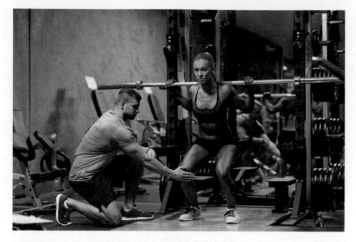

© Syda Productions/Shutterstock

Certified Athletic Trainer

The certified athletic trainer (ATC) is a health care professional with a minimum of a baccalaureate degree who works mainly with sports injuries. Athletic trainers can become certified by the National Athletic Trainers' Association Board of Certification (NATABOC). The certification examination administered by NATABOC consists of a written portion with multiple choice questions, an oral/practical section that evaluates the skill components of the domains within athletic training, and a written simulation test, consisting of athletic training–related situations designed to approximate real-life decision making. When the athletic trainers pass the certification exam, they can use the designation Certified Athletic Trainer (ATC). Usually, the ATC works under the supervision of a physician, providing injury prevention, and treatment and rehabilitation to a patient after an injury. The ATC also can work in colleges and universities, secondary schools, private or hospital-based rehabilitation clinics, and professional athletic associations. As per the U.S. Department of Labor, "between 2012 and 2022, the job growth for athletic trainers will be at a rate of 19 percent."[40]

Physical Therapy Aide

The physical therapy aide is a nonlicensed worker specifically trained under the direction of a PT, or when allowable by law, under a PTA. The aide can function only if he or she is supervised directly (on-site) and continuously by the PT, or when permissible by law by the PTA. Direct personal supervision requires that the PT, or where allowable by law, the PTA, be physically present and immediately available to direct and supervise tasks that are related to patient/client management. The direction and supervision is continuous throughout the time these tasks are performed. The physical therapy aide can perform routine designated tasks related to the operation of physical therapy services such as patient transportation, equipment cleaning and maintenance, secretarial duties, or housekeeping duties. A physical therapy aide cannot perform tasks that require the clinical decision making of the PT or the clinical problem solving of the PTA. The APTA opposes certification or credentialing of physical therapy aides and does not endorse or recognize certification programs for physical therapy aides.

Physical Therapy Volunteer

The physical therapy volunteer is a member of the community interested in assisting physical therapy personnel with departmental activities. He or she may take telephone calls and messages, transport patients from their rooms to the rehabilitation department in acute care hospital settings, and file patients' charts. The volunteer cannot provide direct patient care.

Physical Therapist Student and Physical Therapist Assistant Student

PT and PTA students perform duties commensurate with their level of education. The PT or PTA clinical instructor (CI) is responsible for all actions and duties of the PT or PTA student in the clinical settings. The CI is a PT or PTA at the clinical site who directly instructs and supervises students during their clinical learning experiences. The CIs are responsible for facilitating clinical learning experiences and assessing students' entry-level performances. All students' documentation must be co-signed by the CI. The PTA cannot be a CI for a PT student, but can be a CI for a PTA student. Patients must be informed that they will be treated by a student and have the right to refuse treatment.

Home Health Aide

The home health aide (HHA) is a nonlicensed worker who provides personal care and home management services. Some HHAs are certified in their jurisdictions. The HHA assists the patient in his or her home setting with bathing, grooming, light housework, shopping, and cooking. After receiving instruction and supervision from the PT or the PTA, the HHA may provide supervision or assistance to a patient performing a home exercise program (HEP).

Discussion Questions

1. While working in a skilled nursing facility, the PTA has been asked to attend a care team meeting for a resident. Who will be attending the meeting and what role do they play on the team?
2. Utilizing Appendix E, review the Problem Solving Algorithm Utilized by PTAs in Patient/Client Intervention document. Discuss the role of the PT and PTA in clinical care.

Learning Opportunities

1. Utilizing the APTA webpage (www.apta.org), review the *Value-Based Behaviors for the Physical Therapist Assistant*. Locate the section PT/PTA Collaboration and create strategies to promote the PT/PTA relationship.
2. Interview a health care professional, such as a PT, OT, SLP, or SW. Create a class presentation about the function, role, and interactions of this health care professional.
3. Create a class presentation about who PTAs are and what they do.

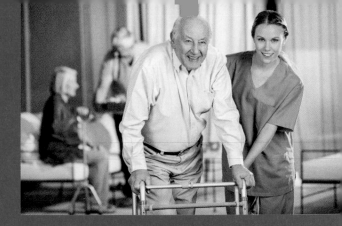
© Tyler Olson/Shutterstock

CHAPTER 3

Physical Therapist Clinical Practice

OBJECTIVES

After studying this chapter, the reader will be able to:

1. Identify when to use the *Guide to Physical Therapist Practice*.
2. Describe the purposes, significance, and utilization of the Guide in clinical practice.
3. Discuss the five elements of patient/client management included in the Guide.
4. Compare and contrast physical therapy and medical diagnosis.
5. List examples of procedural interventions included in the Guide.
6. List employment settings for physical therapists and physical therapist assistants.
7. Compare and contrast the three types of skilled nursing facilities.
8. Discuss employment and physical therapy clinical practice issues such as interviews, policy and procedure manuals, meetings, budgets, quality assurance, and risk management.
9. Describe contemporary clinical trends regarding wellness, health promotion, and disease prevention.

KEY TERMS

medical diagnosis
physical therapy diagnosis

policy
procedure

Patient and Client Management in Clinical Practice

The physical therapist (PT) and physical therapist assistant (PTA) work together (and when appropriate with other individuals) using various physical therapy techniques and procedures to produce changes in the patient/client's condition. As indicated previously, the PT performs the initial examination/evaluation of the patient/client. The PTA helps to gather specific data (requested by the PT) and acknowledges the delegated tasks within the limits of his or her capabilities and considering legal, jurisdictional, and ethical guidelines. This collaborative relationship between the PT and the PTA takes place through all phases of patient/client management including examination, evaluation, diagnosis, prognosis, interventions, and outcomes. Regardless of the setting in which the physical therapy service is provided, the following responsibilities must be borne solely by the PT: (1) interpretation of referrals when available; (2) initial examination, evaluation, diagnosis, and prognosis; (3) development or modification of a plan of care (POC) based on the initial examination or reexamination and which includes the physical therapy goals and outcomes; and (4) determination of when the expertise and decision-making capability of the PT requires the PT to personally render physical therapy interventions and when it may be appropriate to utilize the PTA. The PT shall also determine the most appropriate utilization of the PTA that provides for the delivery of service that is safe, effective, and efficient.

Guide to Physical Therapist Practice

In 1997, the American Physical Therapy Association (APTA) introduced clinical guidelines for PTs in the first edition of the *Guide to Physical Therapist Practice*. The Guide represented 5 years of combined efforts by the APTA's leaders and grassroots members. The development of the Guide started in 1992, was approved by the board of directors in 1995, was reviewed between 1995 and 1996 by more than 200 selected reviewers, and was combined into a two-volume document in 1997. Two APTA task forces, four panels, a project advisory board, a board of directors' oversight committee, and more than 600 reviewers participated in the process of creating the Guide.

Over the years, the Guide has been revised based on research evidence and the suggestions of the APTA's members. In 1999 and 2001, a second edition of the Guide was published. In 2014, the *Guide to Physical Therapist Practice 3.0* was published in an online format and several significant changes occurred. The Guide language changed to be more consistent with the *International Classification of Functioning, Disability, and Health* (ICF) language and preferred practice patterns were removed from the text. The preferred practice patterns are still available online as an educational tool, but no longer serve to inform the public or payer sources.[41]

The Guide, as the result of collaboration among hundreds of PTs, continues to be a resource for both daily physical therapy practice and professional education of PTs and PTAs. All PT education programs utilize the Guide for the education of PTs; in addition, certain PTA programs utilize the Guide for the education of PTAs. PTA students should become familiar with the Guide, using it as a study book in their learning process and as a clinical guideline in physical therapy practice.

THE PURPOSES OF THE GUIDE

The Guide has multiple purposes; however, the most significant ones are:[41]

- To describe PT practice
- To outline the roles of the PT and PTA in a variety of settings and practices
- To describe the settings where physical therapy is practiced
- To standardize physical therapy terminology
- To review the education of PTs and PTAs
- To delineate the clinical decision-making process that occurs as part of patient and client management
- To describe examination and evaluation processes including tests and measures
- To describe interventions and the process of choosing appropriate interventions
- To describe the utilization of outcome measures

THE SIGNIFICANCE OF THE GUIDE

The Guide describes the patient and client management model to help inform and guide the examination, evaluation, diagnosis, prognosis, intervention, and outcomes that a PT might employ. Clinicians can use the Guide to help organize their management process and choose the most helpful pieces of data to collect and analyze during the examination process.

HOW TO USE THE GUIDE

PTs and PTAs can use the Guide in different ways:

- For experienced clinicians, the Guide *confirms* they are making the right choice in examination or selection of interventions.
- For less experienced clinicians, the Guide may offer other *options* to consider that are not regularly used in their day-to-day practice.
- The Guide can serve as a *framework* for clinical decision making for the experienced and the new practitioner.

- The Guide is important for the *terminology* and the *thought processes* behind examinations and interventions. These treatment patterns can be used in case studies instruction.

- For faculty and students, the Guide can be utilized as a *tool* in their teaching and learning methods.

- The Guide is an excellent instrument that *interprets* the physical therapy practice.

- The Guide also can be used as a *reference* to help providers and third-party payers to make informed decisions about patient care and reimbursement.

- The Guide can also suggest to PTs methods to *educate* their patients about long-term outcomes and specific interventions necessary to achieve these outcomes.

- The Guide *promotes research* by establishing consistent terminology and structuring physical therapy practice into answerable research questions about physical therapy interventions. The Guide encourages physical therapy practice that can be validated by evidence-based research.

ELEMENTS OF PATIENT AND CLIENT MANAGEMENT INCLUDED IN THE GUIDE

The Guide uses the World Health Organization's model of understanding health as a combination of a person's anatomy and physiology, socioeconomic resources, and psychological well-being. The *International Classification of Functioning, Disability, and Health* focuses on a person's well-being and function, not just his or her disease or illness. The APTA's House of Delegates also has chosen to use this model and its definitions to describe physical therapy for this exact reason. In addition, the Guide emphasizes that prevention services programs for promoting health, wellness, and fitness and programs for maintaining function are extremely significant to current physical therapy practice.

DESCRIPTION OF THE PRINCIPLES OF PATIENT AND CLIENT MANAGEMENT OF THE *GUIDE TO PHYSICAL THERAPIST PRACTICE*

The first section of the Guide describes the ongoing process of patient and client management that includes working with others who are managing the patient, consultation services, direction and supervision of personnel, and referrals for other services. This section also describes clinical practice where the PT puts together the following six elements of patient/client management:[41]

- Examination
- Evaluation
- Diagnosis
- Prognosis
- Intervention
- Outcomes

Based on these elements, the PT establishes a POC that identifies goals and outcomes and describes the proposed intervention, including frequency and duration.

General Terminology Used in the Guide

In regard to patient and client management, the Guide uses the following terminology:

- A *patient* is an individual who receives health care services including physical therapy direct intervention.

- A *client* is an individual who is not necessarily sick or injured but who can benefit from a PT's consultation, professional advice, or services. Examples of a client can be a student in a school system or an employee in a business.

- The *examination* is the process for gathering subjective and objective data about the patient/client. It is also a comprehensive screening and specific testing process leading to diagnostic classification or, as appropriate, to a referral to another practitioner. Physical therapy examination has three components: the patient/client history, the systems review, and tests and measures.

- The *evaluation* is a dynamic process in which the PT makes clinical judgments based on data gathered during the examination.[41] The evaluation results in the determination of the diagnosis, prognosis, and interventions. The evaluation reflects the severity of the current problem, the presence of preexisting conditions, the possibility of more than one site involvement, and the stability of the condition.

- *Interventions* are skilled techniques and activities that make up the treatment plan.[41]

- *Discharge* is defined as the process of discontinuing interventions in a single episode of care.[41]

- *Goals* are functional activities that are the intended response to the physical therapy intervention and are set by the PT, the patient, and the patient's family/caregivers.
- *Outcome* is defined as the actual functional activity that is achieved by the physical therapy episode of care. By measuring pre-intervention and post-intervention outcomes, the value of physical therapy can be documented.[41]

Components of Physical Therapy Examination and Evaluation Used in the Guide

In regard to physical therapy examination and evaluation, the Guide uses the following terminology:

- The *patient/client history* is an account of the patient/client's past and current health status.[41] The history is obtained by gathering data from the patient/client, immediate family, caregivers, other members of the patient/client's family, and other interested persons such as an employer or a rehabilitation counselor.
- The *systems review* is a short examination providing additional information about the general health of the patient/client.[41] The systems review can include cardiopulmonary status, musculoskeletal status, or communication abilities.
- *Tests and measures* are selected by the PT to be able to acquire additional information about the patient's condition, the physical therapy diagnosis, and the necessary therapeutic interventions.[41] Sometimes tests and measures are not necessary, and at other times, are extensively required. The Guide puts tests and measures into 26 different categories including:

Because of the electronic nature of the Guide, each section is hyperlinked to a document that provides clinical indications, further describes the measure, offers examples of tests and measures, and recommends documentation strategies.

- *Diagnosis* or *physical therapy diagnostic process* includes the following: obtaining relevant patient/client history, performing systems review, selecting and administering specific tests and measures, and organizing and interpreting all data.[41] Physical therapy diagnosis describes the system(s) affected by the alteration in function. It identifies not only the specific patient complaint but the overall effect on the person.[41]
- *Impairments* are abnormalities or dysfunctions of the bones, joints, ligaments, tendons, muscles, nerves, or skin, or problems with movement resulting from pathology in the brain, spinal cord, cardiovascular, or pulmonary systems.[39] Examples of impairments can be muscle weakness, inflammation of the tendon or ligament, muscle spasms, or edema.
- *Functional limitations* are inabilities of a patient/client to function adequately in his or her environment.[39] Examples of functional limitations can be inability to ambulate or inability to perform activities of daily living (ADLs) such as brushing the hair, washing the face, or dressing. Besides impairments and functional limitations, the PT takes into consideration in the examination and evaluation process the patient's or the client's disability.
- *Disability* is the inability to perform or participate in activities or tasks related to a person's work, home, or

Aerobic Capacity/Endurance	Anthropometric Characteristics	Assistive Technology
Balance	Circulation (Arterial, Venous, Lymphatic)	Community, Social, and Civic Life
Cranial and Peripheral Nerve Integrity	Education Life	Environmental Factors
Gait	Integumentary Integrity	Joint Integrity and Mobility
Mental Functions	Mobility (Including Locomotion)	Motor Function
Muscle Performance (Including Strength, Power, Endurance, and Length)	Neuromotor Development and Sensory Processing	Pain
Posture	Range of Motion	Reflex Integrity
Self-Care and Domestic Life	Sensory Integrity	Skeletal Integrity
Ventilation and Respiration	Work Life	

community.[39] Disability affects individual and societal functioning. Examples of disability are the inability to perform occupational tasks, school-related tasks, home management (that can be a disability for a homemaker), caring for dependents, community responsibilities, or service.

- *Prognosis* is a judgment of the PT about the level of optimal improvement the patient/client may achieve and the amount of time needed to reach that level.[41]

- *Interventions* are defined by the Guide as the purposeful and skilled interaction of the PT with the patient/client and, when appropriate, with other individuals involved in patient/client care to produce changes in the condition consistent with the diagnosis and prognosis.[41] Besides the PT, the other individual also involved in patient/client care is the PTA. The interventions are provided in such a way that directed and supervised responsibilities are commensurate with the qualifications and the legal limitations of the PTA. The interventions are altered in accordance with changes in response or status of the patient/client. The interventions are provided at a level that is consistent with current physical therapy practice.

Physical Therapy Diagnosis Versus Medical Diagnosis Described in the Guide

The physical therapy diagnosis is different from the medical diagnosis.

DEFINITION OF MEDICAL DIAGNOSIS

A *medical diagnosis* is determined by a physician (medical doctor [MD] or doctor of osteopathy [DO]) who identifies an illness or disorder in a patient through an interview, physical examination, medical tests, and other procedures.[41] Consequently, the medical diagnosis recognizes a disease and finds out its cause and its nature of pathologic conditions.

Data from American Physical Therapy Association. *Guide to Physical Therapist Practice 3.0*. Alexandria, VA: APTA; 2014.

DEFINITION OF PHYSICAL THERAPY DIAGNOSIS

A *physical therapy diagnosis* is determined by the PT. Consequently, the physical therapy diagnosis is defined as the end result of evaluating information obtained from the examination, which the PT organizes to determine the functional losses and to help determine the most appropriate intervention strategies.[41]

Data from American Physical Therapy Association. *Guide to Physical Therapist Practice 3.0*. Alexandria, VA: APTA; 2014.

The Importance of Physical Therapy Diagnosis

Diagnosis is an essential part of PTs' practice in order to provide proper physical therapy interventions. PTs diagnose with respect to PT practice as authorized by state law.[42] In diagnosing a patient's condition in accord with such law, PTs are not in conflict with the diagnosis provisions of state laws governing the practice of medicine. No states prohibit a PT from performing a diagnosis.

As indicated in the definition of physical therapy diagnosis, PTs utilize the diagnostic process prior to making a patient/client management decision. They establish a diagnosis for the specific conditions in need of the PT's attention. The purpose of the physical therapy diagnosis is to guide the PT in determining the most appropriate intervention strategy for each patient/client. In the event the diagnostic process does not generate an identifiable cluster, disorder, syndrome, or category, physical therapy intervention may be directed toward the alleviation of symptoms and remediation of impairment, functional limitation, or disability.

During the diagnostic process, PTs can obtain additional information, including diagnostic labels, from other health professionals.[42] As the diagnostic process continues, PTs may identify findings that should be shared with other health professionals (including referral sources) to ensure optimal patient/client care. When the patient/client is referred with a previously established diagnosis, the PT should determine that the clinical findings are consistent with that diagnosis. If the diagnostic process reveals findings that are outside the scope of the PT's knowledge, experience, or expertise, the PT should refer the patient/client to an appropriate practitioner.

Physical Therapy Intervention Described in the Guide

Physical therapy intervention has three large components: coordination, communication, and documentation; patient/client-related instruction; and direct interventions. Coordination, communication, and documentation and patient/client-related instruction are provided for all patients/clients, and may include the following:

- Case management
- Coordination of care with the patient/client, family, or other health care professionals
- Computer-assisted instruction
- Periodic reexamination and reassessment of the home program
- Demonstration and modeling for teaching, verbal instruction, and written or pictorial instruction

Direct interventions are based on the following elements:

- Examination and evaluation of data
- The diagnosis and the prognosis (including the POC)
- The anticipated goals and expected outcomes for a particular patient in a specific patient/client diagnostic group[41]

Through coordination, communication, documentation, and patient/client-related instruction, the PT ensures appropriate, coordinated, comprehensive, and cost-effective physical therapy services and patient/client integration in the home, community, and workplace.

The Guide organizes PT interventions into nine categories:

1. Patient or client instruction (used with every patient and client).
   Patient instruction can be provided by the PT and some portions by the PTA. Patient/client-related instruction may include instruction, education, and training of patients/clients and caregivers regarding current condition (pathology, pathophysiology, impairments, functional limitations, or disabilities); enhancement of performance; health, wellness, and fitness; POC; risk factors (for pathology, pathophysiology, disease, disorder or condition, impairments, functional limitations, or disabilities); patient/client's transitions across settings; and patient/client's transitions to new roles.
2. Airway clearance techniques (such as breathing, positioning, and/or manual/mechanical techniques).

Examples of breathing exercises include paced breathing and pursed-lip breathing. Examples of positioning include techniques to maximize ventilation and pulmonary drainage (of specific lobes). Examples of manual/mechanical techniques include chest percussion and vibration and mechanical suctioning.

3. Assistive technology
   The assistive technology category includes the prescription, application, and fabrication/modification of assistive devices. This can be divided into locomotion aids (wheelchairs, walkers, canes, etc.), orthoses (braces and splints), prostheses, wheelchair seating systems, positioning devices (prone and supine standers or upper extremity supportive wheelchair trays), and other technologies that improve safety (home modification devices, slide boards, and mechanical transfer assists).
4. Biophysical agents include electrotherapeutic modalities.
   Examples of electrotherapeutic modalities include utilizing electrical stimulation such as high-voltage pulsed current (HVPC), transcutaneous electrical nerve stimulation (TENS), and neuromuscular electrical stimulation (NMES). Physical agents and mechanical modalities also fit under this heading. Examples of physical agents include cold packs, ice massage, hot packs, paraffin baths, and hydrotherapy (whirlpool tanks or pools). Examples of mechanical modalities include standing frames, tilt tables, or mechanical motion devices such as a continuous passive motion (CPM) knee device.
5. Functional training in self-care and domestic, work, community, social, and civic life.
   Functional training in self-care and home management includes ADLs and instrumental activities of daily living (IADLs). Examples of ADLs are bathing, bed mobility and/or transfer training, developmental activities, dressing, eating, grooming, and toileting. Examples of IADLs include caring for dependents, household chores, shopping, yard work, structured play for children, and home maintenance. Functional training in work (job/school/play), community, and leisure integration or reintegration includes IADLs, work hardening, and work conditioning. Examples of functional training in work (which can take place as back schools, job coaching, or simulated work environments) include

injury prevention or reduction, education during work, safety awareness training, or use of devices and equipment.

6. Integumentary repair and protection techniques
   An example of integumentary repair would be wound or burn care. Protection techniques include aseptic and isolation procedures.

7. Manual therapy techniques
   Manual therapy techniques include mobilization and/or manipulation (such as of soft tissue or spinal and peripheral joints).

8. Motor function training
   Motor function training involves interventions to improve balance, motor control, perceptual awareness, gait training with or without the use of an assistive device, postural awareness, strength and control, and vestibular training.

9. Therapeutic exercise
   Therapeutic exercise includes aerobic conditioning and endurance training, flexibility, coordination, strength and power training, and relaxation strategies.[41]

The electronic version provides further descriptions of each of these categories including possible intervention choices within the category and potential outcomes from employing the intervention.[41]

The PT's POC identifies a plan for discharge of the patient/client, taking into consideration achievement of anticipated goals and expected outcomes, and provides for appropriate follow-up or referral.

Discharge from Physical Therapy and Discontinuation of Physical Therapy Services Described in the Guide

The Guide defines discharge as, "the process of ending physical therapy services that have been provided during a single episode of care, when the anticipated goals and expected outcomes have been achieved."[41] Discharge does not occur with a transfer (when the patient is moved from one site to another site within the same setting or across settings during a single episode of care). Discharge is based on the PT's analysis of the achievement of anticipated goals and the achievement of expected outcomes.

Discontinuation is described as the process of discontinuing interventions that have been provided during a single episode of care when: (1) patient/client, caregiver, or legal guardian declines to continue interventions;

(2) patient/client is unable to continue to progress toward anticipated goals and expected outcomes because of medical/psychosocial complications or financial/insurance resources have been expended; or (3) PT determines that patient/client will no longer benefit from physical therapy.[41] When termination of physical therapy services occurs prior to achievement of anticipated goals and expected outcomes, patient/client status and the rationale for discontinuation should be documented.

Indications for patient/client's discharge include the following:

- The patient/client's desire to stop treatment
- The patient/client's inability to progress toward goals due to medical or psychosocial complications
- The PT's decision that the patient/client will no longer benefit from physical therapy[41]

Data from American Physical Therapy Association. *Guide to Physical Therapist Practice 3.0.* Alexandria, VA: APTA; 2014.

The PT reexamines the patient/client as necessary during an episode of care to evaluate progress or change in patient/client status and modifies the POC accordingly or discontinues physical therapy services. The PT, in consultation with appropriate individuals and considering the anticipated goals and expected outcomes, plans for discharge or discontinuation and provides the appropriate follow-up or referral.

PREFERRED PRACTICE PATTERNS

The original Guide included preferred practice patterns in musculoskeletal, neuromuscular, cardiovascular/pulmonary, and integumentary systems. The most recent edition does not include these patterns; however, they are available on the APTA website for educational purposes. In an effort to guide professionals to provide effective, efficient, evidence-based practice, the APTA has a new initiative to support the development of Clinical Practice Guidelines (CPGs). The CPGs are developed by the APTA sections for specific diagnoses and interventions. A list of currently developing CPGs is available on the APTA website.[45]

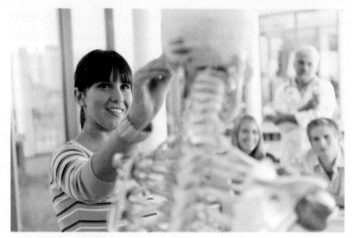
© CandyBox Images/Shutterstock

Physical Therapy Clinical Settings

Typically, PTs and PTAs work together in the same clinical facilities. These facilities range from acute care to extended care in skilled nursing facilities (SNFs) and private practices.

ACUTE CARE FACILITIES

Acute care physical therapy is practiced in hospitals, where patients usually remain for a short period of time. The average length of stay for a patient is less than 30 days. Acute care physical therapy practices are very demanding for PTs and PTAs because of the wide variety of patients having diverse and sometimes critical pathophysiological impairments and functional limitations. For example, in acute care hospitals, after the physical therapy examination and evaluation, the PTAs may need to provide physical therapy treatments for patients who had major surgical procedures such as heart or liver transplants. Additionally, other major surgeries are performed by highly specialized physicians and surgeons in technologically equipped hospitals. These hospitals are increasingly looking to information technology solutions to help deliver better quality patient care while containing costs. Consequently, the PTs and PTAs should learn to use the technology in addition to applying expert and focused physical therapy. Furthermore, in regard to the fast and demanding pace of acute care hospitals, the rapid discharge of patients increases the role of the PT and the PTA as a patient/family/caregiver's educator. The health care providers functioning in acute care clinical settings (in addition to PTs and PTAs) include physicians (MDs or DOs), physician assistants (PAs), nurses (RNs, LPNs), occupational therapists (OTs), social workers (SWs), and speech-language pathologists (SLPs).

PRIMARY CARE FACILITIES

Primary care is a type of health care practice provided by a primary care physician (PCP), where PTs and PTAs work on an outpatient physical therapy basis. The primary care physicians can be family practice physicians or specialists such as pediatricians, internists, or obstetricians/gynecologists (OB/GYNs). These physicians provide basic or first-level health care. The PTs support the physicians as part of the primary care team supplying the patient's examination, evaluation, physical therapy diagnosis, and prognosis. The PTAs support the PTs on the primary care team by implementing the treatment plan. The treatment plan is usually implemented after the PT has established a POC.

SUBACUTE CARE FACILITIES

Subacute care is an intermediate level of care for medically fragile patients too ill to be cared for at home. Subacute care is offered within a subacute hospital or a skilled nursing facility (SNF). Typically, SNFs offer rehabilitation services on a daily basis. There are three types of skilled nursing facilities:

- SNFs providing subacute care (a higher level of care than in extended care)
- SNFs providing transitional care (hospital-based SNFs)
- SNFs providing extended care

Patients who received health care in a transitional care SNF often are discharged to home, assisted living facilities (ALFs), or extended care SNFs. Extended care SNFs are freestanding or may be part of a hospital. They provide health care services on a daily basis, 7 days per week. In these facilities, rehabilitation services are offered 5 days per week. In extended care SNFs, patients are not in an acute phase of illness, but they require skilled interventions on an inpatient basis. Extended care SNFs need to be certified by Medicare. To comply with Medicare certification, extended care SNFs have to offer 24-hour nursing care coverage, as well as physical, occupational, and speech therapy. In these facilities, the PTAs work within the rehabilitation team that includes PTs, OTs, SLPs, certified occupational therapy assistants (COTAs), social workers, and nurses. The PTAs deliver skilled interventions to patients after the supervising PT establishes the POC. The PTAs also may be involved in delegation and supervision (when allowed by the individual facility or state practice) of nonskilled tasks performed by the rehabilitation aides.

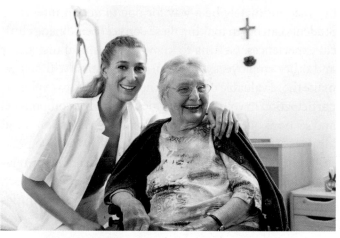
© Kzenon/Shutterstock

OUTPATIENT CARE FACILITIES

A large area of employment for PTs and PTAs includes outpatient care centers (or ambulatory care). These facilities provide outpatient preventive services, diagnostic services, and treatment services. Outpatient care centers are located in medical offices, surgery centers, and outpatient clinics. The health care providers are MDs, PAs, nurse practitioners, PTs, OTs, PTAs, and other rehabilitation personnel. The services in outpatient centers are less costly than in inpatient centers and are favored by managed care insurance companies. The PTAs implement the treatment programs after the PTs complete the POC.

REHABILITATION HOSPITALS

Rehabilitation hospitals are facilities that provide rehabilitation, social, and vocational services to patients who have a disability, facilitating their return to maximal functional capacity. The PTAs implement all or part of the physical therapy POC as delegated by the PTs. The PTAs work as a team with other health care providers, participating in team meetings, and when necessary perform patient and family education.

CHRONIC CARE FACILITIES

Chronic care facilities or long-term facilities provide services to patients who need to stay 60 days or longer. Medical services are offered to patients who have permanent or residual disabilities caused by a nonreversible pathological health condition. The rehabilitation services in these facilities may need to be specialized considering the type of patient pathology involved. The PTAs deliver skilled physical therapy interventions to meet the patient's daily living needs. The interventions needed are not necessarily only to maintain the patient's function, but also to improve the patient's function.

HOSPICE CARE FACILITIES

A hospice care facility is a health care facility that offers care for patients who are terminally ill and dying. The care is offered in an inpatient setting or at home. The health care team includes nurses, social workers, chaplains, physicians, and volunteers. Rehabilitation services are optional. Medicare and Medicaid insurance companies require that most of the health care (80 percent) is to be provided in the patient's home.

HOME HEALTH CARE

Home health care is typically provided to patients and patients' families in their home environments. Home health care can be financially sponsored by the government, private insurance, volunteer organizations, or nonprofit or for-profit organizations. To be eligible, the patient has to be homebound, meaning that he or she requires physical assistance to leave home. Also, eligibility for home health care requires skilled interventions from at least one of the following disciplines: nursing, physical therapy, occupational therapy, or speech therapy. In addition, a physician has to certify that skilled interventions are necessary. If physical therapy is needed, the PT has to reevaluate the patient every 3 to 6 weeks or periodically, depending on the patient's rehabilitation needs. Every visit and reevaluation needs to be documented by the PT or the PTA.

The patient's safety is the main concern for home health care physical therapy. An ongoing patient's environmental assessment takes place during the PT's or the PTA's visits. The PT or the PTA must report any information in regard to substance abuse by the patient or physical abuse of the patient. In home health care physical therapy, the PTA provides skilled interventions in the areas of bed mobility training, transfer training, gait training, and implementation of a home exercise program (HEP). State regulations differ in the use of the PTA in home health care. Some states require 1 year of experience as a PTA, and some do not allow a PTA to practice at all in home health care environments. If the PTA is allowed to practice home health care, the PT needs to examine and evaluate the patient, develop a POC, establish treatment goals, and discuss the patient's program with the PTA before the PTA's first visit. The PT should always be accessible to the PTA by way of telecommunications. Ongoing conferences between the PT and the PTA must occur on a weekly or biweekly basis, and supervisory visits by the PT have to be made every 4 to 6 weeks, or sooner at the PTA's request.

SCHOOL SYSTEM

School system physical therapy takes place in school settings. The PTA works in collaboration with the PT and with teachers and teacher aides in improving the student's function in school. The PT develops an individual education plan (IEP) for the student who has a disability. The IEP focuses on increasing the student's function in school and in the classroom. The PTA provides the necessary interventions for the goals to be achieved and whenever delegated by the PT. Examples of physical therapy recommendations for a student would be to help the student's functional mobility by having the student use a computer or improving a student's mobility in the school building by use of an assistive device (such as a walker).

PRIVATE PRACTICE FACILITIES

Private practice physical therapy is provided in a privately owned physical therapy facility. The private practice can be offered as outpatient services or as contract services for SNFs, schools, or home care agencies. Insurance reimbursement is allowed with a provider number. The provider needs to be a PT. The PTA works with the PT to provide physical therapy services under the PT's supervision (as allowed by the state practice acts). The PT needs to examine and evaluate the patient and provide a POC. Documentation describing the treatment must take place for every visit, and a complete reevaluation by the PT is necessary every 30 days.

Physical Therapy Employment

After completing PTA programs and passing the licensure examination, PTAs are ready to enter the physical therapy workforce. Students should begin their academic preparation with this end goal in mind. Several strategies will assist the student in gaining employment.

NETWORKING

Students may underestimate the value of making relationships to their ability to find employment. Creating relationships with PTs and PTAs not only provides the graduate with a possible reference when applying for a job, but may ultimately be a way for one to get an interview. Students can begin making these connections during clinical experiences. Getting to know their clinical instructor and other employees within an organization will help to make those valuable contacts. Another avenue to explore is participation in volunteer activities within the components and sections of the APTA. Students will meet national and local leaders within the profession and may find job prospects through these relationships. If students form relationships during their academic preparation, it is much more likely that as graduates, they will have opportunities to interview with the employers of their choice.

COVER LETTER

A cover letter is an opportunity to introduce you to a potential employer. Prior to creating a cover letter, a graduate should do his or her homework. A cover letter should be specific to each job or each employer to which the graduate is sending it. This will require research to determine to whom to direct the letter: human resource manager, physical therapy department supervisor, clinic owner, etc. If possible, the letter should be directed to a specific person. In addition, the graduate should learn about the philosophy and mission of the employer. Using this information will help to identify how the graduate can contribute to the employer's success. Graduates should also identify any connections that they have to the company. An example might be that the graduate was encouraged to contact them by a clinical instructor or that the graduate read an article about the company's great work in a trade magazine. Creating a good cover letter can be the difference between getting an interview or not.[46]

RESUME

The resume contains a brief written summary of personal information, educational information, professional qualifications and experience, and references.[46] Resumes can be provided prior to an interview if a cover letter is not used. It is also acceptable to send a resume with a cover letter; or, an applicant may provide it at an interview. It is best to inquire which the employer would prefer.[44] As a statement, the resume must be perfect, computer typed, and printed on a high-quality paper (such as 20-pound white bond). It should not be sloppy with spelling mistakes, be handwritten, or be written on a typewriter.[44]

WHY DO YOU NEED A RESUME?

- To show a desire to work and work ethics by describing that you were able to work and hold a job while in high school or during the PTA program
- To show flexibility by describing that you were able to work in various shifts or weekends or attended evening or weekend classes
- To express ambition by describing previous work experience or advancement in school or in a local chapter of the physical therapy professional organization
- To express dedication by describing membership in the APTA or the state professional organization or long-term employment

There are two types of resumes: chronological and functional.[43] A chronological resume lists experiences in reverse order with the most recent one first. It is the more common type of resume. A functional resume lists the skills a prospective employee possesses. It is not typically utilized by health care professionals.

A chronological resume is divided into the following sections:

- *Identification:* Includes the PTA's name and address.
- *Career objective:* Includes the PTA's desire for growth or to work with a special patient population such as geriatric, pediatric, or orthopedic. This section is important for a new graduate PTA who has no experience in the profession but wants to work with a certain patient population.
- *Work experience:* Includes all full-time positions and relevant part-time positions, education, activities, and honors.

- *Education:* Includes names and addresses of the educational institution, dates of attendance, degree earned (or anticipated to be earned), date the degree was earned, honors obtained, licensure number, special course work, and seminars. Grades and grade point averages are not typically included in the resume. Prospective employers should ask for the prospective employee's consent to obtain academic records, educational program information, and references.
- *Activities:* Includes professional, civic, and/or volunteer activities demonstrating positive work habits, leadership, and acceptance of responsibility. For a new PTA graduate, the honors section may be omitted if all honors are academic.

REFERENCES

References can describe the PTA's clinical and professional experience (and achievements) and his or her character. References describing clinical and professional experience can be provided by faculty members, clinical instructors, clinical supervisors, and/or former employers. References describing a PTA's character can be provided by family, friends, or clergy.

INTERVIEW

Although interviewing as a selection tool is generally considered an unsuccessful method for picking the best worker, interviews remain the main selection tool in the health care industry. The literature indicates that the best way of selecting someone for a position is based on a person's credentials and not the interview.[43] The strengths and weaknesses displayed during an interview are perceived to be the strengths and weaknesses that the person will display as an employee.[44]

The requirements that some health care managers look for in a job applicant include the following:

- Neat and clean appearance
- Showing a pleasant personality

(continues)

- Exhibiting a desire to work and work ethics
- Describing him- or herself as flexible, ambitious, and dedicated
- Having the best presentation[43]
- Having an understanding of the company and what the applicant might contribute as an employee[44]

Similar to health care in general, in physical therapy, during an interview employers look for decision-making style, communication skills, poise, tact, ability to work with others, leadership skills, achievement record, and a sense of personal direction. In physical therapy, interviews can be conducted by a physical therapy director (or supervisor or manager), or a member of the personnel department. The purpose of the interview is to meet with the prospective employee, exchange questions and answers, and obtain enough information about the prospective employee to make an informed decision.

How should you prepare for the interview?

- *Professional preparation:* Education, experience, and professional activities
- *Physical preparation:* Resume, references, attire, and communication skills
- *Mental preparation:* Knowing the information in the resume and the cover letter, and being able to ask and answer questions

Professional Preparation for the Interview

Professional preparation for the interview involves the PTA's education, experience, and activities. For a PTA, professional preparation starts in the PTA program by conscientiously studying the material, applying learned information at school and in clinical settings, and joining the national professional organization (the American Physical Therapy Association) and the state physical therapy professional organization. In addition, participating as a student and as a licensed graduate in seminars and meetings at

the local chapter or national level increases the professional network, ultimately helping with the interview process.

Physical Preparation for the Interview

Physical preparation for the interview involves the PTA's resume, cover letter, portfolio of work, follow-up correspondence, and physical appearance.

ATTIRE AND COMMUNICATION SKILLS

Physical preparation for the interview also involves dressing professionally and using appropriate verbal and nonverbal communication. Clothing must be clean, neat, and conservative. Typically, a business suit or a sport jacket is appropriate for men or women. Trendy hairstyles, makeup, jewelry, and scents should be kept at a minimum. Be particularly sensitive to breath odor; avoid the smell of smoke or alcohol. Tattoos should be covered if possible and piercings removed if distracting.

Verbal communication should show interpersonal skills such as poise and tact. Be courteous to everyone at the business including administrative assistants, professional personnel, custodial staff, and so on. Nonverbal communication should show confidence and consistency in verbal and nonverbal cues. Some appropriate nonverbal communication signs include sitting upright (with both feet on the floor) and slightly forward in the chair, looking straight at the interviewer, using a firm handshake, and maintaining focus and interest in the interview. Signs of nervousness such as fidgeting, restlessness, or chewing gum can be detrimental to the interviewee.

Mental Preparation for the Interview

Mental preparation means being prepared for the interview, knowing the information in the resume and the cover letter, and being able to answer questions. It also includes knowing personal information, answers to typical interview questions, and information about the prospective employer. Questions are typically informational, encouraging discussions. Answers such as yes or no are not appropriate. Answer the interviewer's questions clearly and directly. Do not interrupt the interviewer. Whenever possible, prepare specific examples of the strengths that you have so that the interviewer has a clear understanding of when the graduate has displayed a particular trait.[44] An example of this might include a specific time when the graduate faced a difficult clinical decision and how he or she handled the situation. A prospective employer should not ask questions about a person's age, religion, race, marital status, political interests, social interests, national origin, whether renting or owning a home, training not related to the job, birthplace, height and weight, native language, spouse's occupation, sexual preferences, and number of dependents. In situations when such types of questions are asked, the interviewee should use tactful answers.

> Questions to ask a prospective employer during the interview:
> - Advantages and disadvantages of working for the organization
> - Available benefits
> - Work hours
> - Vacation, sick, and personal leave time
> - Salary range and description of job requirements
> - Provision of professional liability insurance by the employer

After a person is hired, the employer can ask questions related to insurance to obtain the following information:

- Whether the person is able to work legally in the United States
- Person's age
- Spouse's information
- Dependent information
- Citizenship information
- Membership in professional organizations (although this information should be in the resume)
- Minority status for affirmative action plans
- Religious holidays to make work accommodations

Follow-up Activities

Regardless of being hired or not, the PTA graduate should send a thank you note the same day as the interview or as soon as possible. A personal phone call thanking the interviewers for the opportunity to meet with them and expressing continued interest in the position a few days after the interview can be a powerful tool also. The potential

of standing out from the other applicants for a position should not be left to chance and the graduate should show appreciation for the opportunity to interview.[44]

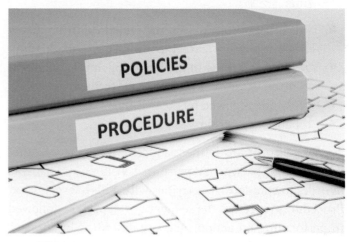

© vinnstock/Shutterstock

POLICY AND PROCEDURE MANUAL

Soon after being employed in a facility, PTAs are required to become acquainted with the facility/departmental policy and procedure manual. The general purpose of a policy and procedure manual is to familiarize the employees with the practice's specific mission, culture, expectations, and benefits. Although the manual is not a contract, it provides a clear, common understanding of the practice's goals, benefits, and policies, as well as what is expected with regard to the employee's performance and conduct. The manual also contributes to the employee's level of comfort because it spells out what is expected of him or her in order to comply with practice guidelines and fit in with the practice culture.

> The purposes of the policy and procedure manual include the following:
> - It provides extensive information on what should be done and how it should be done in a physical therapy department.
> - It is required by the Joint Commission, Commission on Accreditation of Rehabilitation Facilities (CARF), and other physical therapy accrediting agencies.

A **policy** is defined as a broad statement that guides the decision-making process. A policy represents a principle, a law, or a decision that guides actions. Examples of policies in a physical therapy department include the following:

- Time off, leave of absence, and sabbaticals for military service, maternity leave, medical issues, and jury duty
- Vacation according to the length of employment and seniority; vacation is paid time off from work
- Dress code required by the facility
- Probationary period

Procedures are defined as specific guides to job functions for all departmental personnel, visitors, and patients in order to standardize activities with a high level of risk. Procedures represent the sequence of steps to be followed in performing an action typically described in a policy. Procedures are also criteria for the way in which things are done. Procedures can assist employees in dealing with situations that may arise during the daily operations of practice. Examples of procedures in a physical therapy department include the following:

- Equipment management, cleaning, and maintenance; safety inspections; and training requirements
- Safety and emergency procedures
- Hazardous-waste management
- Disciplinary procedures for actions such as violation of the dress code or a patient's confidentiality

Content of the Policy and Procedure Manual

The policy and procedure manual has an introduction that may include things such as the employee welcome message and introductory statement, and an employee acknowledgement form. This section is written in a friendly, conversational style designed to make the employee welcome and comfortable, and provides basic information about the practice and its operating philosophy. The remaining sections of the manual contain very detailed and precise language regarding the rights and obligations of both the employee and the employer, and should be reviewed by a legal counsel to ensure compliance with federal and state laws.

The policy and procedure manual must be guided by various state and federal laws and organizations, such as the Equal Employment Opportunity Commission (EEOC), the Americans with Disabilities Act (ADA), the Family and Medical Leave Act (FMLA), the Fair Labor Standards Act (FLSA), the Occupational Safety and Health Administration (OSHA), the Health Insurance Portability and Accountability Act (HIPAA), and the Center for Medicare and Medicaid Services (CMS). An example of federal legislation included in the policy and procedure manual is the Family and Medical Leave Act (FMLA). The FMLA requires employers with 50 or more employees to allow up to 12 workweeks of unpaid leave in any 12-month period for the birth, adoption, or foster care placement of a child, or serious health condition of the employee, spouse, parent, or child, provided the leave is taken within 12 months of such event. The policy and procedure manual must include all the necessary information related to the FMLA.

DEPARTMENTAL MEETINGS

PTAs participate in facility and departmental meetings. The following types of meetings occur in the physical therapy department:

- Staff/departmental meetings: These are held regularly to discuss departmental (or hospital or management) business.
- Team meetings: Scheduled weekly and involving the interdisciplinary team members, such as the physician, nurse, PT, PTA, OT, COTA, SLP, social services, and other members of the team. The purpose of team meetings is to discuss and coordinate patient care services, set patients' goals, discuss goal achievement necessary for patients' discharge, and discuss discharge plans and continuum of care including equipment needs or home health services.
- Supervisory meetings: These take place regularly between the supervisor and the staff. The supervisory meetings' purpose is to discuss patient care issues. Sometimes, a supervisory meeting can be a one-on-one meeting between a staff member (such as the PTA) and the supervisor (such as the PT) to discuss the immediate needs of the staff member in regard to patient care. The goal of the supervisory meetings is to achieve positive outcomes.
- Strategic planning meetings: These provide an organizational/departmental planning process for the future. These meetings discuss the results of the strategic planning process that was included in the strategic plan. They also make a statement about the mission and the philosophy of values of the organization/department before implementation of the

strategic plan. Strategic planning meetings also can reveal the organizational/departmental strengths and weaknesses and the course of action for achieving future goals. In addition, strategic planning meetings can provide the following:

- Directions on how to achieve the organization's/department's goals
- Identification of the people responsible for developing and carrying out the strategic plan (such as staff members and/or the supervisor)
- Information to external parties (such as the accrediting agencies) about the organization/department
- Analysis of the progress toward the strategic plan goals

The strategic plan goals are time-related and can be for 1 year, 2 years, or 5 years. Analysis of progress toward the goals is generally done quarterly by the supervisor (or director/manager) of the organization/department.

Fiscal Management of a Physical Therapy Service

BUDGETS

Physical therapy services are fiscally managed by a budget. A budget is defined as a financial projection for a specific time period of the amount of funds allocated to cover specific aspects of operating a physical therapy department or a private practice.

Budget periods vary from 1 year for personnel and supplies to 5 years (or longer) for capital expenses (purchase expenses). Budgets need to be revised when conditions in the organization/department change.

The purposes of a budget include the following:

- Explains in detail anticipated income and expenditures (expenses) in regard to personnel, buildings, equipment, supplies, and/or space
- Represents an integral aspect of the planning process
- Provides a mechanism of assessing the success of the practice, programs, or projects

The various types of budgets include the following:

- *Operating expense budget:* A financial projection related to the daily organizational/departmental operation. Examples include salaries, benefits (such as sick days or vacation days), utilities (such as electricity, gas, or telephone), supplies (such as ultrasound gel, changing gowns, or gloves), linen, housekeeping, maintenance, and continuing education.
- *Capital expense budget:* A financial projection related to the purchase of large items for future use. An example is physical therapy equipment to be utilized for more than a year (such as an ultrasound machine).
- *Accounts receivable budget:* A financial projection assessing expected benefits from future operations; includes money owed to a company such as a physical therapy private practice for providing physical therapy services. An example could be money to be received from Medicare for physical therapy services provided to Medicare patients.
- *Accounts payable budget:* A financial projection assessing money owed to a creditor that provided services or equipment to the company; it is the part of the budget where debts are listed. An example could be money to be paid to a company that regularly services physical therapy equipment.

COSTS

In physical therapy, there are four different costs associated with providing physical therapy services:

- Direct costs: Costs directly related to the provision of physical therapy services. Examples include salaries, equipment, treatment supplies, or continuing education.
- Indirect costs: Costs related to the provision of physical therapy services in an indirect way. Examples include housekeeping, utilities, laundry, or marketing.
- Variable costs: Costs related to the provision of physical therapy services that are not fixed and can vary depending on the volume of services. Examples include linen costs or utilities costs, which will increase with an increase in the number of patients' visits.

- Fixed costs: Costs related to the provision of physical therapy services that are fixed regardless of the changes in the volume of services. An example is rent, which will not increase regardless of an increase in the number of patients' visits.

Quality Assurance

Quality assurance (QA) is defined as activities and programs designed and implemented in a clinical facility to achieve high-quality levels of care. In physical therapy, quality assurance is responsible for the following:

- Monitoring the quality of physical therapy services
- Monitoring the appropriateness of patient care
- Resolving any identified problems related to quality of service and patient care

UTILIZATION REVIEW

Quality assurance can be implemented in a clinical facility by using a utilization review, which is the evaluation of the necessity, quality, effectiveness, or efficiency of medical services, procedures, and facilities. For example, in a hospital, utilization review includes the appropriateness of admission, services ordered, services provided, length of stay, and discharge practices. In physical therapy, utilization review can be implemented through a written plan for reviewing the use of resources and determining their medical necessity and cost efficiency. For example, utilization review can analyze the cost and the outcome of using interferential electrical stimulation for patients diagnosed with posterior disk impingement. If the patients' outcomes were positive, it means the use of interferential electrical stimulation was appropriate and the cost of the treatment was efficient.

PEER REVIEW

Utilization review can be applied in clinics by using peer review. As a general definition, peer review means the evaluation of the quality of the work effort of an individual by his or her peers. In addition to the clinical quality of medical care administered by an individual, group, or hospital, peer review is also used to evaluate articles submitted for publication in different scientific journals.

In physical therapy peer review, PTAs can review the work of other PTAs, and PTs can review the work of other PTs. In general, peer review is not punitive but educational. The goal of peer review is to improve the quality of care and to evaluate how well physical therapy services are performed when delivering care.

Types of peer review in physical therapy clinical settings include the following:

- Retrospective peer reviews are conducted after physical therapy services were rendered. They are used to determine whether physical therapy services were necessary, appropriate, and comprehensive in regard to patients' needs.
- Concurrent peer reviews are conducted during physical therapy treatments. They are used to immediately improve the quality of physical therapy treatments and to determine current patients' outcomes and satisfaction.

Peer review also can be performed in physical therapy clinical facilities by different accrediting agencies or third-party payers such as Medicare, Medicaid, or managed care plans. In these situations, the peer review is done by professional review organizations (PROs). An example of such an organization is the Professional Standards Review Organization (PSRO), which performs peer review at the local level as required by Public Law 92-603 (started in 1973) of the United States for the services provided under the Medicare, Medicaid, and Maternal and Child Health programs funded by the federal government.

The major goals of the PSRO are the following:

- To ensure that health care services are of acceptable professional quality
- To ensure appropriate use of health care facilities at the most economical level consistent with professional standards
- To identify lack of quality and overuse problems in health care and improve those conditions
- To attempt to obtain voluntary correction of inappropriate or unnecessary practitioner and facility practices, and if unable to do so, recommend sanctions against violators

RISK MANAGEMENT

Quality assurance also can be implemented in a clinical facility by using risk management. As a general definition, risk management means methods utilized by health care organizations to defend their assets against the threats posed by legal liability. Risk management includes the following:

- Identification of health care delivery problems in an institution (as evidenced by previous lawsuits and patient or staff complaints)
- Development of standards and guidelines to enhance the quality of care
- Anticipation of problems that may arise in the future

For example, risk management issues found in a hospital could include breaches of patients' privacy, failure to disclose risks and alternatives to treatment, intubation errors during anesthesia, or infant trauma or death during childbirth. In physical therapy, risk management can identify, evaluate, and correct against risk to staff or patients. Examples of risk management found in physical therapy could include delegating issues, such as PTs delegating to PTAs or PTAs delegating to physical therapy aides. In such situations, the PTs and the PTAs must consult their individual state practice acts. Another risk management issue in physical therapy could be providing quality care for managed care patients or Medicaid patients. For example, if a managed care company does not provide for enough visits, and the patient needs the additional visits, the PT may need to ask the managed care company for more visits or to ask the owner of the facility to allow free-of-charge services to the patient.

General purposes of physical therapy risk management include the following:

- To decrease risks in physical therapy practice by maintaining equipment safety and providing ongoing staff safety education in the use of equipment
- To identify potential patient or employee injuries
- To identify potential property loss or damage
- To implement procedures to properly clean the equipment and prevent contamination
- To increase patient and staff safety by reporting all incidents, documenting incidents by making reports, reviewing incident reports by a supervisor, identifying all risk factors in regard to patient care and safety, and having all staff certified (and recertified annually) in cardiopulmonary resuscitation (CPR)

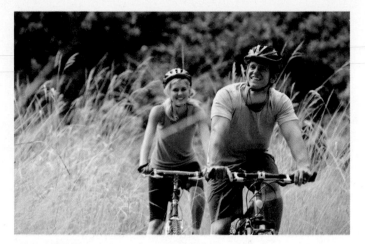
© Warren Goldswain/Shutterstock

Clinical Trends

Wellness and disease prevention are physical therapy goals included in the 2020 Vision Statement. The APTA took the initiative to promote health by being a member of the Healthy People Consortium, assisting with the Healthy People 2010 and Healthy People 2020. Both Healthy People programs are leading the way to eliminate health disparities and attain years of healthy life. PTs' educational and practice guidelines emphasize inclusion of health promotion, wellness, and disease prevention in schools' curricula and physical therapy practice. The Guide also stresses the importance of providing prevention and promoting health, wellness, and fitness for patients/clients. Physical therapy goals for the twenty-first century include prevention of diabetes (and prediabetes), obesity, arthritis, stroke, and falls in older adults.[47] In addition, the goals incorporate promotion of regular physical activity. Encouraging children and adults to adopt a healthy lifestyle using exercises and activities is very important. It is well established that regular physical activity can enhance health and prevent disease.[47] One way to promote physical activity is for PTs to provide individualized assessments and exercise programs for patients/clients who are overweight and need to lose weight. PTAs can assist PTs in this quest for promotion of a healthy lifestyle through physical activity.

WELLNESS AND HEALTH PROMOTION

The concept of wellness is the patient/client's capacity to be in good physical and emotional health and appreciate and enjoy high-quality health. This notion of wellness also means having a harmonious relationship between a patient/client's internal and external environments. Health promotion is the science and art of helping patients/clients change their lifestyle and attain optimal health. Both wellness and health promotion can guide a patient/client toward a healthy lifestyle. In clinical practice, PTs can use patient education to increase a patient/client's health awareness and his or her ability to maintain good health. Examples of health promotion could be the PT's assessments of a patient/client's:

- Behavioral health risks (such as smoking or drug abuse)
- Level of physical fitness
- Psychological function (such as memory, reasoning ability, depression, anxiety, or memory)
- Social activities
- Other clinical findings (such as nutrition or hydration)

Many variables are involved in a patient/client's wellness and health promotion, including the patient/client's own health beliefs and values, personal expectations, and/or physical and social environments.

DISEASE PREVENTION

Disease prevention is an activity that can reduce a patient/client's mortality and morbidity from disease.[47] Disease prevention can help a patient/client avoid possible risk factors that may cause disease, disorder, or injury. In physical therapy clinical practice, PTs can educate patients/clients to identify the risk factors and provide protective measures. Typically, the prevention of risk factors is implemented at three levels, primary, secondary, and tertiary. The most cost-effective prevention method is primary because it occurs prior to the onset of the disease/disorder. For example, in clinical settings, PTs/PTAs have the ability to provide primary prevention to patients/clients by using patient education about guarding against accidents while performing basic ADLs. Secondary prevention concentrates on

early detection of health problems, trying to stop or slow down the progression of the disease.[47] Tertiary prevention attempts to minimize the negative effects of the disease.[47]

Discussion Questions

1. Discuss the terminology found in the *Guide to Physical Therapist Practice* related to physical therapy interventions.
2. List the five elements of patient/client management and identify components that the PTA may participate in.
3. Brainstorm at least three questions that an employer might ask during an interview.
4. Brainstorm three questions that a PTA might ask a potential employer.
5. Develop and share with the group a list of healthy lifestyle tips for a patient who has a chronic health condition such as diabetes mellitus or heart disease.
6. Describe three recommendations for a patient to prevent falls at home.

Learning Opportunities

1. Write a resume.
2. Interview a classmate or be interviewed by a classmate.
3. Use the *Guide for Physical Therapy Practice* to identify the impairment, functional limitation, and disability for a patient who has a rotator cuff tear pathology.
4. A 24-year-old man was involved in a motorcycle accident and has a diagnosis of a traumatic brain injury. Using the *Guide to Physical Therapy Practice* online practice patterns, identify the practice pattern that matches the pathology and list the portions of the examination and intervention that could be designated to the PTA.
5. Write at least one policy and one procedure.

Summary of Part I

Part I of this book, "The Profession of Physical Therapy," discussed the history of rehabilitation treatments in ancient civilizations and in the United States and the history of the physical therapy profession. The organizational structure of the APTA was included, as well as the supervisory role of the PT on the health care team. The collaborative path between the PT and PTA, the health care teams, and the members of the rehabilitation team and their responsibilities were also discussed. The employment settings for PTs and PTAs were listed. Part I concluded with a general description of the *Guide to Physical Therapist Practice* and its use, and explanations of employment and clinical practice topics such as interviews, the policy and procedure manual, meetings, budgets, quality assurance, and risk management. Contemporary clinical trends in wellness, health promotion, and disease prevention also were included.

References (Part I)

1. Smith, W. *A Dictionary of Greek and Roman Antiquities.* 3rd ed. London, England: J. Murray; 1914.
2. Berryman, KW, Park, RJ. *Sport and Exercise Science: Essays in the History of Sports Medicine.* Urbana, IL: University of Illinois Press; 1992.
3. Andry, N. *Orthopedia: Or, the Art of Correcting and Preventing Deformities in Children.* Editors: Raney, RB, Orr, HW. Notes from the Editors. Birmingham, AL: The Classics of Medicine Library, Division of Gryphon Editions; 1980.
4. Braun, MB, Simonson, SJ. *Introduction to Massage Therapy.* Baltimore, MD: Lippincott, Williams & Wilkins; 2007.
5. Gilman, MD. *The Bibliography of Vermont; Or, a List of Books and Pamphlets Relating in Any Way to the State. With Biographical and Other Notes.* Burlington, VT: Free Press Association; 1897.
6. Zander, G. *Mechanico-Therapeutics and Orthopedics by Means of Apparatus.* New York: Mechanico-Therapeutic and Orthopedic Zander Institute; 1891.
7. Albee, HF. in *Journal of the Medical Society of New Jersey.* 1920; Vol. XVII. Accessed online at: http://books.google.com; December, 2009.
8. Cheney, M, Uth, R, Glenn J. *Tesla, Master of Lightning.* New York: Barnes & Noble Books; 1999.
9. Miller, PD. *Disabled Sports USA. Fitness Programming and Physical Disability.* Champaign, IL: Human Kinetics; 1995.
10. Zwecker, M, Zeilig, G, Ohry, S. Professor Heinrich Sebastian Frenkel: A forgotten founder of rehabilitation medicine. *Spinal Cord.* 2004; 42: 55–56.
11. Wilson, DJ. *Living with Polio: The Epidemic and Its Survivors.* Chicago, IL: University of Chicago Press; 2005.
12. Neumann, DA. Polio: Its impact on the people of the United States and the emerging profession of physical therapy. *Journal of Orthopaedic and Sports Physical Therapy.* 2004; 34(8): 479–492.
13. DeLisa, IA. *Physical Medicine and Rehabilitation: Principles and Practice.* 4th ed. Philadelphia, PA: Lippincott Williams & Wilkins; 2005.
14. White, L, Duncan, G. R2 Library (Online Service). *Medical-Surgical Nursing, an Integrated Approach.* Albany, NY: Delmar Thomson Learning; 2002.
15. Kodish, BI. *Back Pain Solutions: How to Help Yourself with Posture—Movement Therapy and Education.* Pasadena, CA: Extension Publishers; 2001.
16. Leithauser DJ. *Early Ambulation and Related Procedures in Surgical Management.* Oxford: Blackwell Scientific Publications; 1947. In *Journal of Bone and Joint Surgery.* 1948; 30B(4). Accessed September 5, 2009, at: www.jbjs.org.uk/cgi/reprint/30-B/4/739-a.
17. Delorme, TL, Watkins AL. *Progressive Resistance Exercise. Technic and Medical Application.* New York: Appleton-Century-Crofts Inc.; 1951. In *Journal of Bone and Joint Surgery.* Accessed September 5, 2009, at: www.jbjs.org.uk/cgi/reprint/34-B/4/722.
18. Houglum, PA. *Therapeutic Exercise for Musculoskeletal Injuries.* 2nd ed. Champaign, IL: Human Kinetics; 2005.
19. Moffat, M. The history of physical therapy practice in the United States. *Journal of Physical Therapy Education.* 2003; 1: 1–50. Accessed September 5, 2009, at: http://findarticles.com.
20. Murphy, W. *Healing the Generations: A History of Physical Therapy and the American Physical Therapy Association.* Alexandria, VA: American Physical Therapy Association; 1995.
21. Stevens, R. *American Medicine and the Public Interest.* New Haven, CT: Yale University Press; 1971.
22. Vogel, EE. The beginnings of modern physiotherapy. *Physical Therapy.* 1976; 56: 15–22.
23. Goldstein, M. Positive employment trends in physical therapy: APTA surveys find decreases in the unemployment rates for PTs and PTAs. Accessed June 2004 at: www.apta.org/pt_magazine/July01/reliableres.html.
24. American Physical Therapy Association. Members of Congress support physical therapists, patients on affordable rehabilitation services under Medicare: Members of Congress to reintroduce legislation on financial cap repeal. Accessed March 2005 at: www.apta.org/rt.cfm/news/newsreleases.

25. American Physical Therapy Association. 2013 American Physical Therapy Association annual report. Accessed July 2014 at: www.apta.org.

26. American Physical Therapy Association. Working operational definitions of Elements of Vision 2020. From the Task Force on Strategic Plan to Achieve Vision 2020. Accessed September 2009 at: www.apta.org.

27. American Physical Therapy Association. New Michigan law means all 51 US jurisdictions allow direct access to PTs. Accessed July 2014 at: www.apta.org/PTinMotion /NewNow/2014/2014/7/1/MichiganDirectAccess.

28. American Physical Therapy Association. PTA caucus. Accessed July 2014 at: www.apta.org.

29. American Physical Therapy Association. Membership benefits for students. Accessed July 2014 at: www.apta.org.

30. American Physical Therapy Association. Demographic profile of physical therapist members 2013. Accessed July 2014 at: www.apta.org.

31. American Physical Therapy Association. Demographic profile of physical therapist assistant members. Accessed July 2014 at: www.apta.org.

32. American Physical Therapy Association. Report of the 2014 House of Delegates. Accessed September 2014 at: www .apta.org.

33. Commission on Accreditation in Physical Therapy Education (CAPTE). Accessed July 2014 at: www.capteonline.org.

34. American Board of Physical Therapist Specialists. About ABPTS. Accessed July 2014 at: www.abpts.org.

35. Federation of State Boards of Physical Therapy. NPTE. Accessed July 2014 at: https://www.fsbpt.org.

36. American Physical Therapy Association. PT-PAC [Physical Therapy Political Action Committee]. Accessed July 2014 at: www.apta.org.

37. Commission on Accreditation in Physical Therapy Education (CAPTE). About CAPTE. Accessed July 2014 at: http://www.capteonline.org.

38. American Physical Therapy Association. Minimum required skills of physical therapist assistant graduate at entry-level. Accessed July 2014 at: http://www.apta.org.

39. American Physical Therapy Association. Direction and supervision of the physical therapist assistant. Accessed July 2014 at: www.apta.org.

40. U.S. Department of Labor, Bureau of Statistics. Home page. Accessed July 2014 at: www.bls.gov.

41. American Physical Therapy Association. *Guide to Physical Therapist Practice 3.0.* Alexandria, VA: APTA; 2014.

42. American Physical Therapy Association. Frequently asked questions on physical therapists' services provided without referral. Accessed December 2009 at: www.apta.org.

43. Drafke, MW. *Working in Health Care: What You Need to Know to Succeed.* Philadelphia, PA: F.A. Davis Company; 2002.

44. Bolles, RN. *What Color Is Your Parachute? 2010. A Practical Manual for Job-Hunters and Career-Changers.* New York City, NY: Ten Speed Press; 2010.

45. American Physical Therapy Association. Clinical practice guidelines. Accessed April 2015 at: www.apta.org.

46. Yate, M. *Knock'em Dead Cover Letters.* 9th ed. Avon, MA: Adams Media; 2010.

47. Dreeben, O. *Patient Education in Rehabilitation.* Sudbury, MA: Jones & Bartlett Publishers; 2009.

PART II

Physical Therapist Practice

This part is divided into two chapters:

- CHAPTER 4: Examination, Evaluation, and Plan of Care
- CHAPTER 5: Physical Therapy Practice Areas

These two chapters describe the process of examination of patients, the evaluation of the data, and the development of the plan of care for the patient. By understanding the process and terminology within the patient record, the physical therapist assistant will be more effective in treating the patient. This portion of the book also identifies practice areas that are common in physical therapy: musculoskeletal, neurologic, cardiopulmonary, pediatric, geriatric, and integumentary. Although physical therapists can specialize in cardiovascular and pulmonary, clinical electrophysiologic, geriatric, neurologic, orthopedic, pediatric, and sports physical therapy, the clinical practices may include more than one of these specialties. For example, musculoskeletal (orthopedic) physical therapy clinical practices may contain physical therapy for rheumatologic conditions, orthopedic rehabilitation, sports injuries and treatments, manual therapy, low back pain, or aquatic physical therapy. Geriatric and pediatric patients can also be treated for musculoskeletal disorders in a musculoskeletal physical therapy practice.

However, as a specialty, musculoskeletal (orthopedic) physical therapy specializes in treating patients who have orthopedic disorders including sports injuries. Neurologic physical therapy specializes in treating patients who have neurologic disorders. Cardiopulmonary physical therapy specializes in treating patients who have cardiac and pulmonary conditions. Pediatric physical therapy specializes in treating children who have developmental dysfunction and specific pediatric disorders. Geriatric physical therapy specializes in treating older individuals who present with musculoskeletal and neuromuscular conditions and dysfunction common to the older adult. Integumentary physical therapy specializes in treating patients who have skin disorders including wounds and burns.

CHAPTER 4

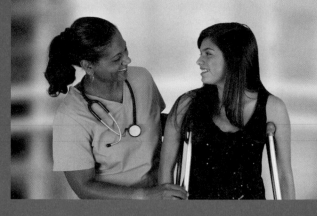

Examination, Evaluation, and Plan of Care

OBJECTIVES

After studying this chapter, the reader will be able to:

1. Discuss the elements of a physical therapy examination.
2. Compare and contrast examination and evaluation.
3. Identify the elements of patient history.
4. Compare the two types of pain scales used frequently in physical therapy practice.
5. List the forms of data collected during the examination.
6. Describe specialized examinations for orthopedic, neurologic, cardiopulmonary, pediatric, geriatric, and integumentary specialty practice areas.
7. Describe the purpose of a plan of care.

KEY TERMS

APGAR screening
congestive heart failure (CHF)
dementia
dyspnea
dystonia
edema
evaluation
examination
flaccidity

hypertonia
hypotonia
kinesthesia
Numerical Rating System (NRS)
proprioception
rigidity
spasticity
Visual Analog Scale (VAS)

Physical therapy care must always begin with the physical therapist (PT) making a physical therapy diagnosis. "A diagnosis is a label encompassing a cluster of signs and symptoms commonly associated with a disorder or syndrome or category of impairments in body structures and function, activity limitations, or participation restrictions."[1] The PT uses the examination and evaluation process to develop a physical therapy diagnosis and create an individualized plan of care for the patient that includes intervention, prognosis, and expected outcomes.

Examination and Evaluation

Examination and evaluation are performed by the PT. Specific data collection can be performed, at the request of the PT, by the physical therapist assistant (PTA).

> **WHAT IS AN EXAMINATION?**
>
> An **examination** is the process of obtaining a history, performing relevant systems reviews, and selecting and administering specific tests and measures.

> **WHAT IS AN EVALUATION?**
>
> An **evaluation** is a dynamic process in which the PT makes clinical judgments based on data gathered during the examination.

The examination is a very comprehensive process that needs to be carried out in a proper and systematic manner. The purpose of the examination is for the physical therapist to understand fully the patient's problems, from the patient's perspective as well as the clinician's perspective. PTs often customize the data that they collect based upon the patient's referral diagnosis or patient's area of concern. It is important that the PT consider the patient as a whole complex being. This means that an orthopedic patient should also have some neurologic and cardiovascular examination and that the neurologic patient should be examined for biomechanical and orthopedic concerns. The process of creating a physical therapy diagnosis hinges on thoughtful consideration of all aspects of the patient's health and consideration towards possible medical concerns that would warrant referral to another health care professional.

EXAMINATION

Initial information from a patient is often collected prior to the PT meeting the patient for the first time. This may occur by reading the medical chart in the acute care setting or by reviewing intake sheets given to the outpatient when registering in an outpatient setting. A patient history is a complete medical history of the patient's chief complaints, present illness, past history, allergies, current medications, lifestyle and habits, social history, vocational and economic history, and family history.

The data obtained will include:

- Medical diagnosis and any precautions related to physical therapy
- Patient's chief complaint, including the patient's description of his or her condition and the reason seeking assistance; identification of patient's primary problem
- Patient's present illness, including the symptoms associated with the patient's primary problem such as location of the problem (may use a body chart), severity, nature (such as aching, burning, or tingling), persistence (constant versus intermittent), and aggravated by activity versus relieved by rest
- Onset of the patient's primary problem, including mechanism of injury (if traumatic), sequence and progression of symptoms, date of the initial onset and status up to the current visit, prior treatments and results, and associated disability
- Patient's past history, including prior episodes of the same problem; prior treatments and responses; other affected areas (or body parts); familial, developmental, and congenital disorders; general health status; medications; and x-rays or other pertinent tests
- Personal information, including the patient's age, gender, and occupation
- Patient's lifestyle, including profession or occupation, assistance from family or friends, occupational and family demands (spouse, children, job expectations), ADLs (hobbies, sports), and patient's concept of the impact of functional (including cosmetic) and socioeconomic factors

PAIN DESCRIPTION

Pain description is part of the patient's history, and includes the location of the pain, extension or radiation, intensity, duration, onset, frequency, progression, aggravating or relieving factors, and previous test results in regard to the pain. Two major pain measurements are used in physical therapy:

- The **Visual Analog Scale (VAS)** consisting of a 10-cm unmarked line, either vertical or horizontal, with verbal or pictorial anchors indicating a continuum from no pain at one end to severe pain at the other. The patient is asked to mark on the line the pain he or she is experiencing (e.g., How bad is your pain?). This mark is then measured with a ruler and expressed in centimeters, with 10 centimeters representing severe pain.

- The **Numerical Rating System (NRS)** is easier to use than the VAS. The NRS uses a range of numbers (e.g., 0–5, 0–10) to reflect increasing degrees of pain. The patient is asked, "If zero is no pain and 10 the worst pain imaginable, how would you rate your pain?"

The pain description measurements should be taken prior to and after treatment in order to assess the patient's response to physical therapy interventions for pain. These treatments may include physical modalities and agents, relaxation training, and patient education for behavioral modification (such as reinforcing proper body mechanics during activities of daily living).

DATA COLLECTION

Objective data collection is an important function of the examination to create a clear picture of the patient's problems. This data collection may include the following:

- *Sensory Examination:* Tests for superficial, deep, and combined sensations are included in the sensory examination in physical therapy. First, the superficial responses need to be assessed. Then, if impairments are found, the deep and combined sensations are to be noted. Superficial sensations consist of pain, temperature, light touch, and pressure. Deep sensations consist of **kinesthesia**, **proprioception**, and vibration.[2] Combined sensations consist of tactile localization, two-point discrimination, barognosis, stereognosis, graphesthesia, and recognition of texture.[2] Further neurological tests may include the testing for spinal nerve integrity. Dermatomes, which are specific areas of the skin that are innervated by nerve roots and myotomes, which are specific muscles that are innervated by a nerve root and deep tendon reflexes (DTRs) indicate the ability of a nerve to respond to a stimulus.

- *Cranial Nerve Integrity:* A cranial nerve examination is an examination of the function of the 12 pairs of cranial nerves that are distributed to the head and neck, except for one nerve (cranial nerve 10, called the Vagus nerve) that is distributed to the thorax and abdomen. Cranial nerve examination is recommended for patients who may have lesions of the brain, brainstem, and cervical spine.

- *Vital Signs:* In addition to other neurologic examinations, an investigation of the cardiopulmonary system is essential to examine the patient's vital signs such as heart rate, respiration, and blood pressure and to note any sign of cardiac decompensation. Cardiopulmonary deficits found through the examination of vital signs can interfere with physical therapy interventions and the recovery process. Vital signs also can show the patient's aerobic capacity and endurance.

- *Anthropometrics:* Measurements that give information about the length, girth, and volume of a patient's body are included in the anthropometric examination. This information is important to identify the equality of a patient's legs or the amount of edema a patient may have in a limb. Patient's height, weight, and body mass index (BMI) are also assessed in this area.

- *Mentation, Hearing, and Vision Examination:* The PT has to evaluate the patient's ability to concentrate and respond by examining the patient's attention, orientation, and cognition. The patient's attention is defined as the patient's awareness of the environment or the ability to focus on a specific stimulus without distraction. The patient's orientation refers to his or her awareness of time, person, and place. A patient's cognition is a complex process that examines the following: thinking skills such as language use and calculation, perception, memory awareness, reasoning, judgment, learning, intellect, social skills, and imagination.[2] Three categories from the above elements of cognition are typically used to test a patient. For example, a patient's memory can be assessed for both long-term memory and short-term memory. Long-term memory is recall of experiences or information gained in the distant past. Short-term memory is recall of experiences or information gained in the immediate past. Neurologic diseases or injuries to any of the memory regions found in the brain impair an individual's ability to incorporate new memories or recall and use prior ones.

Hearing and vision impairments may be present with aging, diseases, or trauma, interfering with the patient's communication and quality of life. A gross examination of hearing can be performed by observing the patient's response to conversation. A gross visual examination can assess the patient's visual acuity and peripheral field vision.

- **Range of Motion:** Range of motion (ROM) examination evaluates the amount of excursion through which a joint or a series of joints can move. The ROM is measured in degrees of a circle using an instrument called a goniometer (see **FIGURE 4-1**).
- **Manual Muscle Testing:** Manual muscle testing (MMT) examination (see **FIGURE 4-2**) evaluates the relative strength of specific muscles and identifies patterns of muscle weakness. Rating categories and values for the MMT include: Normal (5), Good (4), Fair (3), Poor (2), Trace activity (1), and Absent activity (0).
- **Muscle Tone:** Abnormalities of muscular tone are common in neurological disorders. These can range from **spasticity** to **rigidity** to **flaccidity**. Tone in general is defined as the resistance of muscles to passive elongation or stretch. Tone can also be thought of as how much tension a muscle has when it is at rest. Tonal abnormalities can be categorized into three large groups: **hypertonia**, **hypotonia**, and **dystonia**. For example, immediately after a stroke, also called a cerebral vascular accident (CVA), patients can have flaccidity on the side of the body opposite to the brain lesion. Flaccidity is a lack of tension when the muscle is at rest and so the patient has poor or no ability to create enough tension in the muscle to move. Patients also can have spasticity on the side of the body opposite to the brain lesion a few hours (or a few days or weeks) after the stroke. Spasticity is an excessive contraction in

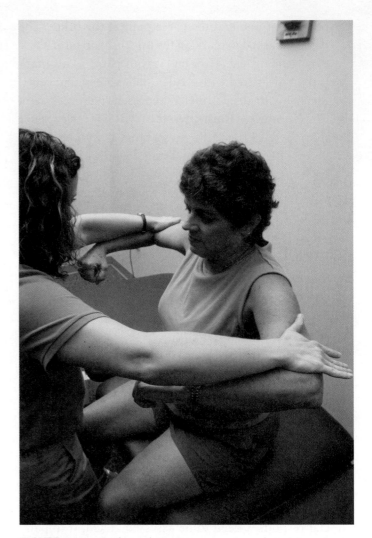

FIGURE 4-2 Manual muscle testing.
© wavebreakmedia/Shutterstock

response to the stretch of a muscle that can occur when the patient is actively moving or being passively moved.

- **Postural Analysis:** Postural examination evaluates the position maintained by the body when standing and sitting in relation to space and other body parts. The patient must be assessed from all angles: the front, the back, and the sides.
- **Balance and Control:** Postural control and balance examination involves the patient's ability to control positions of the body and body parts using skeletal muscles with respect to gravity. For example, a patient who has had a stroke may not be able to maintain balance while sitting, standing, or walking. As a result, the patient's body may lean toward his or her affected side. Standardized examinations of balance include the Berg Balance Test, the Timed Up and Go (TUG)

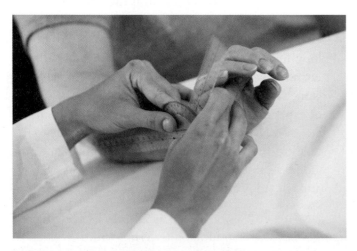

FIGURE 4-1 Measuring ROM using a goniometer.
© aceshot1/Shutterstock

Test, and the Tinetti Performance Oriented Mobility Assessment (POMA).

- **Function:** Functional examination determines the effect of the condition or injury on the patient's daily life. Human functional activities or activities of daily living (ADLs) are divided into: basic activities of daily living (BADLs) such as dressing, transfer activities, walking, or bed activities, and instrumental activities of daily living (IADLs) such as meal preparation, light housework, shopping, or driving the car. Functional examination is performed using different functional tools, such as the following: the Barthel Index, which tests for self-care and patient mobility; the Katz Index of Independence in Activities of Daily Living or the Functional Status Index.

- **Gait Examination:** The PT or the PTA can assess the gait from the front, from behind, and from the side, in each instance observing the patient from the pelvis and lumbar spine down to the ankle and foot. Also, movements in the trunk and upper limbs should be watched. The PT/PTA must also observe the activities that occur in gait from the moment the patient's one lower extremity touches the ground to the moment the same lower extremity contacts the ground again. The activities observed are called a gait cycle. Each portion of the gait cycle involves specific movements and control. The PT or PTA must understand the terminology and practice this examination and documentation process. During gait examination it is also important to examine the patient's footwear and feet to observe any wearing down of the heels and socks and any callus formation, blisters, corns, and bunions. The patient needs to be observed walking with shoes and without shoes, with and without assistive devices, and with prosthetic/orthotic devices, on level ground and on different surfaces, as well as on stairs. If the patient is unable to walk independently, the amount of assistance required must also be identified (see **FIGURE 4-3**).

- **Outcomes Measures:** The use of these standardized tests and measures at regular intervals during a patient's physical therapy episode of care is an important way to objectify the patient's function and abilities. The measures look at the patient's functional abilities and identify if the physical therapy intervention is moving toward the predicted outcomes. This assists the PT in making adjustments in the plan of care.

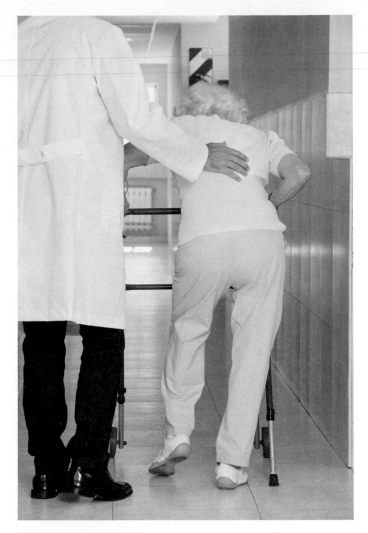

FIGURE 4-3 Gait examination.
© Tyler Olson/Shutterstock

Specialized Examinations

Physical therapy settings have specific examination techniques that are appropriate for specialized patient populations. PTs and PTAs should become familiar with a variety of options for examination to provide the most comprehensive care possible for the patient.

ORTHOPEDIC EXAMINATION

PTs, who work specifically with patients who have orthopedic conditions, utilize special tests that examine the integrity of musculoskeletal components. Joint play movements examine the amount of passive motion available within a joint and help to differentiate what structures may be injured. Other special tests, such as the Neer Test,

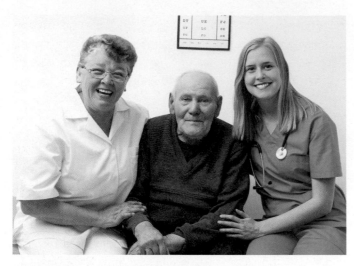

FIGURE 4-4 Man with Parkinson's disease.
© Barabasa/Shutterstock

can help to identify specific pathology In the case of the Neer Test, a positive sign indicates an impingement of shoulder structures.

NEUROLOGIC EXAMINATION

While performing neurologic examinations, the PTA works as a member of the rehabilitation team (see **FIGURE 4-4**). In that position, the PTA has to consider both the therapeutic interventions and the psychosocial aspects of rehabilitation. In general, these aspects include the patient's psychological and social well-being. Specific psychosocial aspects of patient care in neurologic physical therapy may include:

- Patient's adaptation to disability
- Patient's and patient's family's stages of adjustment to the disease and disability
- Effects of impairments, functional limitations, and disability
- Effects of limitations in patient's participation
- Patient's reintegration into environment, family, work, and life

CARDIOPULMONARY EXAMINATION

Cardiopulmonary physical therapy treats patients with cardiac and pulmonary conditions that require physical therapy. In cardiopulmonary rehabilitation, the PTA must be able to reassess the patient as necessary, to monitor the patient in regard to treatment, to monitor the patient's vital signs, and to provide appropriate interventions to the patient. The clinical presentations of cardiovascular

disease are diverse. The most common cardiac diagnoses that are referred for direct physical therapy interventions are coronary artery disease (CAD) and **congestive heart failure (CHF)**.

Pulmonary rehabilitation is a continuum of services directed toward patients who have pulmonary diseases and their families, usually by an interdisciplinary team of specialists. The goals are to achieve and maintain the individual's maximum level of independence and functioning in the community. Chronic obstructive pulmonary diseases (COPDs) and asthma are the most common chronic lung diseases for which pulmonary rehabilitation is needed.

Elements of Cardiac Examination

The cardiovascular examination performed by the PT includes evaluation of the patient's medical status and history, physical examination, assessment of extremities, and the results of diagnostic tests. The patient's medical status and history assessment contains the patient's symptoms of pain including the differentiation among the types of pain. The types of pain can be chest pain, angina, or myocardial infarction pain. Other patient symptoms can be **dyspnea** or shortness of breath, feelings of fatigue or generalized weakness, palpitations such as heart rhythm abnormalities, dizziness, and **edema**. Physical examination of the patient with cardiac disorders assesses the patient's pulses, such as radial pulse, femoral pulse, popliteal pulse, and pedal pulse. It also includes listening to the patient's heart sounds, taking the patient's blood pressure (BP), and counting the respiratory rate (respiration).

Cardiovascular signs and symptoms may include the following:

- Diaphoresis, which is excess sweating associated with decreased cardiac output.
- Decreased or absent pulses associated with peripheral vascular disease (PVD).
- Cyanotic skin, which is associated with decreased cardiac output; or pallor, which is associated with PVD.
- Skin temperature may indicate a lack of blood flow when it is cold.
- Skin changes such as pale, shiny, dry skin with loss of hair associated with PVD.

- Bilateral edema can be an indication of congestive heart failure. Unilateral edema indicates thrombophlebitis or PVD.

The results of diagnostic tests such as an electrocardiogram (ECG) can provide information about the heart rate, rhythm, conduction, areas of ischemia and infarct, increase in size of the heart, and electrolyte imbalances. Electrolytes are mineral salts that conduct electricity in the body.

Elements of Pulmonary Examination

The pulmonary examination (see **FIGURE 4-5**) performed by the PT provides a means of evaluating the patient through interviewing the patient about his or her chief complaints such as decreased ability in performing ADLs due to discomfort in breathing such as dyspnea. The patient's history in regard to his or her occupation needs to be assessed to evaluate, for example, for exposure to asbestos or silicon in his or her prior or present job. The PT must inquire about the patient's habits, such as smoking, alcohol consumption, or taking street drugs. The pulmonary physical therapy examination is similar to the cardiac examination, with the addition of inspection and palpation of the neck and thorax and listening to abnormal inspiration and expiration sounds. These sounds can be crackles (that may indicate a collapsed lung or pulmonary edema) or wheezes (that may indicate asthma or COPD). Evaluation of the patient's chest x-rays can detect the presence of abnormal

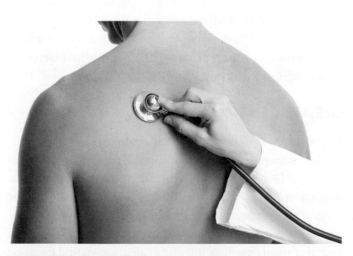

FIGURE 4-5 PT performing auscultation of breath sounds.
© Andrey_Popov/Shutterstock

material such as blood or a change in the lungs such as collapse or fibrosis. Other test results such as a ventilation perfusion scan or laboratory blood gases need to be considered in the initial examination and evaluation.

PEDIATRIC EXAMINATION

In the pediatric examination, evaluation, and interventions, the PT and the PTA need specific knowledge about theories of child development, motor control, and motor learning, such as behavioral theories, principles of motor development, fetal sensorimotor development, pediatric examination, developmental sequence, preterm infant development, and pediatric pathophysiologies. As in all settings, the PTA works in pediatric settings under the supervision of the PT. The PTA's supervision in pediatric settings varies according to the state's practice laws, reimbursement policies and procedures, the settings, the PTA's experience, and the circumstances. If requested by the PT, the PTA supports the PT in collecting data for pediatric examinations; however, the evaluation, or the interpretation of the examination results, as in other physical therapy specialties is performed solely by the PT.

Pediatric Screening Tests

The pediatric examination consists of the patient history in regard to the child's mother's pregnancy and birth history, and the child's medical history. The PT has to be familiar with the results of different pediatric screening tests for infants and children. Some of these screening tests, usually administered by physicians and nurse practitioners, are the **APGAR screening** for newborns at 1 and 5 minutes after birth, the Denver Developmental Screening Test, and the Bayley Scales of Infant Development, just to mention a few. The PT also uses examination tools that are standardized on typically developing children without pathology or dysfunction. Some of these evaluation tools are the Neonatal Behavioral Assessment Scale (NBAS), Movement Assessment of Infants (MAI), and Gross Motor Function Measure (GMFM).

ELEMENTS OF EXAMINATION OF NEWBORNS, INFANTS, AND TODDLERS

For a newborn or an infant patient, the PT performs a neurologic examination including stages of consciousness, skeletal system and ROM examinations, posture, and neonatal reflexes that are present at birth and disappear later in the child's normal development. Examples of neonatal development reflexes

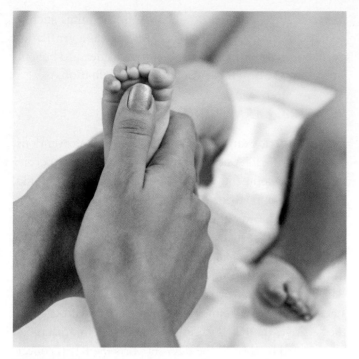

FIGURE 4-6 PT checks plantar grasp reflex.
© Dmytro Vietrov/Shutterstock

are: flexor withdrawal reflex, crossed extension reflex, sucking reflex, plantar grasp reflex (see **FIGURE 4-6**), and symmetrical tonic neck reflex (STNR). For example, the STNR, which is normal for an infant between 6 and 8 months, tests whether bending the infant's head forward causes the arms to bend and legs to straighten, and if straightening of the infant's head causes the arms to straighten and legs to bend. If the STNR persists beyond 8 or 9 months, the infant will have difficulty propping on elbows while lying on the stomach and using the arms and legs in different positions.

Other examinations performed by the PT include newborn, infant, and toddler developmental milestones in the areas of gross motor development, fine motor development, social development, language development, cognitive development, and adaptive skills.

Examples of developmental milestones for a 4- to 5-month-old infant may include the following:

- Rolls from lying on the stomach to the side and face up
- Holds the head steady while sitting supported
- Reaches for toys
- Reacts to music and his or her name

- Plays for 2 or 3 minutes with one toy
- Eats pureed foods
- Takes naps two to three times per day

Examples of developmental milestones for 3- and 4-year-old toddlers may include the following:

- Throws a ball overhead
- Hops 2 to 10 times on one foot
- Stands on tiptoes
- Draws a recognizable human figure
- Enjoys making friends and helping with adult activities
- Has a large (up to 1,000-word) vocabulary
- Learns entire songs
- Identifies colors and shapes
- Uses the toilet without help
- Brushes teeth with supervision

ELEMENTS OF EXAMINATION OF CHILDREN AND ADOLESCENTS

Older children with neurologic disorders may also be examined using observation and standardized tests. Older children are examined for ongoing health needs such as monitoring of progressive diseases such as muscular dystrophy or scoliosis; mobility needs that need to "grow" as the child grows such as walkers and wheelchairs; and functional changes as the child's growth may change the way he or she is able to accomplish school tasks and ADLs. A variety of standardized tests are available to compare the older child's functional abilities, such as the Peabody Developmental Motor Scales or the Bruininks-Oseretsky Test of Motor Proficiency (see **FIGURE 4-7**).

GERIATRIC EXAMINATION

Geriatric physical therapy specializes in treating older individuals who present with musculoskeletal and neuromuscular conditions and dysfunction common to older adults. Similar to other specialized physical therapy areas, geriatric rehabilitation requires understanding of the patient's individuality and his or her unique developmental issues. The initial clinical examination and evaluation should focus on careful and accurate examinations (see **FIGURE 4-8**).

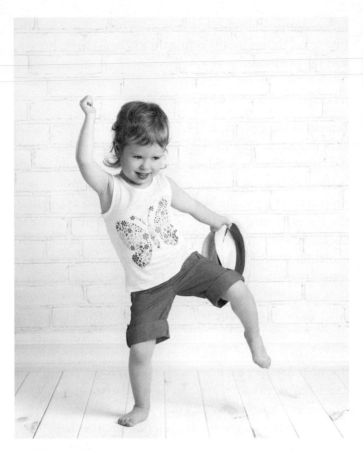

FIGURE 4-7 Preschool child learning to stand on one foot.
© Evgeny Atamanenko/Shutterstock

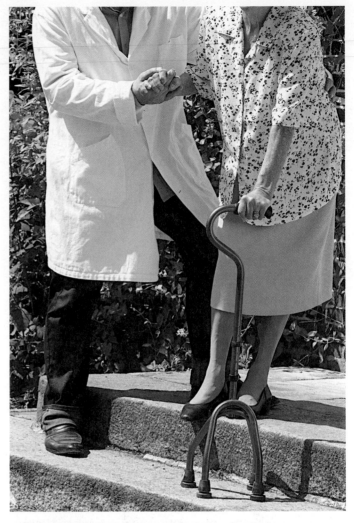

FIGURE 4-8 Older adult being assessed for safe mobility.
© JPC-PROD/Shutterstock

The PT and the PTA help elderly patients to be in control of their own decisions whenever possible. Cultural and ethnic sensitivities are also significant aspects in geriatric rehabilitation. The whole patient should be considered, and social support has to be integrated into the rehabilitation, as well as the demands for continuity of care. In geriatric physical therapy, the PTA's role is important not only for delivering treatments, but also for ongoing reexaminations to determine the following:

- The patient's capacity for safe function
- The effects of inactivity on the patient versus activity
- The effects of normal aging on the patient versus disease pathology

ELEMENTS OF EXAMINATION OF OLDER ADULTS

The geriatric physical therapy examination and evaluation focus mostly on the geriatric patient's level of functioning and his or her ability to remain independent. The plan of care in the initial examination is developed in conjunction with the patient and/or the caregiver.

The elements of a geriatric initial examination and evaluation include the following:

- Patient and or family/caregiver interview
- Pain assessment
- Physical examinations dependent on the patient's pathology (which can be orthopedic, neurologic, and/or cardiopulmonary)
- Psychosocial assessment including depression and **dementia** examinations
- Functional examination
- Environmental examination for the patient's home or for the institution where the patient resides

A psychosocial assessment may include a mini-mental state examination, a mental questionnaire, a depression assessment, and a stress assessment scale. The mini-mental state examination checks the patient's cognitive changes in the areas of orientation, attention, mathematical calculation, recall, and language.[2] The Mental Status Questionnaire (MSQ), composed of 10 questions, has been used in the rehabilitation field for a long time, and is quick and easy to administer.[2] In addition, there are several depression-screening instruments used in physical therapy that assess depression in the older population. Some, such as the Geriatric Depression Scale, are considered to have better sensitivity than others.

The geriatric patient's function is examined in terms of the whole individual and not specific impairments. For example, the patient's function may be examined and evaluated for the following:[3]

- Physical function, including sensory and motor
- Mental function, including intelligence, cognitive ability, and memory
- Social function, including the patient's interaction with family members and the community, as well as economic considerations
- Emotional function, including the patient's ability to cope with stress and anxiety, and the patient's satisfaction with life

Physical therapy intervention goals are geared toward the patient as a whole person and the patient's functionality within the care environment. The geriatric patient's optimal health is contingent on health-conducive behaviors, prevention of disability, and compensation for health-related losses and impairment of aging. The PTA works closely with the PT and is involved in ongoing reexamination of the geriatric patient.

ENVIRONMENTAL EXAMINATION

Environmental examination is done for the patient's home or for the institution where the patient lives. For example, the institutional environmental examination checks the patient's room for clutter or unsafe furniture, whether the lighting is bright enough for reading, and dangerous areas such as bathtubs that need skid-proof surfaces.[2] The environmental examination also checks the outside environment for steps that need to be clearly marked, walkways in good repair, or adequate lighting in all public areas.[2] The

home examination checks the exterior of the home and the interior of the home, including the kitchen, the bathroom, and the bedroom.[2]

INTEGUMENTARY EXAMINATION

Integumentary physical therapy treats patients who have skin disorders. The PT and the PTA treating skin disorders have to be knowledgeable in the function and examination of the integumentary system and common skin disorders. During the skin examination and evaluation, the PT assesses the patient for pruritus (itching), rashes, excessive skin dryness, edema (swelling), unusual skin growths, changes in skin color and temperature, sensory integrity, pain, and soreness. The skin examination may indicate other system disorders, such as changes in skin color showing cyanotic skin, characterized by bluish-gray discoloration, verifies a lack of oxygen and excess carbon dioxide in the blood, which may be caused by a respiratory disorder. Another example, such as edematous skin, can be caused by circulatory, cardiac, or renal diseases.

For example, a positive examination for excessive skin dryness indicates system dysfunction such as diabetes or thyroid problems. Changes in skin color showing cyanotic skin, characterized by bluish-gray discoloration, verifies a lack of oxygen and excess carbon dioxide in the blood, which may be caused by a respiratory disorder. Another example, such as edematous skin, can be caused by circulatory, cardiac, or renal diseases.

In addition to treating skin disorders, a large part of integumentary physical therapy treats wounds and burns (see **FIGURE 4-9**). The role of physical therapy in

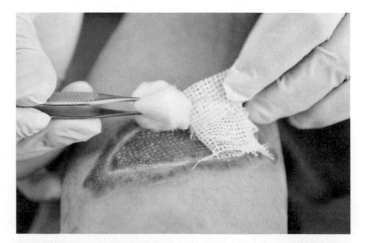

FIGURE 4-9 PT assessing a wound.
© Anukool Manoton/Shutterstock

the management of individuals with chronic wounds is expanding. The practice of managing hospitalized patients who have wounds by using whirlpool baths and dressing changes has extended to the development of wound care centers within physical therapy departments.

Many PTs specialize in wound management. Also, many private physical therapy outpatient clinics offer wound care as the primary practice specialty. Physical therapy wound examination and evaluation are complex processes resulting in information that is critical in determining the diagnosis and prognosis and developing the plan of care. The American Physical Therapy Association's (APTA's) *Guide to Physical Therapist Practice* provides a documentation template that delineates the type of information to be gathered in the initial examination and evaluation of a wound in regard to patient history, systems review, and tests and measures.[4] Examples of tests and measures used to establish wound characteristics include the following:[4]

- Location of the wound
- Size, depth, and drainage of the wound
- Skin changes
- Involved tissue's color and temperature
- Involved extremity's girth, tissue, and sensation

The wound needs to be described using anatomical landmarks. For the wound size, the PT or the PTA can use a film grid or a clear plastic sheet to measure the length and width of the wound. Wound depth is assessed by inserting the tip of a sterile cotton swab into the deepest part of the base of the wound. Wound drainage is indicative of wound healing or infection. For example, clear and shiny watery-like (serous) drainage shows wound healing.[5] By contrast, bright yellow, thicker watery-like (serous) drainage, with a slightly foul smell, shows wound infection.[5] Monitoring the healing process also involves tracking skin changes of the wound and around the wound during healing. For example, black skin over and around a wound identifies tissue death, or necrosis.[5] By contrast, red or pink skin identifies healthy tissue healing.

Burn examination and evaluation performed by the PT is also a complex examination because it takes into consideration the pathophysiology of the type of burn wound. For example, a burn wound has three zones: (1) the zone of coagulation, where the cells are dead; (2) the zone of stasis, where the cells are injured and can die without specialized treatment; and (3) the zone of hyperemia, where the injury is minimal and the cells can recover.[2] In addition, the degrees of burns need to be classified by the severity of the damaged tissue. They are classified as first degree (or superficial), second degree having superficial partial thickness or second degree having deep partial thickness, third degree (or full thickness), and fourth degree (or subdermal).[5] For example, a common first-degree burn is sunburn. The damage in the sunburn is limited to the outer layer of the skin, or epidermis, and is marked by tenderness, redness, and mild pain. The extent of the burned area is ranked using the rule of nines for estimating the percentage of body surface areas.

The rule of nines for an adult:[5]

- The head represents 9 percent.
- Each upper extremity is 9 percent.
- The back of the trunk is 18 percent.
- The front of the trunk is 18 percent.
- Each lower extremity is 18 percent.
- The perineum is the remaining 1 percent.

Different percentages are used to classify children's burns. In addition, there are also classifications regarding percentages of body area burned as related to possible patient complications such as respiratory involvement, smoke inhalation, and destruction of skin.

Plan of Care

After the PT completes the examination and evaluation, the plan of care can be developed. The PT develops a problem list from the evaluation and identifies the interventions to help improve the problem (see **TABLE 4-1**). In addition, functional long-term goals are written to identify the proposed outcome for the patient's episode of physical therapy care. As a requirement of Medicare, the federal insurance plan for Americans older than 65 years of age, the plan of care must also include the physical therapy diagnosis, the type of therapy to be provided, the potential of the patient to reach the functional goals and the intensity, frequency, and duration of the plan of care. This plan will guide the PTA working with the patient. The PTA is not allowed to change the plan of care.

TABLE 4-1   Plan of Care

Patient: John Smith		Date: July 5, 2015
Dx: R Total Knee Arthroplasty June 20, 2015		
Current Functional Limitation:	**Goal:**	**Intervention:**
Patient is unable to ascend or descend stairs independently without safety concerns due to weakness, decreased ROM, and ineffective motor control.	Patient will be able to ascend and descend 7 steps independently with a railing to allow patient to enter and exit his home safely, in 3 weeks.	Therapeutic exercises to include strength and flexibility. Neuromuscular activities to improve motor control. Therapeutic activities to improve functional mobility and safety.
Duration and Frequency:	**Discharge Plan:**	
2 times per week for 3 weeks	Patient will be discharged from physical therapy when he has met his goals, it has been determined that he has plateaued, or it is the patient's desire to discontinue PT services.	

Discussion Questions

1. The patient is returning home after a cerebrovascular accident (stroke). He is able to walk independently with a walker, but has difficulty with stairs. His home has the same layout and conditions as your current home. What changes will need to be made to create a safe home for this patient?

2. Make a list of examination categories and discuss how these will be assessed. Identify any examination skills that people in your group already know how to perform.

3. Discuss the components of the plan of care and how the PTA will utilize this information with a patient.

Learning Opportunities

1. The PTA is creating an intake form for new patients. Create a list of questions to obtain a patient history.

2. Observe a PTA performing examination activities. Interview the PTA about the rationale for collecting the information and describe how the information will be used.

3. Perform an Internet search to identify websites or videos that can assist the PTA in learning examination skills such as obtaining blood pressure, assessing skin sensation, and performing standardized balance examinations.

CHAPTER 5

Physical Therapy Practice Areas

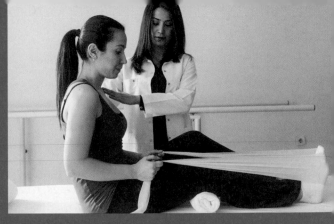

OBJECTIVES

After studying this chapter, the reader will be able to:

1. Describe physical therapy practice areas.
2. Discuss the types of therapeutic exercises used in physical therapy including a home exercise program.
3. Describe basic physical agents used in physical therapy.
4. Discuss patient education.
5. Describe neurologic physical therapy treatments to improve motor control and motor learning.
6. Name interventions used in cardiovascular and pulmonary physical therapy.
7. Describe interventions common in pediatric physical therapy.
8. Describe major physical therapy interventions for wound and burn care.

KEY TERMS

bloodborne pathogens
cryotherapy
duration
electrotherapy
flexibility exercises
frequency

hydrotherapy
orthosis
prosthesis
therapeutic exercises
thermotherapy

Upon entering a physical therapy educational program, students are instructed in all practice areas in order to become competent members of the health care workforce. Upon graduation, physical therapists (PTs) and physical therapist assistants (PTAs) may find employment in practices that require a variety of skills or they may find themselves in an area of focused practice. Each practice area has the opportunity for further education and study that allows for specialization. Currently, the American Board of Physical Therapy Specialties offers board certification to PTs in eight specialty areas of physical therapy: cardiovascular and pulmonary, clinical electrophysiology, geriatrics, neurology, orthopedics, pediatrics, sports, and women's health.

Practice Areas

ORTHOPEDIC PHYSICAL THERAPY

Musculoskeletal or orthopedic physical therapy can be practiced in a variety of clinical settings, treating patients of different ages with a variety of medical and physical problems. For example, young people may present with various orthopedic injuries such as a ligament tear of the knee causing pain and difficulty in walking. An older adult may require rehabilitation after a total knee arthroplasty. The physical therapy approaches to treatments are diverse depending on the patient's needs, the clinical setting, and the clinical experience of the PT and PTA. Goals in orthopedic physical therapy include maximizing the patient's function, alleviating pain, decreasing abnormal stress on joints, ensuring the patient's use of proper posture and promoting tissue healing, range of motion, and flexibility.

NEUROLOGIC PHYSICAL THERAPY

Neurologic physical therapy specializes in treating patients who have neurologic disorders affecting the structure and function of their nervous systems. Neurologic physical therapy can be practiced in acute care hospitals, skilled nursing facilities, rehabilitation hospitals, outpatient centers, or home care. Neurologic physical therapy approaches to treatments are dependent on the disease pathology and concentrate mostly on the treatment of the patient's signs and symptoms. Impairments found in neurologic physical therapy are pain, impaired balance and postural stability, impaired postural control, incoordination, delayed motor development, abnormal tone, and ineffective functional movement strategies.

CARDIOVASCULAR AND PULMONARY PHYSICAL THERAPY

Cardiovascular and pulmonary physical therapy treats patients with cardiac and pulmonary conditions that need physical therapy. In cardiovascular and pulmonary rehabilitation, the PTA must be able to reassess the patient as necessary, to monitor the patient in regard to treatment, to monitor the patient's vital signs, and to provide appropriate interventions to the patient. The clinical presentations of cardiovascular disease are diverse. The most common cardiac diagnoses that are referred for direct physical therapy interventions are coronary artery disease (CAD) and congestive heart failure (CHF). Pulmonary rehabilitation is a continuum of services directed toward patients who have pulmonary diseases and their families, usually by an interdisciplinary team of specialists. Chronic obstructive pulmonary diseases (COPDs) and asthma are the most common chronic lung diseases for which pulmonary rehabilitation is needed. The goals of cardiovascular and pulmonary physical therapy are to achieve and maintain the individual's maximum level of independence and functioning in the community.

PEDIATRIC PHYSICAL THERAPY

Pediatric physical therapy specializes in the treatment of children who have developmental dysfunctions and specific pediatric disorders. The pediatric PT is a direct care provider of pediatric physical therapy for children in hospital settings, in early intervention programs (EIPs), and school settings. EIPs are programs mandated by law to provide comprehensive, multidisciplinary interventions for infants and toddlers (from birth to 3 years old) who have disabilities. Individualized educational plans (IEPs) are programs that mandate comprehensive, multidisciplinary interventions for school-aged children up to the age of 21. The pediatric PT may also act as a consultant to schools by instructing teachers and teacher's assistants to facilitate attainment of educational goals for children (from 3 years old to 21 years old) who have disabilities. Pediatric physical therapy services are dependent on the needs of the child in the type of setting that the physical therapy is being provided; for example, physical therapy will be different in an acute care hospital as compared to a school environment.

The pediatric PT and the PTA are always members of a team that includes the pediatric patient's family, physicians, nurses, social workers, psychologists, occupational therapists, speech and language pathologists, certified occupational therapist assistants, special educators, and teachers.

GERIATRIC PHYSICAL THERAPY

Geriatric physical therapy specializes in treating older individuals who present with musculoskeletal and neuromuscular conditions and dysfunction common to older adults. Similar to other specialized physical therapy areas, geriatric rehabilitation requires understanding of the patient's individuality and his or her unique developmental issues. Generally, geriatric physical therapy focuses on the patient's functional goals, promoting optimal health, and restoring and maintaining the patient's highest level of function and independence within the environment.

INTEGUMENTARY PHYSICAL THERAPY

PTs may specialize in the care of people who have open wounds or burns. Specialized courses of study increase the knowledge of PTs and PTAs in this area. PTs and PTAs may become Certified Wound Care Specialists through several different agencies including: the National Alliance of Wound Care and Ostomy and the American Board of Wound Management. In addition to healing the wound or burn, goals include maintaining functional movements and strength and the prevention of further skin damage due to disease or pressure.

Interventions

Interventions in physical therapy may include therapeutic exercises, patient education, physical agents and modalities, gait training, and use of orthotics and prosthetics, neurologic techniques, and specialized techniques in cardiovascular and pulmonary rehabilitation and integumentary care.

THERAPEUTIC EXERCISES

Therapeutic exercises are major treatments used by PTs and PTAs in physical therapy practice in general and in musculoskeletal physical therapy practice in particular.

> **WHAT ARE THERAPEUTIC EXERCISES?**
>
> **Therapeutic exercises** are interventions that use muscular contraction, bodily movement, posture, and physical activities to improve the overall function of an individual and to help meet the demands of daily living.

Depending on the patient's needs, specific therapeutic exercises or activities can be used to achieve different goals, such as increasing strength and endurance, maintaining flexibility, or promoting functionality. Therapeutic exercises incorporate a variety of activities, actions, and techniques. Therapeutic exercise programs are designed by PTs and are individualized to each patient/client's specific needs (see **FIGURE 5-1**).

Home Exercise Program

The exercise goals can be reinforced with a home exercise program (HEP) by using an exercise booklet or customized

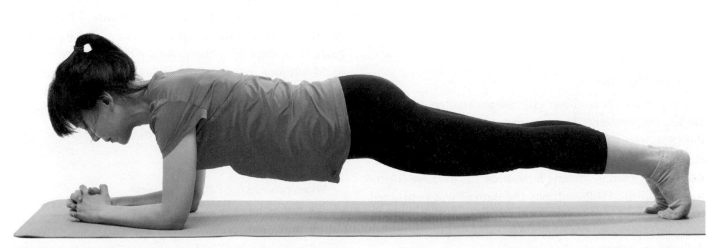

FIGURE 5-1 Patient exercising to improve trunk strength and stability.
© Adam Gregor/Shutterstock

written or computer-generated instructions and drawings with an explanation of the purpose of each exercise.

An example of an HEP for a patient who had a right total hip replacement 1 week ago could be:

EXERCISE 1: ANKLE PUMPS

Slowly push your foot up and down. Do this exercise several times a day for 5 or 10 minutes.

EXERCISE 2: HEEL SLIDES

Slide your right heel toward your buttocks, bending your right knee and keeping your heel on the bed. Do not let your knee roll inward. Repeat this exercise 10 times three times a day.

EXERCISE 3: QUADRICEPS SETS

Lying on the bed with your right leg straight and your left leg bent, press the back of your right knee into the bed (or into a rolled towel as we do in the clinic) by tightening the muscles on the top of your thigh. Count out loud to 10 while holding this position. Relax 1 minute. Repeat this exercise five times twice a day.

Your home exercise program is an important part of getting better and stronger. Please, do these exercises every day. Perform the exercises slowly. If you have any pain, stop the exercises immediately, and call our office. Do not increase the number of repetitions or sets without checking with the PT or the PTA.

Exercise Parameters

The PT and PTA establish exercise parameters appropriate for each patient. The parameters include frequency, duration, repetitions, sets, intensity (or difficulty of the exercise), and the mode or type of activity or exercise. **Frequency** of exercise means how often the exercise is performed. In the HEP example, the patient was instructed to perform ankle pumps several times a day. **Duration** of exercise represents the time period the exercise is necessary. In the HEP example, the patient was instructed to perform the exercises every day, which means the patient was instructed to do the exercises simultaneously with

physical therapy treatments as a supplement to physical therapy sessions. Repetitions and sets of exercise refer to how many exercises need to be performed and how many sets.

Classification of therapeutic exercises:
- Range of motion exercises to preserve flexibility and mobility of joints
- Exercises to increase strength
- Exercises to increase endurance
- Cardiovascular fitness exercises
- Exercises to increase coordination and control
- Exercises to increase speed
- Exercises to promote relaxation

RANGE OF MOTION EXERCISES

Range of motion (ROM) exercises can be defined as exercises that move a joint through the extent of its limitations. These exercises can help promote function, strength, and endurance. ROM exercises are classified as: passive range of motion exercises, active range of motion exercises, and active assistive range of motion exercises.

Passive Range of Motion Exercises

Passive range of motion (PROM) means that a joint is moved by the PT, the PTA, or a mechanical device without any muscle contraction by the patient (see **FIGURE 5-2**). An example of a mechanical device that produces PROM is the continuous passive motion (CPM) device, which passively moves a desired joint continuously through a controlled ROM without patient effort for as long as 24 hours per day. Manual PROM exercises can be applied to the patient by the PT, the PTA, a family member, the patient him- or herself, or a member of the nursing staff.

When can you use PROM exercises?
- When the patient is unable to move a joint
- When active range of motion (AROM) is prohibited
- After surgery or injury and in cases of complete bed rest, paralysis, or coma

- To maintain the mobility of joint connective tissue
- To maintain the elasticity of the muscle
- To increase the synovial fluid for joint nutrition
- To assist circulation
- To prevent joint contracture
- To decrease pain
- To help in the healing process

contract the muscle of a given joint without any restriction of the normal ROM of that joint.

When can you use AROM exercises?

- To increase muscular strength
- To promote bone and soft-tissue integrity
- To promote coordination and motor skills
- To prevent deep vein thrombosis (DVT) after surgery or immobilization
- To increase blood circulation
- To prepare for functional activities such as ambulation or activities of daily living

Active Assisted Range of Motion Exercises

Active assisted range of motion (AAROM) exercises are used when the patient needs help to complete the AROM. In these exercises, the patient is able to assist in the desired motion, but cannot perform the motion independently, without manual or mechanical assistance. The manual assistance can be given to the patient by the PT or the PTA. The mechanical assistance can be given to the patient by a wand or a cane, a finger-ladder device, or overhead pulleys.

STRENGTHENING EXERCISES

There are three large groups of strengthening exercises. These include the following:

- Isometric exercises develop tension in the muscle without visible joint movement and changes in muscle length. These exercises are recommended when joint motion is contraindicated because of pain, inflammation, or surgery. An example of isometric exercises is quadriceps sets.
- Isotonic exercises develop tension in the muscle through dynamic concentric or eccentric muscular contractions (see **FIGURE 5-3**). Concentric muscular contraction causes the muscle to shorten, whereas eccentric muscular contraction causes the muscle to lengthen. Isotonic exercise is a dynamic exercise with a constant load (such as a weight), but uncontrolled speed of movement. An example of isotonic exercises is a biceps curl.

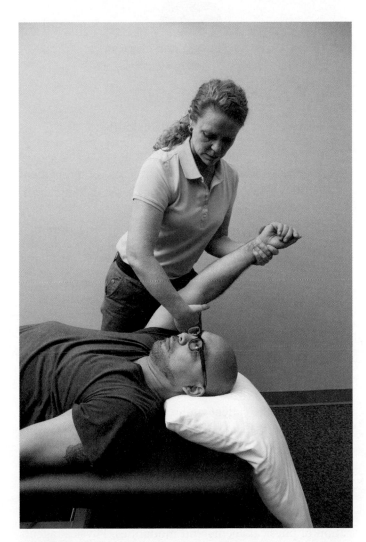

FIGURE 5-2 Patient receiving passive range of motion to his shoulder.
© Photographee.eu/Shutterstock

Active Range of Motion Exercises

Active range of motion (AROM) means that the ROM movement is performed actively by the patient. AROM exercises are used when the patient is able to voluntarily

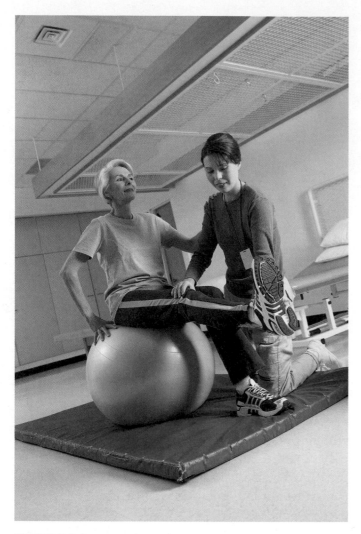

FIGURE 5-3 Patient performing an isotonic exercise with her leg.
© Tyler Olson/Shutterstock

- Isokinetic exercises are dynamic exercises having a predetermined velocity of muscle shortening or lengthening, so that the force generated by the muscle is maximal through the full ROM. Isokinetic exercises take place at a constant speed. Isokinetic exercises are performed using specialized machines such as Cybex, Kincom, or Biodex.

What are flexibility exercises?

Flexibility exercises describe any therapeutic maneuver that increases mobility of soft tissues and improves ROM by elongating structures. Structures that need to be stretched have become shortened and hypomobile (having little mobility).

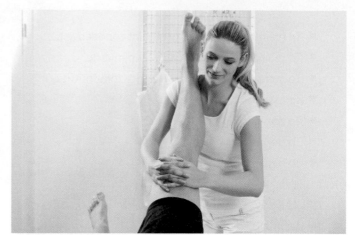

FIGURE 5-4 PT stretching patient's hamstring muscles.
© Kzenon/Shutterstock

FLEXIBILITY EXERCISES

There are several ways to stretch, including:

- Manual passive stretching is the manual application of an external force to move the involved body segment slightly beyond the point of tissue resistance and available ROM (see **FIGURE 5-4**).
- Self-stretching is a type of stretching procedure that the patient can perform independently after receiving instruction from the PT or the PTA.
- Ballistic stretching is a forceful, rapid, intermittent stretch that is high speed and high intensity.

PATIENT EDUCATION

Patient education is an important form of intervention in physical therapy practice. The PTA should utilize a positive regard toward the patient while communicating clearly and simply. Patient education will assist patients in becoming healthy and help them in managing their health in the future.

PHYSICAL AGENTS AND MODALITIES

Another type of physical therapy intervention is the application of physical agents and modalities. Physical agents and modalities use physical energy for their therapeutic effect. Physical agents and modalities may include **thermotherapy**, **cryotherapy**, **hydrotherapy**, **electrotherapy**, manual techniques, and traction.

Because of the passive nature of most of the physical agents or modalities, they are not prescribed by the PT indiscriminately. The modalities are given for only a short period of time as an adjunct, not as a substitute,

Why are physical agents and modalities used?

- To reduce or eliminate soft-tissue inflammation
- To speed the healing time of a soft-tissue injury
- To decrease pain
- To modify muscular tone
- To remodel scar tissue
- To increase connective tissue extensibility and length

to active interventions such as therapeutic exercises and patient education (see **FIGURE 5-5**).

MANUAL THERAPY

Manual techniques are used often in orthopedic physical therapy. They include massage, manipulation, and mobilization. Massage is a systematic, mechanical stimulation of the soft tissue of the body by means of rhythmically applied pressure and stretching for therapeutic purposes. In addition to massage, other kinds of soft-tissue techniques are used in the treatment of musculoskeletal disorders, such as cross-fiber massage, connective tissue massage, soft-tissue mobilization, myofascial release, and acupressure. Manipulation and mobilization are skilled passive, mechanical movements of high or low velocity applied to a specific joint or to a joint segment to restore its motion or extensibility and to reduce pain. As per the American Physical

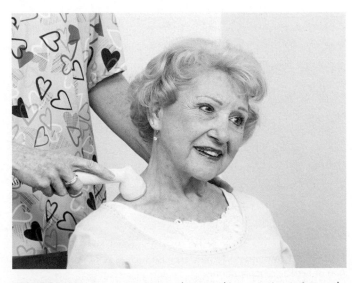

FIGURE 5-5 Patient receiving an ultrasound intervention to her neck.
© Lisa F. Young/Shutterstock

Therapy Association, spinal and peripheral manipulations and mobilizations are among the interventions that should be performed exclusively by the PT; however, these procedures are regulated differently by the individual states' physical therapy boards.

GAIT TRAINING

Because some patients with musculoskeletal pathologies may not be able to walk without assistive devices (or ambulatory aids), the PTA needs to teach these patients gait patterns and gait sequences that use assistive devices such as walkers, crutches, or canes. The gait patterns are non–weight bearing (NWB), partial weight bearing (PWB), weight bearing as tolerated (WBAT), and full weight bearing (FWB). Gait sequences or patterns are called three-point gait, two-point gait, four-point gait, swing-to, and swing-through.

ORTHOTICS AND PROSTHETICS

Other forms of physical therapy interventions for musculoskeletal disorders are the use of orthotic and prosthetic devices. An **orthosis** (or brace) is an external device applied to body parts to provide support and stabilization, improve function, correct flexible deformities, prevent progression of fixed deformities, and reduce pressure and pain by transferring the load from one area to another. A **prosthesis** is an artificial substitute for a missing body part. Prostheses are used for patients who have had amputations.

MOTOR CONTROL AND MOTOR LEARNING

In neurologic physical therapy, there are specific neurologic treatments to improve a patient's motor control and motor learning (see **FIGURE 5-6**). Motor control is the ability of the central nervous system to control or direct the neuromotor system in purposeful movement and postural adjustment.[6] Motor learning is the acquisition of skilled movement based on previous experience.[6]

Neurologic treatments to improve motor control have been developed taking into consideration a compensatory training approach, remediation and facilitation approaches, and functional task-oriented strategies.[6] A compensatory training approach is the resumption of functional independence by using the uninvolved or less involved extremity for function. Remediation and facilitation techniques, also called neurophysiologic approaches, focus on therapeutic exercises and special facilitation techniques to reduce sensory and motor deficits and improve patients' function.

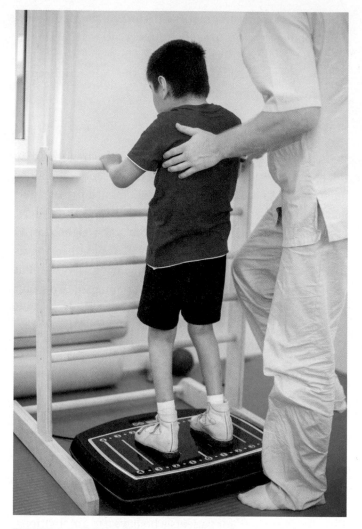

FIGURE 5-6 Child working on a balance platform with a PT.
© Pavel L Photo and Video/Shutterstock

Neurophysiologic Approaches

Four major traditional types of neurologic interventions were developed initially for stroke, cerebral palsy, and polio rehabilitation:

- *Neurodevelopmental treatment (NDT), developed by Drs. Karl and Berta Bobath:* The treatment aims to improve posture, movement, and daily function using inhibition of abnormal patterns and facilitation of automatic reflexes.

- *Proprioceptive neuromuscular facilitation (PNF), developed by Dr. Herman Kabat and Maggie*

Knott (and later expanded by Dorothy Voss): The treatment aims to restore function using specific sensory stimulation techniques of joint position and auditory and/or visual stimuli.

- *Sensory stimulation techniques, based mostly on the work of Margaret Rood:* The treatment aims to facilitate function by using specific positioning techniques of movement control (such as mobility, stability, control mobility, and skill).

- *Movement therapy in hemiplegia, developed by Signe Brunnstrom:* The treatment aims for voluntary activation of muscular control using abnormal flexor and extensor synergistic movements.

CARDIOVASCULAR AND PULMONARY INTERVENTIONS

In physical therapy practice, cardiac rehabilitation (or cardiac rehab) is a specialized intervention for patients who have had myocardial infarction, unstable angina, or heart transplants. Cardiac rehab is multidisciplinary and may include the physician, nurse, PT, PTA, occupational therapist, certified occupational therapist assistant, social worker, nutritionist, and exercise physiologist. Cardiac rehab starts in the hospital and extends indefinitely into the maintenance phase (see **FIGURE 5-7**).

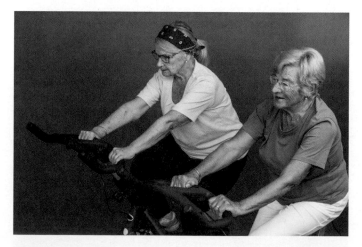

FIGURE 5-7 Monitored aerobic exercise such as stationary biking is part of cardiac rehabilitation.
© karelnoppe/Shutterstock

Phases of Cardiac Rehabilitation

The phases of cardiac rehabilitation include the following:[7]

- Phase I takes place in the hospital. Examples of interventions in phase I of cardiac rehab are patient education about life changes, encouraging the patient's family to provide positive family support, and teaching the patient bed mobility skills, the use of gentle exercises to return to basic activities of daily living, how to transfer with assistance, and gait training.

- Phase II takes place in outpatient settings. Examples of interventions in phase II of cardiac rehab are patient education for self-monitoring of vital signs, ADLs, upper body therapeutic exercises, treadmill activities, and stationary bicycle riding.

- Phase III takes place when the patient is discharged from outpatient programs but continues in a community-based program or voluntary program of his or her choosing. In phase III of cardiac rehab, the patient continues a fitness program and activities of his or her choosing in the community or at home.

Secretion Removal Techniques

Pulmonary physical therapy interventions concentrate on secretion removal techniques. Secretion retention can interfere with ventilation and the diffusion of oxygen and carbon dioxide. Patients retaining secretions need an individualized program of secretion removal techniques directed to the areas of involvement.

Postural drainage techniques (also called chest physical therapy) are positional interventions. The patient is positioned so that the bronchus of the involved lung segment is perpendicular to the ground and gravity assists in the removal of excessive secretions. Postural drainage drains and removes secretions from particular areas of the lungs. In addition to the positioning, a technique called percussion is applied (with cupped hands) by the PTA to a specific area of the patient's chest wall that corresponds to an underlying lung segment to release pulmonary secretions.

PEDIATRIC INTERVENTIONS

Pediatric treatments are dependent on pediatric pathologies. The interventions need to be very functional and effective, and appropriate to the circumstances. Most interventions use neurologic treatments of sensory stimulation to influence the motor response. For example, neurologic interventions such as the neurodevelopmental treatment or the motor control approach are used to influence the inborn postural reflexes and affect the child's functional motor skills. Pediatric orthopedic interventions may use strengthening exercises (as in kicking or swimming). Achievement of functional skills such as walking, feeding, eating, and dressing also is essential for the child and his or her family.

Functional activities are encouraged using mobility and standing positioning devices. Some of the mobility devices in pediatric physical therapy are the rollator walker and posterior rolling walker (see **FIGURE 5-8**). Walkers promote

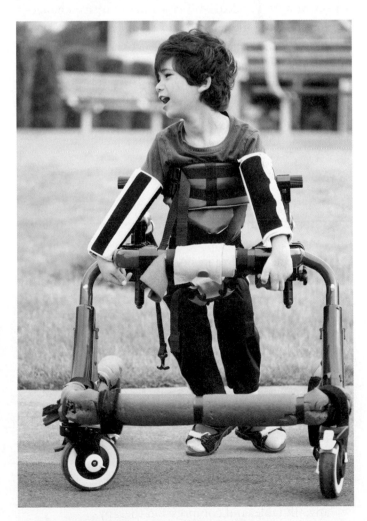

FIGURE 5-8 Child walking using a rolling walker.
© Jaren Jai Wicklund/Shutterstock

independence in mobility skills by strengthening the musculoskeletal system through active weight bearing in the lower limbs. The standing positioning devices are the prone stander, standing frame, and parapodium. The prone stander and the standing frame stimulate the child to hold up the head and trunk and to stand upright. The parapodium allows the child to move in a standing position at the same visual height as his or her peers. Other mobility devices, such as the manual and the power wheelchair and the power scooter, can be used in multiple environments including school and family activities.

GERIATRIC INTERVENTIONS

The interventions used in geriatric physical therapy depend on the disease process. The rehabilitation of the aged adult is very challenging for the PT and the PTA, primarily because it is difficult to separate the physiologic aspect of aging and disability from cognitive changes.[2] To maintain the highest level of function for the longest time, the PT and the PTA need to consider the patient's neurologic decline and physical functioning capabilities. In many situations, the geriatric patient has multiple conditions that need to be treated simultaneously. Multiple diagnoses can imply multiple impairments that complicate ADLs and hinder maximal functional capabilities.

INTEGUMENTARY INTERVENTIONS

Physical therapy interventions depend on the pathophysiology of the skin disorder or dysfunction. For example, for immune disorders of the skin such as psoriasis, physical therapy treatments are performed taking into consideration the patient's medications prescribed by the treating physician (the dermatologist). The physical therapy intervention consists of an ultraviolet light modality. Ultraviolet light is a form of radiant energy from the ultraviolet portion of the electromagnetic spectrum. For other skin disorders, the treatment may consist of the following:

- Patient education about the disorder
- Therapeutic exercises
- Functional training for ADLs and for skin and joint protection
- Modalities such as ultrasound, aquatic therapy, whirlpool, pulsed lavage, heat, paraffin baths, fluidotherapy, tilt table, and compression therapy

Wound interventions need treatments different from those for skin disorders (see **FIGURE 5-9**). Wound care interventions may consist of wound cleansing, wound debridement, wound dressing, and observing the patient's vital signs, nutritional considerations, and positioning (if necessary). Wound cleansing involves removal of cellular debris, bacteria, or fungus utilizing different topical agents. Wound debridement is removal of necrotic tissue, bacteria, and fungus utilizing selective and nonselective debridement procedures. Selective and nonselective debridement procedures performed by the PT and the PTA involve using the whirlpool, pulsed lavage, and medications prescribed by the physician as topical agents, and enzymatic and autolytic debridement agents. As per the American Physical Therapy Association (APTA),[4] in selective debridement procedures, the PT is the only individual who can use sharp and surgical instruments such as scalpels, forceps, and scissors to clean devitalized tissue. Wound dressing, also prescribed by the physician, applies topical medications to the wound, taking into consideration whether the wound is dry, moist, or infected.

Physical therapy for burn care consists of:

- Hydrotherapy using whirlpool or aquatic therapy
- Debridement
- Positioning of the affected body part
- ROM exercises
- Elastic or pressure garments to prevent scarring
- Edema control
- Strengthening exercises
- Breathing exercises
- Functional training

Positioning of the affected extremity to prevent or correct deformities is specific for burn care physical therapy. For example, to prevent deformities in adduction and

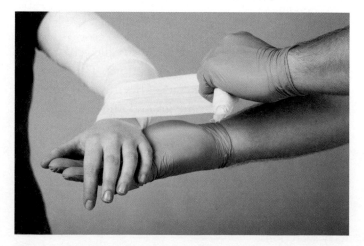

FIGURE 5-9 Wound care bandaging.
© Photographee.eu/Shutterstock

internal rotation of the shoulder, the patient's shoulder and axilla are positioned in abduction of 90° with an airplane-type splint to be worn in the daytime and at night. The airplane splint is an appliance made of plaster of Paris (or plastic or wood) that elevates the shoulder, holding the arm suspended away from the body.

During wound and burn care the PT and the PTA need to follow standards of safety and infection control such as handwashing; wearing gloves, mask, eye protection, and gown; cleaning and discarding patient care equipment; environmental cleaning and disinfection of the work area; and occupational health and **bloodborne pathogens** standards.

Discussion Questions

1. The PTA is teaching the patient about avoiding a recurrence of low back pain. Discuss strategies that will help ensure that the patient understands the information.
2. Discuss with your classmates the different types of therapeutic exercise and how each is used: isometric, isotonic, and isokinetic resistance exercises, flexibility exercises, and ROM exercises (PROM, AAROM, and AROM).
3. Share with your classmates the opportunities and experiences you have had in each of the practice areas of physical therapy: orthopedic, neurologic, geriatric, pediatric, cardiopulmonary, and integumentary.

Learning Opportunities

1. Using the American Physical Therapy Association website and the APTA Section websites (www.apta.org), develop a list of resources to develop skills in the physical therapy practice areas.
2. The PTA is working with a 3-year-old patient who needs an assistive device to stand and ambulate. Utilizing the Internet, explore the options for standing positioning devices and mobility devices.
3. Utilize commercial websites to find examples of different types of assistive devices used for gait: walkers, canes, etc. Consider what would be appropriate for different age groups (pediatric vs. geriatric).

Summary of Part II

Part II of this text discussed the initial physical therapy examination and evaluation, the physical therapy practice areas, and interventions used in physical therapy.

References (Part II)

1. American Physical Therapy Association. Diagnosis by physical therapists. Accessed July 2014 at www.apta.org.
2. O'Sullivan SB, Schmitz TJ. *Physical Rehabilitation: Assessment and Treatment*. 5th ed. Philadelphia, PA: F.A. Davis Company; 2007.
3. Lewis CB, Bottomley JM. *Geriatric Physical Therapy: A Clinical Approach*. East Norwalk, CT: Appleton and Lange; 1994.
4. American Physical Therapy Association. *Guide to Physical Therapist Practice*. 2nd ed. Alexandria, VA: American Physical Therapy Association; 2003.
5. Dreeben O. *Physical Therapy Clinical Handbook for PTAs*. 2nd ed. Sudbury, MA: Jones & Bartlett Publishers; 2013.
6. Shumway-Cook A, Woollacott MH. *Motor Control: Translating Research into Clinical Practice*. Philadelphia, PA: Lippincott Williams & Wilkins; 2007.
7. Rothstein JM, Roy SH, Wolf SL, Scalzitti DA. *The Rehabilitation Specialist's Handbook*. Philadelphia, PA: F.A. Davis Company; 2005.

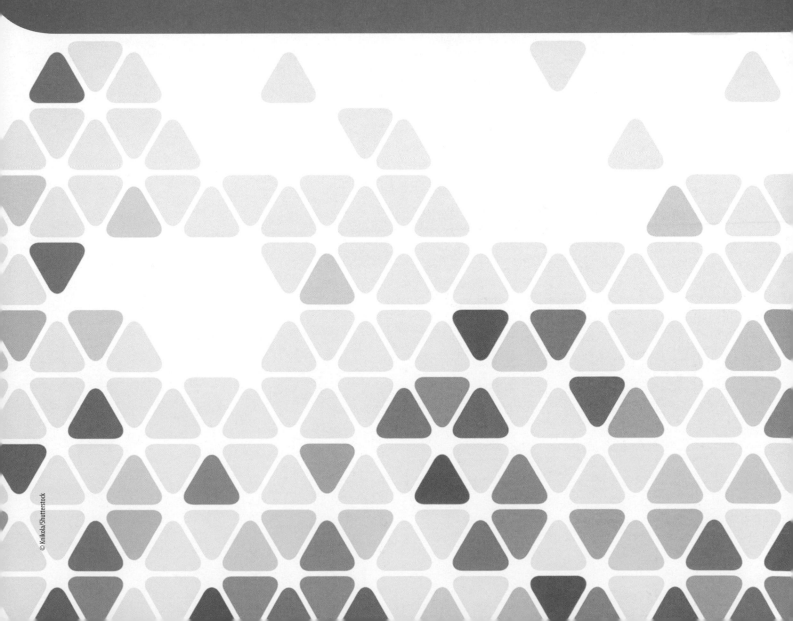

PART III

Ethical and Legal Issues

This part is divided into two chapters:

- CHAPTER 6: Ethics and Professionalism
- CHAPTER 7: Laws and Regulations

These two chapters describe moral, ethical, and legal issues encountered in physical therapy practice. Elements of patient confidentiality, cultural competence, and laws and regulations when working with patients/clients are also addressed.

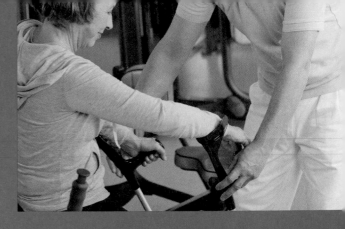

CHAPTER 6

Ethics and Professionalism

© CandyBox Images/Shutterstock

OBJECTIVES

After studying this chapter, the reader will be able to:

1. Define morals and ethics.
2. Delineate the difference between medical law and medical ethics.
3. List six biomedical ethical principles and their roles in health care.
4. Discuss patient confidentiality.
5. Describe the Health Insurance Portability and Accountability Act (HIPAA) of 1996.
6. Discuss the patient's bill of rights and its importance to physical therapy practice.
7. Explain cultural competence in health care and physical therapy.
8. List the elements of full informed consent.
9. Explain the guide for professional conduct that physical therapists are morally bound to follow.
10. Explain the guide for conduct of the affiliate member that physical therapist assistants are morally bound to follow.
11. Identify at least five directive ethical provisions expected of the physical therapist assistant.
12. Discuss the eight value-based behaviors for the physical therapist assistant.

KEY TERMS

autonomy
cultural competence
ethics
ethnocentrism
Health Insurance Portability and
　　Accountability Act (HIPAA)

informed consent
morals
protected health information (PHI)

Medical Ethics Versus Medical Law

Medical ethics and medical law are disciplines with frequent areas of overlap, yet each discipline has unique standards. Medical law and medical ethics share the goal of creating and maintaining social good. They are both dynamic and are in a constant state of change. For example, new legislation and court decisions occur, and medical ethics responds to challenges created by new laws by providing new ethical standards.

MEDICAL ETHICS

Ethics is a system of moral principles or standards governing a person's conduct. Morals are the basis for ethical conduct. They are an individual's beliefs, principles, and values about what is right and wrong. **Morals** are personal to each and every individual. If an individual wants to do the "right thing," he or she tries to act with moral virtue or character. Morals are culture based, culture driven, and time dependent.

Medical ethics is a system of principles governing medical conduct. It deals with the relationship of a physician to the patient, the patient's family, fellow physicians, and society at large. Also, medical ethics refers to how other health care providers conduct themselves in their professional undertakings. For example, in physical therapy, we can say that physical therapy ethics is a system of principles governing a physical therapist (PT) or a physical therapist assistant (PTA). For the PTA, ethics deals with the relationship of a PTA to the patient, the patient's family, PTs, fellow PTAs, associates, and society at large.

Physical therapy ethics for PTs and PTAs is derived through policies of the professional organization, the American Physical Therapy Association (APTA). These ethical policies, or guidelines, set standards of conduct that must be adhered to by the members of the APTA. Generally, the ethics statements are significant professional and moral guides, but are unenforceable by law.

MEDICAL LAW

Medical law is the establishment of social rules for conduct. A violation of medical law may create criminal and civil liability. Lawmakers frequently turn to policy statements including medical ethics statements of professional organizations when creating laws affecting that profession. In this way, health care providers may influence legal standards when creating professional ethics standards.

On many occasions, ethics and law can blend into common standards of professional conduct. Often, a breach of ethics may also constitute a violation of the law, and a violation of the law may also infringe upon specific ethical principles. For example, in physical therapy a breach of the fourth standard of the Standards of Ethical Conduct for PTAs,[1] which states that PTAs shall comply with laws and regulations governing physical therapy, can also cause a violation of the statutory laws. A PTA representing him- or herself as a PT violates the fourth standard of the Standards of Ethical Conduct as well as the professional licensing laws enacted by all states.[1]

Biomedical Ethical Principles

Health care providers are guided by six fundamental biomedical ethical principles: beneficence, non-maleficence, justice, veracity, confidentiality, and autonomy. Health care providers use these ethical principles when working with patients, when conducting clinical research, or when educating students to care for patients. Various clinical situations can cause ethical dilemmas. In our society, adherence to certain biomedical ethical principles can be controversial for some health care providers, depending on their moral values and their social conditioning. Also, ethical principles may be debatable for people from other cultures or people having different religious or civic beliefs. For example, being confronted with the truth about a grave medical condition can be extremely painful and even unacceptable to a patient or to a patient's family coming from another culture. Nevertheless, traditional biomedical ethicists maintain that the ethical dilemmas should be resolved only by applying the most rational and objective rule and principle to each situation.

BENEFICENCE

Beneficence is the ethical principle that emphasizes doing the best for the patient. It means that health care providers have a duty to promote the health and welfare of the patient above other considerations. For PTs and PTAs it means that they are bound to act in the patient's best interests in physical therapy clinical practices. An example of the ethical principle of beneficence for PTs and PTAs would be to genuinely show concern for the physical and psychological welfare of their patients and clients at all times.

NON-MALEFICENCE

Non-maleficence is the ethical principle that exhorts practitioners to not do anything that causes harm to the patient. Hippocrates, who lived around 400 BC and is considered the father of medicine, was the first physician to express ethical principles of beneficence and non-maleficence in his Hippocratic Oath (Appendix A). Hippocrates felt that non-maleficence was one of the most important principles of medical practice. For PTs and PTAs, non-maleficence means that they cannot intentionally cause harm to patients/clients under their care. For example, a breach of the ethical principle of non-maleficence would be exploiting the patient financially by selling the patient an unnecessary assistive device or one at an inflated price.

JUSTICE AND VERACITY

Justice is an ethical principle that mandates that a health care provider distribute fair and equal treatment to every patient. In the context of receiving health care in general, justice requires that everyone receives equitable access to the basic health care necessary for living a fully human life. An example of the ethical principle of justice in physical therapy would be advocating to legislatures, regulatory agencies, and insurance companies the need to provide and improve access to necessary health care services for all individuals (with and without health insurance).

Veracity is an ethical principle that binds the health care provider and the patient in a relationship to tell the truth. The patient must tell the truth concerning history and symptoms in order for the health care provider to apply appropriate care. The health care provider has to tell the truth in order for the patient to exercise personal autonomy. In physical therapy, PTs and PTAs are obligated to provide the patient with ethical and truthful information. For example, a breach of the ethical principle of veracity would be a PTA identifying him- or herself as a PT.

CONFIDENTIALITY

Confidentiality is an ethical principle that requires a health care provider to maintain privacy by not sharing or divulging to a third party privileged or entrusted patient information. Matters discussed by the patient with the health care provider in confidence are held secret except for rare instances when the information presents a clear threat to the well-being of the patient or another person, or when the health of the public may be compromised. Confidentiality is considered a fundamental ethical principle in health care, and a breach of confidentiality can be a reason for disciplinary action.

Maintaining patient confidentiality encourages patients to fully divulge relevant information so that the health care professional can make a proper assessment of the patient/client's condition. Occasionally, there may be circumstances where the interest in maintaining confidentiality is outweighed by the public interest. For example,

in some situations, disclosing confidential information without a patient/client's consent may prevent a crime. This can justify the disclosure of confidential information without consent.

Examples of federal statutes that require disclosure of confidential information (where these would otherwise be breaches of confidentiality):

- The Police and Criminal Evidence Act of 1984 indicates that the police can access medical records for the purpose of a criminal investigation by making an application to a circuit judge.

- The Public Health (Control of Disease) Act of 1984 and Public Health (Infectious Diseases) Regulations of 1988 indicate that a doctor must notify the relevant local authority if he or she suspects a patient of having a notifiable disease. AIDS and HIV are not notifiable diseases. Examples of notifiable diseases (in 2010) include anthrax, botulism, cholera, diphtheria, or gonorrhea.

- The Abortion Regulations of 1991 indicate that a doctor carrying out a termination of pregnancy must notify the relevant chief medical officer, including giving the name and address of the involved patient.

- The Births and Deaths Registration Act of 1953 indicates that a doctor or a midwife normally has a duty to inform the district medical officer of a birth within 6 hours; stillbirths also must be registered. Doctors attending patients during their last illness must sign a death certificate and give a cause of death.

- The Children Act of 1989 regulates many aspects of child care, including a health care professional's duties to report suspicion of child abuse.

In physical therapy, as with any health profession, a patient's information is confidential and should not be communicated to a third party not involved in that patient's care without the prior consent of the patient. A PTA should refer all requests for release of confidential information to the supervising PT. A PT may disclose information to appropriate authorities when it is necessary to protect the welfare of an individual or the community or when required by law.

Even without ethical principles and standards, health care providers are bound by state and federal laws to maintain patient/client confidentiality. A breach of confidentiality can include a disclosure to a third party without patient consent by various media such as oral, written, telephone, fax, electronically, or via email. State and federal laws protecting patients' confidentiality include the following:

- Federal and state constitutional privacy rights
- Federal legislation and regulation governing medical records and licensing of health care providers
- Specific federal legislation designed to protect sensitive information such as HIV test results, genetic screening information, drug and alcohol abuse rehabilitation, and mental health records

---

A patient's written authorization for release of information is required for the following:

- Patient's attorney or insurance company
- Patient's employer (unless a workers' compensation claim is involved)
- Member of the patient's family (except where a member of the family received durable power of attorney for health care agencies)

On rare occasions, when a patient accepts treatment or hospitalization or when the patient is transferred from one practitioner or facility to another, a patient's consent to disclosure of confidential information can be implied from the circumstances. In such situations, disclosure of confidential patient information is necessary to ensure the patient's emergency treatment or continuation of patient care. State and federal laws authorize or require disclosure of medical records to health care providers involved in the patient's treatment or upon transfer of the patient from one facility to another.

Health Insurance Portability and Accountability Act of 1996 (HIPAA)

In 1996, the **Health Insurance Portability and Accountability Act (HIPAA)** created additional patient confidentiality considerations. HIPAA mandates the adoption of federal privacy protections for individually identifiable health information. In response to this mandate, the U.S. Department of Health and Human Services (DHHS) published the privacy rule in the Federal Register on December 28, 2000. Subsequently, on August 14, 2002, the DHHS issued a final rule making modifications to the privacy rule. In addition, the Health Information Technology for Economic and Clinical Health (HITECH) Act was passed in 2009. This law describes how electronic data must be safeguarded under the HIPAA regulations.

PRIVACY RULE

As per the U.S. DHHS,[2] the HIPAA privacy rule establishes national standards to protect individuals' medical records and other personal health information. The privacy rule applies to health plans, health care clearinghouses, and health care providers that conduct health care transactions electronically.[2] The rule requires appropriate safeguards to protect the privacy of personal health information, and sets limits/conditions on the uses and disclosures that may be made of such information without patient authorization. The rule also gives patients' rights over their health information, including rights to examine and obtain a copy of their health records, and to request corrections. However, the rule does not replace federal, state, or other laws that provide individuals even greater privacy protections.

The privacy rule requires covered entities to implement appropriate administrative, technical, and physical precautions to reasonably safeguard protected health information from any intentional or unintentional use or disclosure that violates the privacy rule. Covered entities are health care providers (such as PTs), health plans (such as Medicare or Blue Cross/Blue Shield), and health care clearinghouses (which process nonstandard health information from another entity into a standard format).

In certain situations, a patient or client may ask the covered entity for more protection than the privacy rule affords. The covered entity can agree or disagree with the patient/client's request. If the covered entity agrees with the request to add further restrictions to the privacy rule, the covered entity is bound by HIPAA to add those restrictions to the privacy rule. For example, if the patient/client asks the PT or PTA not to call his or her place of employment about confirmation of an appointment for physical therapy services, the PT/PTA must agree with the patient/client request. If the PT or the PTA inadvertently calls the patient at work, he or she violates HIPAA.

PROTECTED HEALTH INFORMATION (PHI)

What is protected health information?

Protected health information (PHI) includes individually identifiable health information in any form, including information transmitted orally or in written or electronic form.[2] PHI represents information in any form or medium that is created or received by a health care provider, health plan, public health authority, employer, life insurer, school or university, or health care clearinghouse and relates to the past, present, or future physical or mental health of an individual, the provision of health care to that individual, or future payment for the provision of health care to an individual.

PHI is part of standard transactions including the use of electronic media to do the following:

- File claims for reimbursement
- File requests for payments or remittance advice
- Check on a claim's status
- Coordinate benefits
- Check enrollment and disenrollment in a health plan
- Determine health plan eligibility
- Make or receive referral certifications and authorizations
- Make or receive health plan premium payments
- Submit health claims attachments
- File a first report of injury
- Transmit other information (prescribed by the secretary of the DHHS)

NOTICE OF PRIVACY PRACTICES FOR PHI

What is notice of privacy practices?

The privacy rule states that an individual (a patient/client) has a right to adequate notice of how a covered entity (a health care provider) may use and disclose the individual's PHI.[3] The notice of privacy practices must be given to the individual by the covered entity on the first date of service delivery, involving face-to-face exchange with the patient/client.

This means that the PT must give the notice of privacy to the patient/client on the first date of service (usually on the initial examination and evaluation). However, another covered entity such as a radiologist, who did not see the patient/client at all but only read the x-ray, did not have face-to-face contact with the patient/client does not need to give a notice of privacy to the patient/client. The health care provider (such as the PT) must also make a "good faith" effort to get the individual's (patient/client's) written acknowledgment that the privacy notice was received.

The privacy rule does not require an individual's signature to be on the notice. Consequently, the individual (patient/client) can sign a separate sheet or initial a cover sheet of the notice, depending on what he or she chooses.

INCIDENTAL USES AND DISCLOSURES OF PHI

Many health care providers are concerned that they cannot engage in confidential conversations with other providers or patients if there was a possibility that they could be overheard. However, DHHS stated that the privacy rule is not intended to prevent customary and necessary health care communications or practices from occurring. Thus, it does not require that risk of incidental use or disclosure be eliminated to meet the standards.[3] An incidental use or disclosure is permissible if the covered entity (health care provider) has applied reasonable safeguards and implemented the minimum necessary standards. This means that the covered entity must have in place appropriate administrative, technical, and physical safeguards that limit incidental uses and disclosures.

Examples of reasonable safeguards that a covered entity (such as a physical therapy provider) needs to implement may include:

- Avoiding use of the patient's name in public hallways
- Speaking quietly when discussing a patient's condition in the waiting room with the patient/patient's family
- Locking file cabinets or records rooms
- Requiring additional passwords on computers used by all employees working in the facility; this can better protect the patient's identity (see **FIGURE 6-1**)

For example, if a PTA wants to discuss a patient treatment with a PT (or another assistant) in a public area, he or she should move to a more private place and speak softly. When talking to a patient in a semiprivate room, the PTA should pull the curtain, lower his or her voice, and be discreet.

Relative to safeguarding PHI, the DHHS specifies the following:[2]

- Providers (such as PTs) do not need to retrofit their offices, have private rooms, or soundproof walls to avoid the possibility that a conversation would be overheard. In physical therapy, cubicles, dividers, shields, or curtains may constitute reasonable safeguards. Gyms, where several patients receive exercise therapy at the same time, may not constitute reasonable safeguards.
- Providers can leave messages for patients on their answering machines, but they have to limit the amount of information disclosed on the answering machine (such as confirming the patient's appointment by mentioning only the patient's name and no other information related to the type of provider, etc.). The same applies when leaving a message with a person who answers the phone.
- Providers must take safeguards limiting access to areas where the patient's chart is located by ensuring the area is supervised, by keeping the chart facedown or facing a wall if stored vertically, or by escorting non-employees in the area.
- Having patients sign in or calling out patient names in a waiting room is acceptable as long as the information disclosed is appropriately limited. For example, the sign-in sheet should not include the reason for the visit.

The Privacy Rule and Students' Training

The privacy rule does not ban health care providers from sharing patient information with students. Students and trainees are permitted to have access to patient/clients' PHI for training purposes.[2] In the privacy rule, covered entities are allowed to share information when conducting training programs in which students, trainees, or practitioners in areas of health care learn under supervision to practice or improve their skills as health care providers.

For example, in physical therapy, when the academic institution sends PTA students (or PT students) to clinical sites for their training, the clinical site and specifically

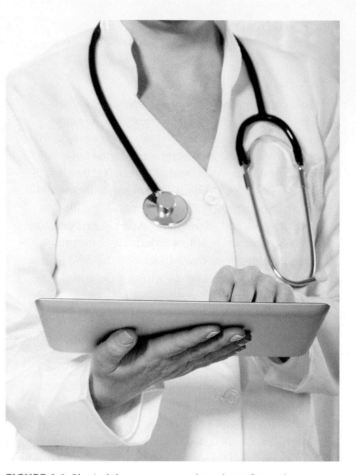

FIGURE 6-1 Physical therapy personnel need to safeguard electronic documentation.
© Rustle/Shutterstock

the clinical instructor is allowed to disclose PHI to the student. According to the privacy rule, student training is included in the clinical site's health care operations, having the same ruling as for treatment and payment. When the student returns to the academic institution, the patient/client information should be de-identified before it is shared.[2] Alternatively, the student could obtain an authorization from the patient/client to utilize (for training purposes) the patient/client's PHI at the academic institution. Covered entities should take reasonable safeguards by encouraging their students to protect the identity of patients/clients during discussions and be mindful of the minimum necessary standard.

The Privacy Rule and Family Members

Under the privacy rule it is permissible for a provider to disclose PHI to a family member or other person involved in the patient's care. Where the patient is present during a disclosure, the provider may disclose PHI if it is reasonable to infer from the circumstances that the patient does not object to the disclosure. This means that the provider may:[2]

- Obtain the patient's agreement
- Give the patient the opportunity to object (and he or she does not object)
- Decide from the circumstances and based on professional judgment that the patient does not object

When the patient is not present (or is incapacitated), the provider may disclose relevant information if (based on professional judgment) the disclosure is in the patient's best interest.[2]

PATIENT/CLIENT AUTHORIZATION FOR USES AND DISCLOSURES OF PHI

Patient/client authorization is needed for research activities. Certain institutional review boards (IRBs) waive the

Patient/client authorization is not needed for the following:

- Patient/client seeking his or her own PHI
- Disclosure to the DHHS
- Uses and disclosures required by laws other than HIPAA (vital statistics, communicable diseases, product recalls, and certain employer reporting of Occupational Safety and Health Administration [OSHA]-related workplace surveillance)
- Victims of domestic violence or elder abuse, as required by law
- Judicial and administrative proceedings (such as court of law orders, court of law subpoena for relevant information)
- Use and disclosure of health oversight activities (such as state licensure, or government benefits programs in Medicare audits)
- Law enforcement activities
- Specialized government functions (such as when the Secret Service needs information about a patient to protect the president of the United States)
- Emergency situations with serious threats to health or safety
- Workers' compensation (exempted only to the extent required by state law)

requirement of written authorization depending on the minimal privacy risks and if the research is impractical if authorization is required. HIPAA's privacy rule for clinical research conducted by universities and government agencies is very complex. The privacy rule states that a researcher may use or disclose PHI from existing databases or repositories for research purposes either with the patient/client's authorization or with a waiver of authorization from an IRB.

MINIMUM NECESSARY STANDARDS FOR DISCLOSURE OF PHI

The privacy rule requires covered entities to make reasonable efforts to limit the disclosure of PHI to the minimum necessary to accomplish the intended purpose.[3]

Exceptions to the minimum necessary rule include:

- Uses or disclosures required by law.
- Disclosures to the individual who is the subject of the information.
- Uses or disclosures for which the covered entity has received an authorization that meets the appropriate necessary requirements; the authorization must identify the minimum necessary requirements.
- Uses or disclosures to requests by a health care provider for treatment purposes; for example, a PT is not required to apply the minimum necessary standards when discussing a patient's plan of care with a PTA.
- Uses or disclosures required for compliance with the regulations implementing the other administrative simplification provisions of HIPAA, or disclosures to DHHS for purposes of enforcing the privacy rule.

PERSONAL REPRESENTATIVES OF PATIENTS/CLIENTS

In situations where the patient/client is not capable of exercising his or her privacy rights, that patient/client may designate another individual to act on his or her behalf with respect to these rights. According to the privacy rule, a person authorized to act on behalf of a patient/client in making health care-related decisions is the patient/client's personal representative. In regard to uses and disclosures, the personal representative must be treated by the covered entities as the patient/client him- or herself by exercising the patient/client's rights. For example, the PT or the PTA must provide to the patient/client's personal representative any requests of disclosure or any authorization for disclosure of the patient/client's PHI.

PARENT'S ACCESS TO A MINOR'S PHI

The privacy rule defers to the state or other applicable law regarding a parent's access to health information about a minor. The state or other applicable law explicitly requires, permits, or prohibits access to PHI about a minor to a parent. Most of the states have the parent as the personal representative of a minor patient/client.

A parent is not the personal representative of a minor patient/client under the following conditions:[2]

- When a court of law determines someone other than the parent will make decisions for the minor

- When state or other law does not require the consent of a parent or other person before a minor can obtain a particular health service, and the minor consents to the health service (for example, there are state laws where a minor can obtain mental health treatment without parental consent)

- When a parent agrees to a confidential relationship between the minor and the physician (or health care provider)

- When the minor has been legally emancipated from his or her parents

---

PATIENT/CLIENT ACCESS TO PHI

An individual (such as a patient/client) has the right to access his or her PHI and any piece of information that reflects a decision the provider makes regarding the patient/client.[2] The patient/client has the right to examine his or her chart and other records, even records the provider thinks the patient will never see. For example, if the provider sends a letter to a collection agency to collect the copayment for a patient/client's visit, the patient/client

has the right, upon request, to get a copy of the letter in 30 days (if the records are on-site) or 60 days (if the records are off-site). The provider can charge a reasonable copying cost. Some state laws require the provider to charge a certain amount per copy per page. A patient/client also has the right to receive an accounting of disclosures of PHI made by the covered entity if the patient/client requests such an accounting.

The patient/client is entitled to receive the following information from a covered entity:[2]

- Protected health information (PHI) that was generated during the 6 years prior to the date of the request

- An accounting of disclosures that includes the date of each disclosure, the name of the entity or person who received the PHI, a brief description of the PHI disclosed, and a brief statement of the purpose of the disclosure

---

The covered entity (health care provider) may charge the patient/client a reasonable cost of accounting the disclosure of PHI if the patient/client requests more than one accounting in a 12-month period. The covered entity cannot terminate the patient for requesting many accountings of disclosure of PHI because it is a federal right of the patient/client, and the provider cannot take retaliatory action.

MARKETING OF PHI

A covered entity cannot use PHI in marketing without prior written and specific authorization from the patient/client. The privacy rule defines marketing as a communication about a product or service that encourages recipients of the communication to purchase or use the product or service.[3] Marketing is also an arrangement where a covered entity discloses PHI to another entity in exchange for direct or indirect remuneration. Marketing is not considered a communication that describes a health-related product or service provided by the covered entity itself. For example, for PTs, a health-related product could be a cervical pillow or a home traction device. Describing in a pamphlet a health-related product to the patient/client does not constitute marketing. Also, a communication made during a face-to-face patient/client encounter, even if it is marketing, does not require an authorization. In addition, giving patients/clients promotional gifts of nominal value (such as pens or magnets) does not require authorization. For example, if the PT gives the patient a sample of therapeutic gel to use at home, it does not require authorization because the communication was face to face and the gel was of nominal value. However, if the PT wants to sell that patient's name to the company that sells the therapeutic gel (so the company can contact the patient to encourage him or her to buy the gel), prior patient authorization is required.

PENALTIES FOR VIOLATION OF HIPAA

HIPAA's privacy rule is overseen and enforced by the U.S. DHHS Office for Civil Rights. Breaking HIPAA's privacy rule means either a civil or a criminal sanction. Civil penalties are imposed for inadvertent violations not resulting in personal gain; they are usually fines. Criminal sanctions involve monetary penalties and jail time.

The enforcement of the transactions and standard code sets is primarily complaint driven. For example, when the Centers for Medicare and Medicaid Services (CMS) receives a complaint about a covered entity, it notifies the entity in writing that a complaint has been filed. The entity has the opportunity to demonstrate compliance or to submit a corrective action plan. Organizations that exercise "reasonable diligence" and make efforts to correct problems and implement changes required to comply with HIPAA are unlikely to be subject to civil or criminal penalties.[2] If the covered entity does not respond to CMS, fines could be imposed as a last resort.

AUTONOMY AND PATIENTS' RIGHTS

Autonomy is an ethical principle that in health care means a form of personal liberty or self-governance. The principle of respect for patient autonomy acknowledges the right of a patient to have control over his or her own life (including the right to decide who should have access to his or her personal information). The patient is free to decide to act upon his or her decisions, and his or her decisions have to be respected. An example of the ethical principle of autonomy in physical therapy would be the PT's obligation not to restrict the patients' freedom to select their provider of physical therapy services.

In our society, a patient's autonomy and ultimate control over treatment is reflected in the patient's bill of rights (Appendix B). The patient's bill of rights was first adopted by the American Hospital Association in 1973 and was revised in 1992. Patient rights were developed with the expectation that hospitals and health care institutions would support these rights in the interest of delivering effective patient care. A patient's rights can be exercised on his or her behalf by a designated surrogate or proxy decision maker if the patient lacks decision-making capacity, is legally incompetent, or is a minor.

In regard to patients' rights in physical therapy practice, the APTA's position states that the individual referred or admitted to the physical therapy service has rights, which include but are not limited to the following:[4]

- Selection of a PT of one's own choosing to the extent that it is reasonable and possible
- Access to information regarding practice policies and charges for services
- Knowledge of the identity of the PT and other personnel providing or participating in the program of care
- Expectation that the referral source has no financial involvement in the service. If that is not the case, knowledge of the extent of any financial involvement in the service by the referring source
- Involvement in the development of anticipated goals and expected outcomes, and the selection of interventions
- Knowledge of any substantial risks of the recommended examination and intervention
- Participation in decisions involving the physical therapy plan of care to the extent reasonable and possible
- Access to information concerning his or her condition
- Expectation that any discussion or consultation involving the case will be conducted discreetly and that all communications and other records pertaining to the care, including the sources of payment for treatment, will be treated as confidential
- Expectation of safety in the provision of services and safety in regard to the equipment and physical environment
- Timely information about impending discharge and continuing care requirements
- Refusal of physical therapy services
- Information regarding the practice's mechanism for the initiation, review, and resolution of patient/client complaints

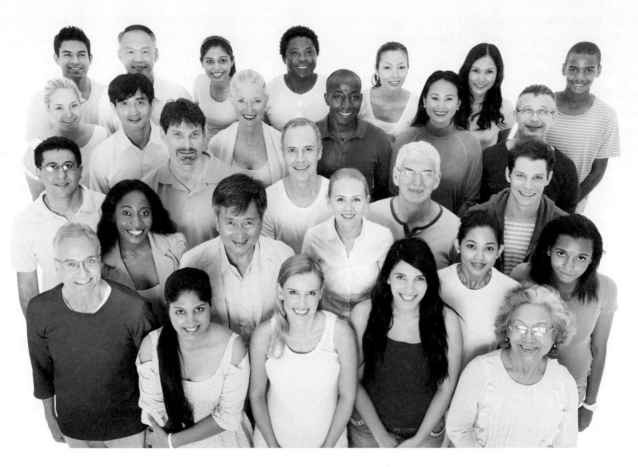

FIGURE 6-2 Cultural diversity requires respect of all people.
© Rawpixel/Shutterstock

Understanding Cultural Competence

The first guideline in the patient's bill of rights is the patient's right to considerate and respectful care. From the **cultural competence** perspective, it means that patients who are racially, ethnically, culturally, and linguistically diverse have the right, the same as other patients, to receive effective, understandable, and respectful care that is provided in a manner compatible with their cultural health beliefs and practices and preferred language (see **FIGURE 6-2**). Patients also have the right to accessible and appropriate health care services, and to evaluate whether health care providers can offer these services. Health care organizations and health care providers can offer accessible and appropriate health care services if they become culturally and linguistically competent.

Cultural and linguistic competence is defined as a set of congruent behaviors, attitudes, and policies that come together in a system, an agency, or among professionals that enables effective work in cross-cultural situations.[5] Culture means the integrated patterns of human behavior that include the language, thoughts, communications, actions, customs, beliefs, values, and institutions of racial, ethnic, religious, and social groups.[5] Culture, learned from the earliest age, enables humans to connect and interact meaningfully with others and the surrounding environment. Through the process of connecting with others, people come to recognize and share knowledge, attitudes, and values, resulting in a shared perception of the world and how to act within it. Culture also can have a profound influence on an individual's values, beliefs, and behaviors.

Cultural competence is also an awareness of, sensitivity to, and knowledge of the meaning of culture.[5] Cultural competence implies having the capacity to function effectively as an individual and an organization within the context of the cultural beliefs, behaviors, and needs presented by consumers and their communities.[5] Cultural competence includes a person's openness and willingness to learn about cultural issues and the ability to understand a person's own biases, values, attitudes, beliefs, and behaviors.

What is cultural competence?
- An evolving process
- An acceptance of and respect for differences
- A continuing self-assessment regarding culture
- Vigilance toward the dynamics of differences
- Ongoing expansion of cultural knowledge and resources
- Adaptations to services

The development of cultural competence depends more on attitude than on specific knowledge of the culture, and the outcome is having respect and sensitivity for other cultures.

ETHICAL AND LEGAL PERSPECTIVES OF CULTURAL COMPETENCE

From an ethical perspective, cultural competence is vital to all levels of health care practice. Ethnocentric approaches to health care practice can be ineffective in meeting the health care needs of diverse cultural groups of patients and clients. Health care providers' cultural and linguistic competence can strengthen and broaden health care delivery systems. The U.S. DHHS Office of Minority Health has issued 14 national standards for culturally and linguistically appropriate services in health care. The national standards, intended to be inclusive of all cultures, are proposed as a means to correct inequities that currently exist in the provision of health services and to make these services more responsive to the individual needs of all patients and clients.[5] Although the national standards are primarily directed at health care organizations, individual health care providers are also encouraged to use the standards to make their practices more culturally and linguistically accessible.

The 14 governmental standards for culturally/linguistically accessible health care service are:[5]

- Patients and clients receive effective, understandable, and respectful care from all staff members that is provided in a manner compatible with their cultural health beliefs and practices and preferred language.

- Health care organizations implement strategies to recruit, retain, and promote at all levels of the organization a diverse staff and leadership that are representative of the demographic characteristics of the service area.

- Health care organizations ensure that staff at all levels and across all disciplines receive ongoing education and training in culturally and linguistically appropriate service delivery.

- Health care organizations offer and provide language assistance services, including bilingual staff and interpreter services, at no cost to each patient/consumer with limited English proficiency at all points of contact, in a timely manner during all hours of operation.

- Health care organizations provide to patients/consumers in their preferred language both verbal offers and written notices informing them of their right to receive language assistance services.

- Health care organizations assure the competence of language assistance provided to limited English-proficient patients/consumers by interpreters and bilingual staff. Family and friends should not be used to provide interpretation services (except on request by the patient/consumer).

- Health care organizations make available easily understood patient-related materials and post signage in the languages of the commonly encountered groups and groups represented in the service area.

- Health care organizations develop, implement, and promote a written strategic plan that outlines clear goals, policies, operational plans, and management accountability and oversight mechanisms to provide culturally and linguistically appropriate services.

(*continues*)

- Health care organizations conduct initial and ongoing organizational self-assessments of culturally and linguistically appropriate services and are encouraged to integrate cultural and linguistic competence into their internal audits, performance improvement programs, patient satisfaction assessments, and outcome-based evaluations.

- Health care organizations ensure that data on the individual patient/consumer's race, ethnicity, and spoken and written language are collected in health records, integrated into the organization's management information systems, and periodically updated.

- Health care organizations maintain a current demographic, cultural, and epidemiological profile of the community as well as a needs assessment to accurately plan for and implement services that respond to the cultural and linguistic characteristics of the service area.

- Health care organizations develop participatory, collaborative partnerships with communities and utilize a variety of formal and informal mechanisms to facilitate community and patient/consumer involvement in designing and implementing culturally and linguistically appropriate services.

- Health care organizations ensure that conflict and grievance resolution processes are culturally and linguistically sensitive and capable of identifying, preventing, and resolving cross-cultural conflicts or complaints by patients/consumers.

- Health care organizations are encouraged to regularly make available to the public information about their progress and successful innovations in implementing the culturally and linguistically appropriate services standards and to provide public notice in their communities about the availability of this information.

As both an enforcer of civil rights law and a major purchaser of health services, the federal government has a pivotal role in ensuring culturally competent health care services. For example, Title VI of the Civil Rights Act of 1964 mandates that no person in the United States shall, on the ground of race, color, or national origin, be excluded from participation in, be denied the benefits of, or be subjected to discrimination under any program or activity receiving federal financial assistance. The standards for culturally and linguistically appropriate services are current federal requirements for all recipients of federal funds. State and federal agencies increasingly rely on private accreditation entities to set standards and monitor compliance with these standards. Both the Joint Commission, which accredits hospitals and other health care institutions, and the National Committee for Quality Assurance (NCQA), which accredits managed care organizations and behavioral health managed care organizations, support the standards for culturally and linguistically appropriate services. In physical therapy, the Commission on Accreditation in Physical Therapy Education (CAPTE) also supports the standards, promoting incorporation of cultural and linguistic competence into physical therapy education curricula. In addition, the Maternal and Child Health Bureau has cultural and linguistic competence training programs that emphasize cultural competency as an integral component of health service delivery.[6]

DEVELOPING CULTURAL COMPETENCE IN HEALTH CARE

The makeup of the American population is changing as a result of immigration patterns and significant increases among racially, ethnically, culturally, and linguistically diverse populations already residing in the United States. It is projected that by 2060 nearly 57 percent of the U.S. population will consist of ethnic minorities.[7] By 2060, the minority subgroups will comprise the majority of the total population.[7] Despite similarities, fundamental differences among people arise regarding nationality, ethnicity, and culture, as well as family background and individual experience. These differences affect the health beliefs and behaviors that both patients and providers have and expect of each other.

The delivery of high-quality primary health care that is accessible, effective, and cost-efficient requires health care practitioners to have a deep understanding of the sociocultural background of patients, their families, and the environments in which they live. Culturally competent primary health services facilitate clinical encounters with more favorable outcomes, enhance the potential for a more rewarding interpersonal experience, and increase the satisfaction of the individual receiving health care services.

Health care providers should realize that addressing cultural diversity means more than knowing the values, beliefs, practices, and customs of Asians, African Americans, Hispanics, Latinos, Alaskan Natives, Native Americans, and Pacific Islanders.

misjudgment. Although it is impossible to learn all there is to know about all cultural subgroups, culturally competent health care providers must be aware of the relevant beliefs and behaviors of their patients/clients and their patient/clients' families, and must be able to adapt to diversity to create a better fit between the needs of the people requiring services and the people meeting those needs.

Cultural diversity can be addressed through awareness/acceptance of the following patient/client characteristics:

- Racial characteristics and national origin
- Religious affiliations
- Physical size
- Spoken language
- Sexual orientation
- Physical and mental disability
- Age
- Gender
- Socioeconomic status
- Political orientation
- Geographic location
- Occupational status

Strategies to improve patient–provider interaction include:

- Providing training to increase cultural awareness, knowledge, and skills
- Recruiting and retaining minority staff
- Providing interpreter services
- Providing linguistic competency that extends beyond the clinical encounter to the appointment desk, advice lines, medical billing, and other written material
- Coordinating evaluations and treatments with traditional healers
- Using community health workers
- Incorporating culture-specific attitudes and values into health promotion tools
- Including family and community members in health care decision making
- Locating clinics in geographic areas that are easily accessible for certain populations
- Expanding hours of operation

Health care providers must continuously strive to achieve the ability and availability to work effectively within the cultural context of a patient/client, the patient/client's family, and the community. The concept of cultural desire involves caring for patients/clients and being open and flexible with them, accepting their differences, and being willing to learn from others about their culture. Health care providers must possess a cultural desire involving commitment to care for all patients and clients, regardless of their cultural values, beliefs, customs, or practices.

A culturally competent health care provider values diversity with an awareness, acceptance, and observance of differences in life views, health systems, communication styles, and other life-sustaining elements. Cultural knowledge must be incorporated into the delivery of services to minimize misperception, misinterpretation, and

Health care providers must focus on enhancing attitudes in the following areas:

- Become aware of the influences that sociocultural factors have on patients, clinicians, and the clinical relationship.
- Be willing to make clinical settings more accessible to patients.
- Be able to accept responsibility and to understand the cultural aspects of health and illness.
- Be able to recognize personal biases against people of different cultures.
- Be able to respect and have tolerance for cultural differences.

- Be willing to accept responsibility to combat racism, classism, ageism, homophobia, sexism, and other kinds of biases and discrimination that occur in health care settings.

Health care providers are continuously striving to increase their cultural competence, responding to the needs of racial and ethnic minorities. The reasons may be the state and federal guidelines that encourage or mandate greater responsiveness of health systems to the growing population diversity, and meeting the federal government's Healthy People 2020 goal of eliminating racial and ethnic health disparities. In addition, many health care systems are finding that developing and implementing cultural competence strategies are good business practices for increasing the interest and participation of both providers and patients in their health plans among racial and ethnic minority populations. As an example, when increasing cultural competence, the most successful efforts of health care providers have been directed at elimination of language and literacy barriers. Bilingual and bicultural services have been developed serving Asian American and Latino communities. Within the Latino community, the use of peer educators (called promotoras) was so successful that more and more ordinary people from other diverse and hard-to-reach populations began to act as bridges between their community and the world of health care. These peer educators learn about health care principles from physicians, nonprofit organizations, or other health care providers, and share their knowledge with their communities. The peer education model is becoming extremely effective in reaching populations that find the health care information more credible coming from someone with a familiar background as opposed to a health care provider.

DEVELOPING CULTURAL COMPETENCE IN PHYSICAL THERAPY

PTs and PTAs need to develop culturally competent communication skills and understandings to effectively interact with patients/clients from diverse cultures. In physical therapy, the primary health care teams working with primary care physicians on an outpatient basis encounter the most cultural diversity. However, all physical therapy clinicians encounter some degree of cultural diversity because culture is so complex, involving not only cultural diversity experiences but also other patient/clients' cultural and socially unique characteristics.

PTs and PTAs can increase their cultural competence by utilizing the following steps:[8]

1. Identify personal cultural biases.
2. Understand general cultural differences.
3. Accept and respect cultural differences.
4. Apply cultural understanding.

Identifying Personal Cultural Biases

Identifying personal cultural biases is the first step in becoming culturally competent. Many people do not realize their own attitudes and values in connection to other people, especially people from diverse populations. Every person has his or her ethnocentrism and personal values and beliefs that contribute to cultural misalignments. **Ethnocentrism** is the act of judging another culture based upon one's own cultural customs and standards. For example, in physical therapy, a PT or a PTA can label a patient "noncompliant" with a physical therapy home exercise program, when in reality the patient did not understand the instructions relating to the exercises. A blind ethnocentric approach to this "noncompliant patient" will not lead to an effective solution. In this example, the misalignment is the attempt of the therapist to simplify a complex world. To manage diversity, people tend to identify similarities and commonalities and ignore the differences. Oversimplification leads to generalization, which may lead to stereotyping, which is an oversimplified conception, opinion, or belief about people. Knowingly or unknowingly, the therapist, as with the majority of health care providers, imposes his or her expectations on the patient in an effort to accomplish the desired task. Rather than labeling the patient as noncompliant, the PT or PTA should identify the language barrier whether it is linguistic, jargon, or comprehension issues.

Understanding General Cultural Differences

Understanding general cultural differences is the second step in becoming culturally competent. It involves actively seeking knowledge regarding different cultures to be able to deal with diverse patient/client populations. This is almost an impossible task when related to knowing all cultures. However, when identifying a patient/client from another culture, the PT and the PTA can refer to appropriate resources to address the situation positively and effectively. For example, consider a patient of Hispanic descent that continuously arrives late for physical therapy treatments. The therapist, whose dominant U.S. culture places great value on timeliness, expects the patient to arrive on time for his or her scheduled appointment. The therapist misinterprets the patient's lateness as disinterest about physical therapy treatment and possibly as noncompliance. In this example, the therapist must refer to the appropriate resources about the Hispanic culture to discover that punctuality is not necessarily a high priority. The therapist may either ignore the patient's lateness or modify the patient's schedule, allowing the patient enough time to arrive late.

Accepting and Respecting Cultural Differences

Accepting and respecting cultural differences is the third step in becoming culturally competent. It involves acknowledging, accepting, appreciating, and valuing diversity. The natural human tendency is to respond to differences with discomfort, apprehension, and fear. People have the tendency to avoid or minimize situations of cultural diversity, and perhaps tolerate them, but not acknowledge and respond to them. To become culturally competent, PTs and PTAs should be able to accept, value, and be equipped to adjust physical therapy care to culturally suitable standards. For example, an elderly Asian American patient is not performing the recommended home exercise program, and is labeled as noncompliant. In reality, the elderly patient, as the "family leader" in Asian American culture, was often not allowed to perform any activity or task without the family helping him or her. In this example, the therapist should discuss the situation with the elderly patient's family, adjusting the home exercise program and incorporating it into the family's activities and tasks.

Applying Cultural Understanding

Applying cultural understanding is the fourth step toward increasing cultural competence, and involves implementing culturally competent health care practices. The PT and the PTA have already identified personal culture and biases, recognized diversity as worthy, acquired an understanding of various cultural differences, and now are prepared to apply cultural competence in physical therapy clinical practice.

When applying cultural competence, we must accept, value, and understand the following:

- The beliefs, values, traditions, and practices of a culture
- The culturally defined health-related needs of individuals, families, and communities
- The culturally based belief systems regarding the etiology of illness and disease and those related to health and healing
- The culture's attitudes toward seeking help from health care providers

The development of cultural competence is an ongoing learning process. During this learning process, in clinical settings, the PT and the PTA may make mistakes; however, the therapist should be able to learn from these mistakes. Research[8] has shown that the acquisition of cultural competency has proven elusive to health care professionals; therefore, clinicians, educators, and students must develop, implement, and promote a strategic plan outlining clear goals, policies, operational plans, and management accountability to provide culturally and linguistically appropriate services. Cultural and linguistic competence is typically incorporated into the PT or PTA's curricula in school and training.

Physical therapy educators can promote the following:

- Increase student awareness about the impact of culture and language on health care delivery.
- Provide education about the importance of recruitment and retention of diverse students to faculty, administrators, and staff.
- Offer continuing education and training about cultural and linguistic competence to faculty, administrators, and staff.

The APTA's resources about cultural and linguistic competence can be found at www.apta.org. The APTA's Minority and Women's Initiatives Department offers bibliographies, videographies, and information on diversity and cultural competence.

Informed Consent

The third principle of the patient's bill of rights states that the patient has the right to receive information from his or her certified health care provider to make an **informed consent** prior to the start of any procedure and/or treatment. The informed consent includes such information as the medically significant risks involved with any procedure and probable duration of incapacitation, and where medically appropriate, alternatives for care or treatment. Informed consent is the process by which a fully informed patient can participate in choices about his or her health care.

> Elements of informed consent to be discussed with the patient/client include:
>
> - The nature of the decision or the procedure (such as a clear description of the proposed intervention)
> - Reasonable alternatives to the proposed intervention
> - The relevant risks, benefits, and uncertainties related to each alternative
> - Assessment of patient understanding
> - The patient's acceptance of the intervention

For the informed consent to be valid, the patient must be considered competent to make the decision, and the consent must be voluntary. Health care providers (such as PTs) should not coerce patients into making uninformed decisions about their health, especially considering that patients feel powerless and vulnerable when facing illness or affliction. PTs should involve the patient in decision making by explaining to the patient that he or she is an active participant in his or her health care resolutions. All the necessary information has to be explained to the patient in layman's terms, and the patient's understanding has to be continuously assessed. In addition, the information must be delivered in terms that the patient is able to understand (including translating the material into another language) and be free of professional jargon.[9] As in any communication with the patient, the PT and the PTA must take into consideration the following basic communication elements:[10]

- Talking clearly and simply (using everyday words)
- Repeating the information as necessary
- Breaking down the information into a series of steps
- Taking into consideration the patient's difficulties in understanding (such as speaking another language, having visual or hearing impairments, and/or having difficulty reading or understanding the material)

In emergency situations when the patient is unconscious (especially when the patient's life is in danger) or is incompetent and no surrogate decision maker is available, the health care provider is obligated to use the principle of beneficence and to act on the patient's behalf. The type of consent used in emergency situations is called *presumed* or *implied consent*.

In physical therapy, the PT has the sole responsibility to provide information to the patient and to obtain informed consent during the first visit, prior to starting the initial examination/evaluation. This process is in accordance with jurisdictional law. When the patient is a minor or an adult who is not competent, a legal guardian (or a designated surrogate) or a parent (in case of a minor) receiving the information has to understand the information and be able to give or refuse informed consent. The PTA also has to provide information to the patient and obtain informed consent when applying reassessments (as directed by the PT) and intervention(s).

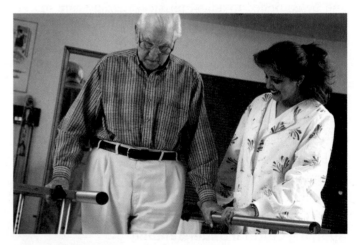

© GWImages/Shutterstock

Ethics Documents for Physical Therapists

The APTA has developed ethical principles to assist PT and PTA members in their understanding of how to act morally and professionally. In addition, the APTA's ethical principles can help PTs and PTAs to:

- Identify and clarify moral issues[9]
- Evaluate moral reasons and form moral viewpoints
- Acquire awareness of alternative viewpoints[9]
- Strengthen attitudes of care and respect for patients/ clients and oneself
- Maintain integrity and act in morally responsible ways[9]

For PTs who are members of the APTA, the Association has created a code of ethics and a guide for professional conduct (Appendix C). The code of ethics for PTs provides ethical principles for maintaining and promoting an ethical practice. The purpose of the guide for professional conduct is to interpret the ethical principles of the code of ethics. The guide contains mostly directive ethical provisions and only eight nondirective ethical provisions regulating the official conduct of member PTs. Currently, the general framework of the guide for professional conduct contains 11 principles having the following topics:[11]

Principle 1: Attitudes of a physical therapist

Principle 2: Patient–physical therapist relationship: truthfulness, confidential information, patient autonomy, and consent

Principle 3: Professional practice, just laws and regulations, and unjust laws and regulations

Principle 4: Professional responsibility, direction and supervision, practice arrangements, and gifts and other considerations

Principle 5: Scope of competence, self-assessment, and professional development

Principle 6: Professional standards, practice, professional education, continuing education, and research

Principle 7: Business and employment practices, endorsement of products or services, and disclosure

Principle 8: Accurate and relevant information to the patient and accurate and relevant information to the public

Principle 9: Consumer protection

Principle 10: Pro bono service and individual and community health

Principle 11: Consultation, patient–provider relationships, and disparagement

These ethical documents govern members within the APTA. While the APTA cannot sanction nonmembers

for ethical violations, these documents provide guidance for best-practice guidelines and can be utilized in legal and regulatory proceedings when ethical and legal issues arise in practice.

Ethics Documents for Physical Therapist Assistants

The APTA also has created standards of ethical conduct and a guide for the conduct of PTAs (Appendix D). The purpose of the standards of ethical conduct is to maintain and promote high standards of conduct for PTAs who are affiliate members of the APTA. The guide for conduct helps PTAs interpret the standards of ethical conduct. Similar to the guide for PTs, the guide for PTAs contains mostly directive ethical provisions and only two nondirective ethical provisions regulating the official conduct of member PTAs. The guide also contributes to the development of PTA students. Currently, the general framework of the guide for conduct of the affiliate member contains seven standards having the following topics:[11]

Standard 1: Attitude of a physical therapist assistant

Standard 2: Trustworthiness, exploitation of patients, truthfulness, and confidential information

Standard 3: Supervisory relationship

Standard 4: Supervision and representation

Standard 5: Competence, self-assessment, and development

Standard 6: Patient safety, judgments of patient/client status, and gifts and other considerations

Standard 7: Consumer protection and organizational employment

Generally, the standards and the guide also promote the following seven ethical principles for PTAs:

- Provide respectful and compassionate care for the patient, including sensitivity to individual and cultural differences
- Act on behalf of the patient/client while being sensitive to the patient/client's vulnerability
- Work under the direction and supervision of the PT
- Comply with laws and regulations governing physical therapy
- Maintain competence in the provision of selected physical therapy interventions

- Make judgments commensurate with one's educational and legal qualifications
- Protect the public and the profession from unethical, incompetent, and illegal acts

All of the guidelines for PTs and PTAs are issued by the ethics and judicial committee of the APTA and are amended to remain current with changes in the physical therapy profession and new patterns of health care delivery.

Other professions such as occupational therapy, orthotics and prosthetics, psychology, respiratory care, and nursing also have ethical guidelines for professional conduct. Most commonly, the codes of ethics within many specialties of the health professions contain vague language as to levels of expected performance. The reason for vague language may be that it is very difficult to include in the code of ethics technical aspects of a profession's medical or clinical practice.

Confronting Ethical Dilemmas

It is likely that at some point in a health care worker's career, he or she will be confronted by an ethical dilemma. It is important to recognize when this occurs and have a plan to work through the process in order to make the best decision based upon legal and ethical principles. An article published by Laura Lee (Dolly) Swisher, PT, PhD; Linda E. Arslanian, PT, DPT, MS; and Carol M. Davis, PT, EdD, FAPTA in the *HPA Review* in 2005 explains a process labeled RIPS. Realm-Individual Process-Situation (RIPS) Model of Ethical Decision Making is a four-step process to considering not just what to do but why (see **TABLE 6-1**).[12]

Professionalism

Professionalism is difficult to define because it involves many variables. In physical therapy, elements of professionalism may include the following values/attributes:

- Ethical principles and reasoning
- Attitudes of the PTs and PTAs
- Decision making
- Behaviors
- Judgments
- The relationship of PTs and PTAs with other professionals, the public, and the physical therapy profession

TABLE 6-1 RIPS Model of Ethical Decision Making

Step 1:	Investigate the Situation
Realm:	There are three realms: individual, organizational, and societal. Individual realm is concerned with the people involved in the situation. For example, the patient, the patient's caregiver, and the PT/PTA may all be affected in an ethical situation. Organizational realm is concerned with the effect decisions will have on the institution. An example of organization is the PT department or the hospital. Societal realm is concerned with how a situation may affect the population as a whole. This could include the local, national, or global society.
Individual Process:	This process requires that the PT/PTA consider what is occurring and what his or her role should be in the situation. There are four questions to be asked. 1. Should I be morally sensitive to the situation? This is a level of awareness of the situation. 2. Should I be making a moral judgment? This requires that a decision be made about what is "right" vs. "wrong." 3. Do I have the moral motivation to do something about the situation? This requires that one place the moral value affecting the situation above other values. 4. Do I have the moral courage to do something about the situation? This requires one to consider whether he/she is willing to do something about the situation.
Situation:	This step in the process requires that the PT/PTA classify the situation. There are five classes: 1. Issue/Problem: Ethical values are part of the situation. 2. Dilemma: There are at least two choices that could be made, both of which may be "right" decisions. 3. Distress: While there is a "right" choice, the power to implement the solution is not yours. 4. Temptation: In this situation, there is a "right" vs. "wrong" choice; however, you may benefit from choosing the "wrong" choice. 5. Silence: No one is speaking out about the situation. This may lead to distress later.
Step 2:	Reflect
	It is important to consider and weigh each aspect of the RIPS in Step 1. Some may carry more weight in the situation and thus will make more of an impact on the decision. One should also consider if the situation is unethical or illegal, "feels" like it is wrong, or could withstand the scrutiny of the public or family.

Step 3:	**Make a Decision**
	If the situation is "right" vs. "wrong," one can go directly to Step 4: Implementation.
	If the situation has more than one "right" choice, the PT/PTA must consider which is the best choice by weighing other factors.
	1. Are there rules that help to make this decision? Examples would be laws, regulatory decisions, policy and procedures, etc.
	2. For each of the choices, make a list of "pros" and "cons" to the decision. This will help you weigh the choices of each for all people affected.
	3. How will this affect the relationships that have been established?
Step 4:	**Implement, Evaluate, and Reassess**
	The steps of implementation will have little value if the person does not follow up with an assessment of its effectiveness. So the PT/PTA should make sure that the implementation has been successful in solving the situation and if not, consider whether or not there was fault in the RIPS process, implementation, or if the situation changed and needs reassessment.

Data from Swisher, L, Arslanian, L, Davis, C. The realm-individual process-situation (RIPS) model of ethical decision making. HPA Resource. October 2005; 1-8. Accessed July 2015, at: www.apta.org.

CORE VALUES

The APTA describes professionalism as a systematic and integrated set of core values.[11] These values are identified as the following (in alphabetical order):[11]

- Accountability
- Altruism
- Compassion/caring
- Excellence
- Integrity
- Professional duty
- Social responsibility

Although the seven core values represent PT professionalism, as members of the physical therapy team, PTAs must also be receptive to these values. As active participants in the professional physical therapy environment, PTAs must employ values for self-assessment, critical reflection, and professional behaviors and attitudes in relation to their colleagues, patients/clients, other professionals, the public, and the profession.

In 2009, the APTA's board of directors created a task force to identify specific behaviors that would be appropriate for PTAs to display. The task force's work created the eight Value-Based Behaviors for the PTA.[13]

1. Altruism
2. Caring and compassion
3. Continuing competence
4. Duty
5. Integrity
6. PT/PTA collaboration
7. Responsibility
8. Social responsibility

Altruism

Altruism is "the primary regard for or devotion to the interest of patients/clients, thus assuming the fiduciary responsibility of placing the needs of the patient/client ahead of the PT's self-interest."[13] Examples of altruism for the PTA may include:[13]

- Placing the patient/client's needs above those of the PTA
- Providing pro bono services (under the direction of the PT)
- Providing physical therapy services to underserved and underrepresented populations (under the direction of the PT)
- Completing patient/client care prior to attending to personal needs (under the direction of the PT)

Caring and Compassion

Compassion (as a precursor of caring) is "the desire to identify with or sense something of another's experience."[13] Caring is "concern, empathy, and consideration for the needs and values of others."[13] Examples of compassion and caring for the PTA may include:[13]

- Respectfully listening to the patient's concerns without judgment and interacting with the patient's needs and desires in mind
- Understanding the sociocultural, economic, and psychological influences on the individual's life in his or her environment
- Understanding an individual's perspective
- Communicating effectively (verbally and nonverbally) with others, taking into consideration individual differences in learning styles, language, and cognitive abilities

- Recognizing and refraining from acting on one's social, cultural, gender, and sexual biases
- Attending to the patient/client's personal needs and comforts
- Demonstrating respect for others and considering others to be unique and of value

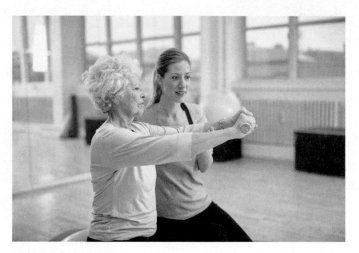

© Ammentorp Photography/Shutterstock

Continuing Competence

Continuing competence requires conscious reflections of the PTA's current abilities and developing a plan for lifelong learning of knowledge, skills, and attitudes that will benefit patient interactions. Examples of continuing competence for the PTA may include:[13]

- Personal self-assessment practices and assessment by a PT to help create a plan for improvement
- Creating a personal goal of lifelong learning through continuing education courses, journal reading, and learning from colleagues
- Creating a plan for career advancement through education and opportunities for growth and advancement
- Engaging in acquisition of new knowledge throughout one's career
- Sharing one's knowledge with others

Duty

Duty is "the commitment to meeting one's obligations to provide effective physical therapy services to patients/clients to serve the profession, and to positively influence the health of society."[13] Examples of professional duty values for the PTA may include:[13]

- Demonstrating beneficence by providing "optimal care"
- Facilitating each individual's achievement of goals for function, health, and wellness
- Preserving the safety, security, and confidentiality of individuals in all contexts related to physical therapy
- Promoting the profession of physical therapy
- Taking pride in being a PTA

Integrity

Integrity is "steadfast adherence to high ethical principles or professional standards; truthfulness, fairness, doing what you say you will do, and 'speaking forth' about why you do what you do."[13] Examples of integrity for the PTA may include:[13]

- Abiding by the rules, regulations, and laws applicable to the profession
- Adhering to the highest standards of the profession (ethics, reimbursement, honor code, etc.)
- Being trustworthy
- Knowing one's limitations and acting accordingly
- Confronting harassment and bias among ourselves and others
- Choosing employment situations that are congruent with ethical standards

PT/PTA Collaboration

"The PT/PTA team works together, within each partner's respective role, to achieve optimal patient/client care and to enhance the overall delivery of physical therapy services."[13] Examples of PT/PTA collaboration may include:[13]

- Promoting understanding of the role of the PTA, education level, state laws, rules and regulations, and APTA guidelines for PTAs
- Creating a respectful working relationship with the PT that utilizes both team members' skills and strengths for the betterment of the patient
- Promoting physical therapy to consumers and community members

Responsibility

Responsibility is the "active acceptance of the roles, obligations, and actions of the PTA, including behaviors that positively influence patient/client outcomes, the profession, and the health needs of society."[13] Examples of responsibility include:[13]

- Understanding personal strengths and weaknesses and practicing ethically within the PTA's abilities
- Working conscientiously to provide accurate and timely care
- Taking responsibility for actions and consequences
- Communicating clearly with all team members (patient, PT, other health care providers)

Social Responsibility

Social responsibility is "the promotion of a mutual trust between the profession and the larger public that necessitates responding to societal needs for health and wellness."[11] Examples of social responsibility values for the PTA may include:[11]

- Advocating for the health and wellness needs of society including access to health care and physical therapy services
- Promoting cultural competence within the profession and the larger public
- Promoting social policy that affects function, health, and wellness needs of patients/clients
- Ensuring that existing social policy is in the best interest of the patient/client
- Advocating for changes in laws, regulations, standards, and guidelines that affect PT service provision
- Promoting community volunteerism
- Participating in collaborative relationships with other health practitioners and the public at large
- Ensuring the blending of social justice and economic efficiency of services

INTEGRITY IN PRACTICE

The APTA has created the Center for Integrity in Practice as part of its Integrity in Practice initiative. The initiative grew out of a recognition of fraud, abuse, and waste that occurs in health care and the desire to educate PTs and PTAs about the issues occurring in practice. The Center provides scenarios to help identify the issues and suggestions for problem resolution. Additionally, the Center has joined with the American Board of Internal Medicine Foundation's Choosing Wisely® campaign to create a list of five things that PTs, PTAs, and consumers should question about physical therapy care.[14]

Discussion Questions

1. Describe behaviors that you would find in a professional.
2. Using the behaviors described in question 1, connect each one to a core value that professionals hold.
3. The PTA works for a skilled nursing facility and is frequently encouraged to bill patients for enough time so that they qualify for the highest Medicare payment allowed. The PT and PTA discuss that one of the patients is unable to effectively work the amount of time that the manager is requesting. What are the ethical dilemmas presented in this scenario and what options do the PT and PTA have regarding this situation?

Learning Opportunities

1. Using the following chart, create a list of things that you can do to develop the professional behavior.

Professional Behavior	Practice or Skill	Core Value
Example: Good judgment	Continuing education	Excellence

2. Utilizing the Internet, find information regarding a cultural group in your area and share your findings with your group. Investigate the culture's beliefs about health and accessing health care providers, the use of alternative health practices, social interactions that may be different from your culture, and so on. Describe how you might respectfully interact with them in a health care setting.
3. Utilize the RIPS steps to analyze the following ethical situation.
   The PT clinic employs two PTs and three PTAs. One of the PTs has gone on maternity leave for 12 weeks and there is no one to cover her caseload and supervise one of the PTAs. The clinic manager states that it shouldn't be a problem for the other PT to supervise all three PTAs because it is only a few weeks. State law restricts the PT to supervising no more than two PTAs at any one time.

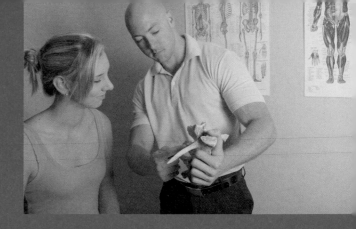

CHAPTER 7

Laws and Regulations

OBJECTIVES

After studying this chapter, the reader will be able to:

1. Identify the four primary sources of law in the United States.
2. Describe the Americans with Disabilities Act of 1990.
3. List the main points of the Americans with Disabilities Act and its effect on businesses and employers.
4. Discuss the Individuals with Disabilities Education Act of 1997.
5. Describe the role of licensure laws.
6. Identify the organization responsible for creating and managing the National Physical Therapy Examination for physical therapists and physical therapist assistants.
7. Explain four minimum standards for licensure/ certification to enter the profession for physical therapists and physical therapist assistants.
8. Describe the Occupational Safety and Health Administration and its role in health care.
9. Discuss the importance of the bloodborne pathogens OSHA standard in health care, including physical therapy practice.
10. Identify the Violence Against Women Act of 2013 and domestic violence issues in the United States.
11. Describe domestic violence responses in health care and physical therapy.
12. Identify two types of malpractice laws that can affect physical therapist assistants.
13. Compare and contrast the principles of negligence and malpractice.

KEY TERMS

Americans with Disabilities Act (ADA)
bloodborne pathogens standards (BPS)
disability
domestic violence
economic abuse
emotional abuse

Occupational Safety and Health Administration (OSHA)
physical abuse
psychological abuse
sexual abuse

Sources of Laws and Examples

There are four primary sources of law and legal obligations in society: constitutional law authority, statutory law authority, common law authority, and administrative or regulatory law authority. Constitutional laws have superiority because they were created from the federal Constitution, which is the supreme law of the land. Most federal constitutional obligations incumbent upon members of society are found in the amendments to the Constitution. The first 10 amendments, or the Bill of Rights, delineate specific individual protections from federal, state, and local governmental overreaching. These rights include the right to be free from unreasonable searches and seizures, protection from being tried twice for the same crime within a single jurisdictional system, and others. State constitutional laws offer to citizens greater rights than federal constitutional laws; however, state constitutional laws are subordinate to federal constitutional laws.

Statutory laws have the second priority after constitutional laws. Congress and state legislatures enact statutes within their spheres of legal authority. Federal statutes are divided by general subjects into titles. Examples of important federal statutes that affect physical therapy practices are Medicare and Medicaid laws, workers' compensation acts, the Americans with Disabilities Act (ADA) of 1990, the 1973 Rehabilitation Act, the Individuals with Disabilities Education Act (IDEA) of 1997, and licensure laws.

Common laws have third priority as legal tenets. Judges created them. In the United States, there are common laws that are still based on early English common laws. Most of the U.S. civil laws related to health care ethical and legal issues are derived from common laws. An example of common law affecting physical therapy practice is the malpractice law.

Administrative or regulatory laws are enacted by administrative or regulatory agencies at the local, state, and federal levels. They promulgate administrative rules and regulations that supplement statutes and executive orders. The administrative or regulatory laws influence business conduct. These administrative or regulatory laws, through regulatory agencies, have a major effect on health care professions in the areas of practice, research, and educational settings. Examples of federal administrative agencies having broad authority over physical therapy business affairs include the Occupational Safety and Health Administration (OSHA) and the Centers for Medicare and Medicaid Services (CMS).

Laws Affecting Physical Therapy Practice

There are typically two large areas of law affecting physical therapy practice. These include the Americans with Disabilities Act (incorporating mostly Titles I to V) and the Individuals with Disabilities Education Act (IDEA) of 1997.

THE AMERICANS WITH DISABILITIES ACT

The **Americans with Disabilities Act (ADA)** is a nondiscrimination law that prevents discrimination against persons with disabilities in the areas of employment, public accommodations (see **FIGURE 7-1**), state and local government services, and telecommunications.[15]

What is **disability** (as per the ADA)?

- Physical or mental impairment that substantially limits one or more major life activities.
- The person with a disability needs to have a record of such physical or mental impairment.
- The person with a disability is regarded as having such impairment.
- The major life activities include, among others, all the important activities of daily living (ADLs) including the ability to see, hear, speak, walk, care for one's self, maintain cardiorespiratory function, perform manual tasks, and engage in formal and informal learning activities.

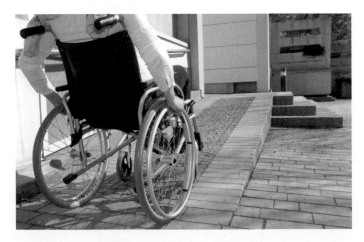

FIGURE 7-1 Accessibility should not be an issue.
© RioPatuca/Shutterstock

The ADA's purpose is to ensure that people with disabilities are able to integrate into U.S. society by ensuring equal access to public accommodations and services and equal opportunities in employment.[15] The ADA was modeled after the Rehabilitation Act of 1973, which prohibits employment discrimination based on disability in federal executive agencies and in all institutions receiving Medicare, Medicaid, and other federal support. The ADA has five sections or titles.

Title I of the ADA

Title I of the ADA protects people with disabilities against employment discrimination. Title I became effective in July 1992 for businesses employing 25 or more people, and on July 1994 for businesses employing 15 or more people. Title I prohibits employment discrimination by private and public employers and employment agencies or union organizations against employees and job applicants who are qualified to perform the essential functions of their jobs. Discrimination applies to an employee's recruitment, selection, training, benefits, promotion, discipline, and retention. The qualified individual with a disability is a job applicant or employee who can perform essential functions with or without reasonable accommodations.[15]

A reasonable accommodation means any change or adjustment to a job, the work environment, or the way things usually are done that would allow a person with a disability to apply for a job, perform job functions, or enjoy equal access to benefits available to other individuals in the workplace.[15] There are many types of accommodations that may help people with disabilities work successfully. Some of the most common types of accommodations include:[15]

- Making physical changes, such as installing a ramp or modifying a workspace or restroom
- Providing sign language interpreters for people who are deaf or readers for people who are blind
- Providing a quieter workspace or making other changes to reduce noisy distractions for someone with a mental disability
- Providing training and creating written materials in an accessible format, such as in Braille, on audio tape, or on CD
- Providing teletypewriters (TTYs) for use with telephones by people who are deaf, and hardware and software that make computers accessible to people with vision impairments or who have difficulty using their hands
- Giving time off to an individual who needs treatment for a disability

The reasonable accommodations must be carried out upon the request of an applicant or employee (or by the employee having a disability), unless the employer can prove that to do so would amount to an undue hardship.

Undue hardship means that the accommodation would be excessively disruptive, very costly, or difficult to implement, or would fundamentally alter the nature of the employer's business operation.[15] For example, if a public hospital were to offer monthly childbirth classes on an upper floor of an older building without an elevator, the hospital has a number of options in how it may make this program accessible without "undue hardship." The hospital's options are to install an elevator, schedule the class in a ground floor classroom in the future, or relocate the class to a ground floor room where individuals who use wheelchairs can register for the class. If the elevator installation constitutes undue hardship, the hospital could utilize the other options.

Titles II, III, IV, and V of the ADA

Title II of the ADA protects against discrimination related to equal access to public services, including public transportation services. Title III of the ADA protects against discrimination related to equal public accommodations, including all private businesses and services. All religious organizations and some private clubs are not included in the group requiring private accommodations. Title IV of the ADA protects against discrimination related to equal access to telecommunications services. Title V of the ADA is a miscellaneous section that discusses the ADA's relationship to other federal statutes, key definitions, and an affirmation that the states cannot claim immunity from the ADA requirements. Included in this section, is the protection from retribution for any individual who advocates for a person with a disability.[15]

Both public and private hospitals and health care facilities such as physical therapy facilities must provide their services to people with disabilities in a nondiscriminatory manner. To do so, they may have to modify their policies and procedures, provide auxiliary aids and services for effective communication, remove barriers from existing facilities, and follow the ADA accessibility standards for new construction and alteration projects. However, when the health care providers need to modify their policies and procedures, the ADA does not require providers to make changes that would fundamentally alter the nature of their services.

Health care providers must also find appropriate ways to communicate effectively with persons who have disabilities affecting their ability to communicate. Various auxiliary aids and services such as interpreters, written notes, readers, large print, or Braille text can be used depending on the circumstance and the individual. However, if provision of any auxiliary aid or services would result in an undue burden or fundamentally alter the nature of services, the ADA does not require the health care provider to acquire these auxiliary aids and services. For example, telecommunication devices for the deaf (TDD) such as teletypewriters (TTYs) must be accessible where a voice telephone is made available for outgoing calls on more than an incidental convenience basis. This includes areas such as inpatient rooms and emergency department or recovery room waiting areas. Outpatient medical and health care facilities (such as physical therapy outpatient facilities) are not required to have TTYs for patients/clients but should be able to rely on relay systems for making and receiving calls from patients or clients with hearing or speech impairments.

INDIVIDUALS WITH DISABILITIES EDUCATION ACT (IDEA) OF 1997

The Individuals with Disabilities Education Act (IDEA) was first introduced in 1975. In 1997, the act was amended by then-President Clinton. IDEA is a law ensuring services to children with disabilities throughout the nation. IDEA governs how states and public agencies provide early intervention, special education, and related services to more than 6.5 million eligible infants, toddlers, children, and youth with disabilities.[16,17] Infants and toddlers (birth to 2 years of age) with disabilities and their families receive early intervention services under IDEA Part C.[16,17] Children and youth (ages 3 to 21 years) receive special education and related services under IDEA Part B.[16,17]

The purposes of the IDEA of 1997 include the following:

- To ensure that all children with disabilities have available to them a free appropriate public education that emphasizes special education and related services designed to meet their unique needs and prepare them for employment and independent living
- To ensure that the rights of children with disabilities and parents of such children are protected

- To assist states, localities, educational service agencies, and federal agencies to provide for the education of all children with disabilities
- To assist states in the implementation of a statewide, comprehensive, coordinated, multidisciplinary, interagency system of early intervention services for infants and toddlers with disabilities and their families
- To ensure that educators and parents have the necessary tools to improve educational results for children with disabilities by supporting systemic change; coordinated research and personnel preparation; coordinated technical assistance, dissemination, and support; and technology development and media services
- To assess and ensure the effectiveness of efforts to educate children with disabilities

Physical Therapy Services for Children with Disabilities

The American Physical Therapy Association (APTA) supports the provision of physical therapy services to children with special needs. Physical therapy contributes to the delivery of services to children with disabilities by developing and implementing cost-effective services within the framework of federally approved state plans.[18] Physical therapy's primary goal is identifying and serving the best interests of children with disabling conditions both within the school setting and in overall quality of life.[18] Physical therapists (PTs) and physical therapist assistants (PTAs) are providing:

- Early physical therapy services for infants and toddlers with disabilities
- Physical therapy services for children with disabilities in educational programs

The PTs examine, evaluate, plan, and implement physical therapy programs for children having a variety of sensory and motor disabilities.[18] These programs help the children attain their optimal educational potential and also benefit from special education.[18] Also, PTs assume a significant role in the development of a child's individualized education program (IEP) or individualized family service plan (IFSP).[16,17]

The PTs' roles in early intervention for infants and toddlers with disabilities include the following:

- Consult with parents, other service providers, and representatives of appropriate community agencies to ensure effective provision of services in that area
- Train parents and others regarding the provision of those services
- Participate in the multidisciplinary team's assessment of a child and the child's family, and in the development of integrated goals and outcomes for the individualized family service plan

Physical therapy may include the following services:

- Screening, evaluation, and assessment of infants and toddlers to identify movement dysfunction
- Obtaining, interpreting, and integrating information appropriate to program planning to prevent, alleviate, or compensate for movement dysfunction and related functional problems
- Providing individual and group services or treatment to prevent, alleviate, or compensate for movement dysfunction and related functional problems

Requirements of regulatory practice acts include the following:

- Requirements for licensure of professionals educated in the United States
- Requirements for licensure of foreign-educated or foreign-trained professionals
- Requirements for continuing professional education
- Requirements for practice within the state pursuant to temporary licensure
- Requirements for periodic relicensure
- Requirements for mandatory reporting of perceived unethical conduct within the scope of permissible practice
- Restrictions, if any, on independent or autonomous practice called *practice without referral*
- Provisions establishing licensure boards to administer professional licensure
- Provisions defining grounds and procedures for disciplinary action

Violations of mandatory licensure laws are punishable as criminal offenses and form the basis for administrative claims and civil health care malpractice lawsuits.

LICENSURE FOR PTs AND PTAs

The APTA established the following policies regarding the licensure of PTs and PTAs in the United States:[19]

- PTs are licensed.
- PTAs should be licensed or otherwise regulated in all U.S. jurisdictions.
- State regulation of PTs and PTAs should at a minimum:
  1. require graduation from a physical therapy education program that is accredited by the Commission on Accreditation in Physical Therapy Education (CAPTE), or
     a. in the case of an internationally educated PT seeking licensure as a PT, a substantially equivalent education, or
     b. in the case of a graduate of an international PTA program seeking licensure, certification, or registration as a PTA, a substantially equivalent education

Licensure Laws

Licensure laws are enacted by all states, giving licensees the exclusive right to practice their professions. Licensure laws protect the consumer against professional incompetence. Health care professionals such as physicians, surgeons, dentists, occupational therapists, PTs, registered nurses, and technically educated health care providers such as PTAs and certified occupational therapist assistants are subject to mandatory licensure requirements for practice. State licensure laws also implement regulatory practice acts that define the requirements of licensed health professional practices such as PTs, occupational therapists, physicians, surgeons, dentists, and registered nurses.

2. require passing an entry-level competency exam
3. provide title protection
4. allow for disciplinary action

- Additionally, PTs' licensure should include a defined scope of practice.
- All PTAs must work under the direction and supervision of the PT.

Physical therapy licensure laws for PTs are enacted in 53 jurisdictions, including the 50 states and the District of Columbia, Puerto Rico, and the U.S. Virgin Islands.[20] PTAs are licensed or certified in 50 jurisdictions.[20] The licensure examination and related activities are the responsibility of the Federation of State Boards of Physical Therapy (FSBPT).[20] The federation also works towards desirable and reasonable uniformity in regulation and standards through a process of strategic planning and ongoing communications between the jurisdictions. The jurisdictions agreed to support one passing score on the national licensure examination for PTs and PTAs. This facilitates mobility of PTs and PTAs across states and at the same time holds all PTs beginning practice in the United States to the same entry-level standard of competence. Each state determines the criteria to practice and issues a license to a PT or a PTA. Additionally, some states require that students take a jurisprudence exam to ensure that they are informed about the laws and regulations governing PTs and PTAs in that state. For more information, please check the FSBPT website at www.fsbpt.org.

Occupational Safety and Health Administration's Federal Standards

The **Occupational Safety and Health Administration (OSHA)** is a federal government regulatory agency concerned with the health and safety of workers.[21]

OSHA's role is defined as to assure safe and healthful working conditions for working men and women by

- Authorizing enforcement of the standards developed under the OSHA Act
- Assisting and encouraging the states in their efforts to assure safe and healthful working conditions

- Providing for research, information, education, and training in the field of occupational safety and health[21]

OSHA's services include establishment of protective standards, enforcement of those standards, and reaching out to employers and employees through technical assistance and consultation programs. OSHA is "determined to use its resources effectively to stimulate management commitment and employee participation in comprehensive workplace safety and health programs."[22]

THE BLOODBORNE PATHOGENS STANDARD

Section 5 of the OSHA Act requires that:[22]

- "Each employer shall furnish to each of his employees employment and a place of employment which are free from recognized hazards that are causing or are likely to cause death or serious physical harm to his employees;
- Each employer shall comply with occupational safety and health standards promulgated under this Act; and
- Each employee shall comply with occupational safety and health standards and all rules, regulations, and orders issued pursuant to this Act which are applicable to his own actions and conduct."

Bloodborne Pathogens Standards Training

OSHA has developed factsheets on the **bloodborne pathogens standards (BPS)**. The OSHA website at www.osha.gov has files that can be downloaded and contact information for regional OSHA offices where questions about compliance and the standard can be answered. Individual employers should have a training program in place to inform their employees about risks and safety standards in their health care setting.[22]

Methods of Infection Control

As per Section 7 of OSHA's Regulatory Impact and Regulatory Flexibility Analysis, limiting worker exposure to bloodborne diseases is achieved through the implementation of the following categories of infection controls:[23]

- Engineering controls
- Immunization programs

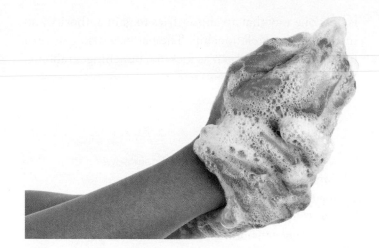

FIGURE 7-2 Safety starts with washing hands.
© Samuel Borges Photography/Shutterstock

- Work practices, such as careful hand washing after each patient contact and procedures for handling sharps (see **FIGURE 7-2**)
- Disposal and handling of contaminated waste
- Use of personal protective equipment, especially gloves, gowns, and goggles
- Use of mouthpieces, resuscitation bags, or other ventilation devices
- Use of disinfectants
- Labeling and signs
- Training and education programs
- Postexposure follow-up

Universal Precautions

Universal precautions represent OSHA's recommendations to control and protect employees from exposure to all human blood and other potentially infectious materials. The BPS require all blood and other potentially infectious materials to be considered infectious regardless of the perceived risk of an individual patient or patient population. For example, a PTA who treats mostly elderly patients in a rural area may feel that the prevalence of human immunodeficiency virus (HIV) and hepatitis B virus (HBV) among these patients is negligible. However, the PTA is required by the standards to use the same universal precautions as when treating patients who are actually infected. Using the precautions can protect the PTA and the patients from potential contamination.

In regard to universal precautions, and respecting OSHA's rules and regulations, health care employees are responsible for the following:[22]

- Make consistent use of protective barriers and procedures in all situations and for all patients.
- Understand that the purpose of practicing universal precautions is to prevent infection from bloodborne pathogens on the job.
- Assume that any patient or bodily fluid is potentially infectious for bloodborne pathogens such as HBV or HIV.
- Understand that potentially infectious materials include semen, vaginal secretions, cerebrospinal fluid, synovial fluid, pleural fluid, pericardial fluid, peritoneal fluid, amniotic fluid, saliva in dental procedures, and any body fluid that is visibly contaminated with blood.
- Comply with the summaries of the universal precautions recommendations.

Universal precautions recommendations include the following:[22]

- Use protective equipment and clothing whenever in contact with bodily fluids.
- Dispose of waste in proper containers using proper handling techniques for infectious waste.
- Dispose of sharp instruments and needles in proper containers.
- Keep the work area and the patient area clean.
- Wash hands immediately after removing gloves and at all times as required by the agency policy.
- Immediately report any exposure to needle sticks or blood splashes or any personal illness to the direct supervisor and receive instructions about follow-up action.

What is domestic violence?

Domestic violence, also called domestic abuse, intimate partner violence (IPV), or battering, occurs between people in intimate relationships and takes many forms including coercion, threats, intimidation, isolation, and emotional, sexual, and physical abuse.

Domestic Violence and Legal Issues

Domestic violence is a significant problem in the United States. Domestic violence statistics are frightening. Although many domestic violence assaults are never reported, the U.S. Department of Justice estimated that more than 12 million women and men are physically abused, raped, or stalked by their intimate partners each year.[23]

Domestic violence often may result in death. For example, in 2011, 926 women died because of intimate partner violence (IPV).[24] In addition to loss of life, medical care and loss of productivity resulting from IPV cost the United States billions of dollars each year. In 2003, the expenditure resulting from IPV was calculated at $8.3 billion.[24]

Domestic violence is not confined to certain groups, and there are no typical victims of domestic abuse. Domestic violence can be found among people of all ages, races, ethnicities, and religions. It occurs in both opposite-sex and same-sex relationships. Economic or professional status does not indicate a likelihood of domestic violence. Abusers and victims can be laborers or college professors, doctors or judges, truck drivers or schoolteachers, store clerks or stay-at-home moms and dads. Domestic violence can occur in the fanciest mansions or the poorest ghettos.

Domestic violence or IPV is a health problem of enormous proportions. It is estimated that in the United States, 27 percent of women and 11.5 percent of men experience physical and/or **sexual abuse** by an intimate partner at some point in their adult lives.[25] Heterosexual women are five to eight times more likely than heterosexual men to be victimized.[25] Research of homosexual partner abuse is less available; however, one recent survey indicated that 39 percent of homosexual men had reported intimate partner violence.[25] Elderly Americans are also victims of domestic abuse. For example, research published in the *American Journal of Public Health* found that one in ten Americans over 60 years of age experienced abuse each year.[26] In addition, children are also exposed to IPV. Research has shown that 15.5 million children in the United States live in a family where partner violence has occurred in the last year.[25]

RECOGNIZING DOMESTIC VIOLENCE PATTERNS

The relationships between the abuser and the person abused differ. In all abuse cases, the abuser aims to have power and control over his or her intimate partner. Anger is only one way that an abuser tries to gain authority and instill fear in a relationship. The batterer also can turn to physical violence such as kicking, punching, grabbing, slapping, or biting.

Methods the abuser may use to gain power and control over the intimate partner include the following:[27]

- Physical violence, such as hitting, kicking, or in general hurting the victim using physical force
- Sexual violence, such as forcing the victim to have sexual intercourse or to engage in other sexual activities against the intimate partner's will
- Using children as pawns, such as accusing the intimate partner of bad parenting, threatening to take the children away, or using the children to relay messages to the partner
- Denial and blame, such as denying that the abuse occurred or shifting responsibility for the abusive behavior onto the partner
- Coercion and threats, such as threatening to hurt other family members, pets, children, or self
- **Economic abuse**, such as controlling finances, refusing to share money, sabotaging the partner's work performance, making the partner account for money spent, or not allowing the partner to work outside the home
- Intimidation, such as using certain actions, looks, or gestures to instill fear, and breaking things, abusing pets, or destroying property
- **Emotional abuse**, such as insults, criticism, or name calling
- Isolation, such as limiting the partner's contact with family and friends, requiring permission to leave the house, not allowing the partner to attend work or school, or controlling the partner's activities and social events
- Privilege, such as making all major decisions, defining the roles in the relationship, being in charge of the home and social life, or treating the partner as a servant or possession

DOMESTIC VIOLENCE AND HEALTH CARE

Domestic violence is a serious crime that has a substantial impact on the health and welfare of adults and children.[28] Physical and sexual assaults by partners can result in a range of injuries including cuts, broken bones, bruises, internal injuries, concussions, internal bleeding, and death. Additionally, mental health consequences of physical, sexual, and/or domestic **psychological abuse** may include posttraumatic stress disorder, depression, suicide, substance abuse, and anxiety disorders.

Physicians and health care professionals can play a major role in helping victims to disclose violence. They also can assure the victim that advice and support is available.[28] Domestic violence can go undetected in health care settings, mostly because a majority of the victims are reluctant to report domestic abuse.

> Reasons health care providers may experience difficulties identifying/helping victims of domestic violence:[28]
>
> - The health care provider's fears or experiences of exploring the issue of domestic violence
> - The health care provider's lack of knowledge of community resources
> - The health care provider's fear of offending the victim and jeopardizing the provider–patient relationship
> - The health care provider's lack of time or lack of training
> - The health care provider's unresponsiveness caused by feeling powerless and not being able to fix the situation
> - The victim's infrequent visits as a patient
> - The victim's unresponsiveness to questions asked by the health care provider

The first step toward ensuring appropriate care is identifying individuals experiencing domestic violence. Health care providers may try the following actions:[28]

- Observe the victim for physical and behavioral clues.
- Question the victim and validate domestic abuse.
- Respect the victim's privacy and utilize confidentiality measures.
- Assess and treat the victim.
- Keep accurate records and concise documentation about the victim's abuse.
- Support and follow up the victim's care.

In many situations, the victim may not realize the health impact of the abuse. The victim may or may not be symptomatic. Also, he or she may not disclose abuse because he or she cannot understand how the violence affects his or her health. Other reasons for not disclosing may be fear of the partner, embarrassment, and fear of talking about the abuse with the health care provider. Consequently, the health care provider's role is to initiate prevention strategies. For example, the health care provider can make available patient education about healthy relationships, parenting skills, and the warning signs of an abusive relationship. Female victims may also be prompted by the health care provider that:[28]

- Social norms are changing.
- Social norms do not promote hostility or violence toward women.
- Men these days are more involved as co-parents.
- The status of women in U.S. society is growing through education and jobs.

It is imperative for health care providers to believe that preventing domestic abuse can reduce other types of interpersonal violence such as child abuse, elder abuse, and the physical and mental health effects of childhood exposure to domestic violence. By educating patients about the broad implications of domestic abuse and the elevated risk for multiple forms of violence in the same household, health care providers can help to end the cycle of family violence.[28]

DOMESTIC VIOLENCE AND PHYSICAL THERAPY

Because control and power are the two main issues of domestic violence, the abuser uses fear and the threat of physical harm to control the victim. The abuser may use physical and economic control to limit the victim's access to medical care, including physical therapy. The victim's regular appointments at a physical therapy clinic can pose a threat to the abuser, giving the victim an opportunity to form a relationship with the PT and the PTA and to possibly reveal the cause of her or his injuries. The abuser may not allow the victim to continue physical therapy by limiting the victim's access to transportation or finances. As a result, the victim/patient may appear noncompliant with physical therapy. Noncompliance can also be caused by the effects of depression or fatigue caused by the abuse.

Recognizable signs of abuse while the victim is accessing physical therapy services may include:[29]

- The abuser accompanying the victim to all appointments and refusing to allow the victim to be interviewed alone; also the abuser can use verbal or nonverbal communication to direct the victim's responses during appointments
- The patient's noncompliance with physical therapy treatment regimens and/or frequently missing appointments
- The patient's statements about not being allowed to take or obtain medications (prescription or nonprescription medication)
- The abuser canceling the victim's appointments or sabotaging the victim's efforts to attend appointments (e.g., by not providing child care or transportation)
- The patient engaging in therapist-hopping
- The patient lacking independent transportation, access to finances, or the ability to communicate by phone

An abuser's tactics to control the health care providers may include the following:[29]

- Intimidating health care professionals with a variety of threats or acts
- Portraying him- or herself as a good provider and caregiver and/or consistently praising health care professionals
- Harassing health care professionals by repeated phone calls, threats of legal action, and/or false reports to superiors about supposed breaches of confidentiality, inappropriate treatment, or rude behavior
- Splitting health care teams by creating divisiveness among professionals

For PTs and PTAs (the same as for other health care providers), recognizing a victim of domestic violence is not easy. Some victims attempt to conceal their injuries from health care providers. However, it is possible that, if asked, the victim may reveal his or her situation. As signs, victims may have more than one injury including short-term injuries such as black eyes, contusions, lacerations, and fractures. Other injuries that can be observed in physical therapy are burns, vision or hearing loss, knife wounds, or joint damage.

Signs that a patient should be screened for domestic abuse may include:[29]

- Chronic pain
- Injuries during pregnancy
- Repeated and chronic injuries
- Exacerbated or poorly controlled chronic illnesses such as asthma, seizure disorders, diabetes, hypertension, and heart disease
- Unattended gynecological problems
- Physical symptoms related to stress, anxiety disorders, or depression
- Hypervigilant signs such as being easily startled or very guarded; experiencing nightmares or emotional numbing
- Suicide attempts
- Eating disorders
- Self-mutilation
- Car accidents where the victim is the driver or the passenger
- Overuse of prescription pain medications and other drugs

PTs and PTAs have an ethical duty to treat victims of domestic violence, addressing the rights and dignity of the victim, confidentiality, compliance with governing laws, and acceptance of responsibility. If a PTA suspects a patient to be a victim of domestic violence, the PTA should report her or his suspicions to the PT of record. PTs and PTAs could work together with other health care providers and their community leaders to establish the following domestic violence guidelines for their organization(s):

- Develop objective criteria for identifying, examining, and treating patients/clients who may be victims of domestic violence.
- Have available legally required notifications and release of information to the proper authorities when evaluating/examining patients/clients who may be victims of domestic violence.
- Screen, evaluate/examine, reevaluate, and care for patients/clients who may be victims of domestic violence.
- Provide in-service training and continuing education about domestic violence to all physical therapy personnel.
- Establish a domestic violence protocol for emergency situations for patients/clients who may be victims of domestic violence.
- Have available a list of appropriate referrals to community agencies for patients/clients who may be victims of domestic violence.

The APTA provides several continuing education courses in the Learning Center to assist PTs and PTAs in identifying victims of family violence.[30] The APTA advises that PTs should routinely screen for domestic violence by asking direct questions about injuries, evasive behavior, and the patient's fear of her or his partner. Patients must be interviewed in private and away from the intimate partner or other family members. For patients who understand terms such as abuse or battered, direct questioning is the best way to elicit a response. For patients who don't understand these terms, indirect questioning may be more appropriate. The best questioning methods are to frame the questions in a context of domestic violence being a common problem in U.S. society. This allows the patient to be more comfortable discussing the subject and to open up about his or her problems as a victim of domestic abuse.

Examples of direct questions for victims of domestic violence include:[29]

- I am concerned about your symptoms, especially because they may be caused by someone hurting you. Has someone been hurting you?
- Your bruise looks painful. Did someone hit you?
- Did your partner hit you?

Examples of indirect questions for victims of domestic violence include:

- You seem concerned about your partner. Are you having problems with your partner?
- What types of problems do you have with your partner?
- How does your partner feel about you having physical therapy? Does your partner resent you coming here?

Questions that PTs or PTAs should never ask victims of domestic violence include:[29]

- Why would you stay with a person like that?
- What could you have done to diffuse the situation?
- Why don't you just leave?
- What did you do to aggravate your partner?
- Did you do something to cause your partner to hit you?

In some states, health care providers are mandated to report when patients are injured by a knife, gun, or other deadly weapon, or if the injury resulted from a criminal act, act of violence, or a nonaccidental act. PTs and PTAs should obtain a copy of their state's statutes and consult with legal counsel regarding individual cases and changes in state and federal laws relating to domestic violence. In cases where the PT or PTA needs to report the abuse, they should be able to work with the patient so that the timing of the report allows for the patient's safety. Specific state-by-state information can be found at the Health and Human Services government website.[31]

When domestic abuse is confirmed, PTs and PTAs must be able to document correctly the abuse in the patient's medical records. Although sometimes a victim may not intend to pursue legal remedies, the victim may change his or her mind and proceed to go to court. The medical records must be admissible in a court of law.

DOMESTIC VIOLENCE AND LEGAL ISSUES

On October 28, 2000, the U.S. Congress passed the Violence Against Women Act (VAWA), which reauthorized

The APTA's documentation guidelines on domestic violence include:[32]

- The medical records must be written in the regular course of business during the examination or the interview.
- The medical records must be legible.
- The medical records must be properly stored and be accessed only by the appropriate staff.
- The medical records must include the following information:
  - Patient's date and time of arrival at the clinic or the treatment site.
  - Patient's name, address, and the phone number of the person(s) accompanying the victim (if possible).
  - Patient's own words about the cause of his or her injuries.
  - A detailed description (with explanations) of injuries, including the type, number, size, location, and resolution; a description of a chronology of the violence asking about the first episode, the most recent, and the most serious episode.
  - Any documentation of inconsistency between the injury and the explanation about the injury.
  - Documentation that the clinician asked about domestic violence and of the patient's response.
  - Color photograph(s) including the patient's informed consent for the photograph(s); photographs should be taken from different angles including the patient's face in at least one picture. Two pictures are necessary for each major trauma area. The photographs must be marked including the patient's name, the location of the injury, and the name of the person taking the pictures.
- If police were called, documentation about the investigating officer's name, badge number, phone number, and any actions taken.
- Documentation about the name of the PT, PTA, physician, or nurse who treated the patient (if applicable).

Data from: American Physical Therapy Association. Documenting domestic violence. Accessed April 2005, at: www.apta.org.

and expanded the 1995 Violence Against Women Act.[27] VAWA 2000 improves legal tools and programs addressing domestic violence, sexual assault, and stalking.[27] VAWA 2000 also reauthorized critical grant programs created by the original Violence Against Women Act and subsequent legislation, established new programs, and strengthened federal laws. For example, VAWA 2000 referred to the definition of dating violence as violence committed by a person who has been in a social relationship of a romantic or intimate nature with the victim. The existence of such a relationship is determined by the length of the relationship, the type of relationship, and the frequency of interaction between the persons involved. In 2013, further reauthorization legislation expanded protections to immigrants, gays, lesbians, and transgender individuals. It also expanded Native American tribal court powers to prosecute perpetrators of violence.[35]

The U.S. Department of Justice, in cooperation with the National Advisory Council on Violence Against Women and the Violence Against Women Office, educates and mobilizes the public about violence against women.[27] These organizations are asking communities to help victims of domestic violence by:[27]

- Engaging the media, community members, and educators
- Ensuring that services are available to those who seek help
- Creating campaigns with a grassroots-organized component
- Forming community partnerships
- Targeting education and awareness campaigns to young people and men
- Creating partnerships with the media so that antiviolence campaigns continue through changes in media ownership and leadership
- Complementing community service campaigns with aggressive free media campaigns
- Seeking corporate support for media campaigns
- Targeting education and awareness campaigns to populations that might not be reached via a general outreach
- Evaluating public education efforts rigorously

Legally, domestic violence can be handled in three different types of courts of law:[27]

- Criminal court, where the state will prosecute the abuser. The possible crimes include abuse of intimate partner, violation of a protection order, elder abuse, murder, rape, assault, kidnapping, false imprisonment, property destruction, vandalism, trespassing, stalking, unlawful possession or concealment of a weapon, intimidating a witness, and many others.

- Divorce or family court, where family violence directly affects divorce proceedings and can be a factor in limiting or prohibiting the abuser's rights to child custody or visitation rights.
- Civil court, where the victim can address a violation of a protection order or sue for money damages. Possible civil lawsuits include sexual harassment or personal injury.

ELDER ABUSE

Elder abuse occurs when someone knowingly, intentionally, or by negligence causes harm to an older adult. This can take the form of **physical abuse**, sexual abuse, negligence, exploitation, emotional abuse, abandonment, or not confronting an older adult's self-neglect.[33] The Elder Justice Act of 2010 established governmental authorities and funding to support Adult Protection Services in all states. Grants are available for training of staff and those who oversee elderly residential facilities in an attempt to better identify instances of elder abuse (see **FIGURE 7-3**). Because PTs and PTAs work closely with patients for extended periods of time, it may be easier for these health care professionals to recognize elder abuse. Each state has resources to assist with reporting these issues by contacting Adult Protective Services of the state in which the person resides.[33]

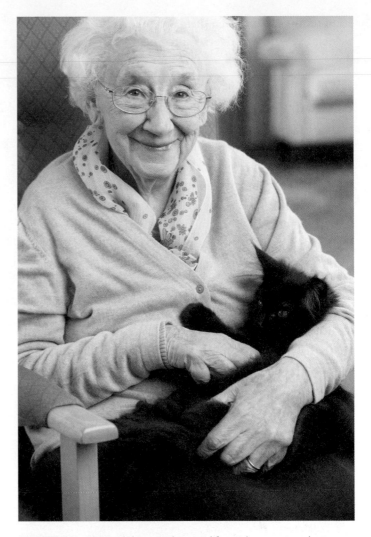

FIGURE 7-3 Older adults must be cared for with respect and concern for quality of life.
© Monkey Business Images/Shutterstock

Harassment

Harassment within the workplace can occur by supervisors, coworkers, and those who are not employees. In the case of health care environments, this can also include patient harassment of personnel.[34] Harassment is described as unwanted conduct and can be directed due to race, color, religion, sex, age, or disability. Harassment becomes illegal when it affects continued employment or is considered intimidating or hostile in nature.[34] Generally, the employee must take steps to mitigate the harassment by expressing his or her feelings to the person directly or to a supervisor. It is the responsibility of the employer to take steps to prevent harassment from occurring.[34] If these steps do not stop the harassment, a criminal case may be made.

PTs and PTAs should consider how they might address patient harassment when it occurs so that they can have a respectful but clear response. An example of this may be a request for a date by a patient. A respectful response may include that it is not legal for practitioners and patients to date. Another example may be an inappropriate comment about the health care worker. A respectful response would include that those comments are not appropriate or necessary for the clinical environment.

Malpractice Laws

Malpractice laws are civil laws derived from common laws. Health care malpractice is defined as liability-generating conduct on the part of a primary health care professional associated with an adverse outcome of patient care.

> Health care malpractice liability may include the following:[36]
>
> - Professional negligence (due to delivery of substandard care)
> - Intentional misconduct
> - Patient injury from abnormally dangerous examination/treatment-related activities
> - Patient injury from dangerously defective examination/treatment-related products

Health care professionals such as PTs can be sued by patients or their legal representatives for treatment-related health care malpractice. A PTA can also be sued, but the liability prevails with the PT of record who was the supervisor of the PTA. A settlement or an adverse judgment against a health care provider for malpractice means possibly practice-related sanctions such as licensure restrictions or licensure fines. In physical therapy, PTs are personally responsible for malpractice acts involving the relationships between the PT and the PTA (or nonlicensed personnel) and between the PT and the patient. Examples of PTs' malpractice acts can be:[36]

- Negligence
- Faulty supervision of PTAs or nonlicensed personnel
- Violation of ethical principles
- Other performances that result in harm to the patient

PTAs are also responsible for malpractice acts involving the relationships between the PTA and the patient and between the PTA and nonlicensed personnel. Examples of PTAs' malpractice acts can be negligence and performances that result in harm to the patient.

NEGLIGENCE

PTs, PTAs, and PTA students are liable for their own negligence. Negligence can be caused by failing to do what another competent practitioner would have done under similar circumstances.[36] It is the failure to give reasonable care or the giving of unreasonable care. A health care practitioner is negligent only when harm occurred to the patient/client. For example, a PTA working in the same clinic with a PT leaves a hot pack on the patient for too long without applying the necessary layers of toweling and without supervising the patient. The hot pack causes burns to the patient. The PTA is liable for negligence because he or she did not do what another PTA would have done in the same circumstances. In this situation, the PTA disregarded the following actions:

- Applying the necessary layers of toweling
- Supervising the patient closely
- Giving the patient a bell to ring if the hot pack was too hot
- Checking the treatment area every 5 minutes

The supervisory PT is also liable for negligence because of faulty supervision of the PTA. Also, PTs and PTAs can be liable for failing to perform "a duty of care," causing harm to the patient. A duty of care is an obligation of a PT or a PTA to prevent harm to the patient/client.[36] The patient/client is protected by the process known as the duty of care. This entitles the patient to safe care by making it mandatory that he or she be treated by meeting the common or average standards of practice expected in the community under similar circumstances.

To prove negligence for a breach of the duty of care, the patient/client must provide evidence that harm resulted from the breach in the duty of care. For example, in the case of the patient who was burned by the hot pack, the patient must be examined by a physician to confirm that the patient actually suffered skin burns from the hot pack.

Negligence, to be proven by the patient as the plaintiff, requires all of the following:[36]

- The health care provider, as the defendant, owed a legal duty of care to the plaintiff.
- The defendant breached, violated, or failed to comply with the legal duty of care owed to the plaintiff.
- The defendant's breach of duty of care caused injury to the person or property or other interest of the plaintiff.
- The plaintiff sustained or suffered legally cognizable damages, for which a court of law will award monetary judgment designed to make the plaintiff as "whole" again as possible.

In regard to negligence, typically the patient must show that he or she was harmed because the health care provider did something wrong or failed to do something that normally should have been done under the circumstances. For example, consider a PTA who is treating a patient who was just examined and evaluated by the PT for physical therapy (postsurgery) for a total hip replacement (THR).

The PTA disregards patient education about THR precautions. After the treatment, the patient doesn't know about THR precautions and ends up with a dislocation of the new hip and an unwanted new THR operation. In this case, the PTA failed to perform a duty of care by not educating the patient about THR precautions. The PTA caused harm to the patient and is personally liable for a malpractice act. Depending on the circumstances and the jurisdictional practice acts, the PT may also be liable for being the PTA's direct supervisor, and perhaps for not educating the patient in the initial examination and evaluation about THR precautions (and/or for not reminding the PTA to educate the patient about the precautions).

There are situations in physical therapy clinical practice when patients may contribute to their own negligence by not following directions from the PTA. For example, if the patient with a THR received education about the THR precautions but tried to perform activities on his or her own and dislocated the hip, the patient contributed to his or her own negligence. In this circumstance, the PT and the PTA have to show proof that the patient received, orally and in writing, education about THR precautions, and understood the precautions. The proof can be a written copy (that was given to the patient) of the THR precautions filed in the patient's records.

There are also situations in physical therapy clinical practice when the institution is negligent if a patient/client was harmed as a result of an environmental problem such as a slippery floor or a poorly lit area where a patient/client can fall. The institution can also be liable if the PT or the PTA was incompetent (or was not licensed) or for allowing a nonlicensed person to perform the duties of a PT or a PTA.

MALPRACTICE ACTS IN PHYSICAL THERAPY

Examples of malpractice acts involving PTs, PTAs, or PT/PTA students include the following:[36]

- Burns due to defective equipment (such as an ultrasound device)
- Utilization of defective equipment (such as wheelchairs or assistive devices)
- Patient falls during gait training
- Exercise injuries
- Any action or inaction inconsistent with the APTA's ethical principles and standards of practice

Patients have a statute of limitations of 1 to 4 years after the injury in which to make a claim. While employers provide malpractice insurance to protect their employees and businesses, individual PTs and PTAs should consider obtaining their own personal policies. This protection is necessary in instances where the employee may have violated company policy, either intentionally or inadvertently.

PTs and PTAs can be asked to testify in a court of law as expert witnesses. To be legally competent to testify as an expert witness, a witness must meet two basic requirements: (1) the expert witness must be knowledgeable concerning the health professional product or service, and (2) the expert witness must have been directly or indirectly involved with the legal standards of care for the defendant's health care discipline at the time that the incident creating the legal controversy took place.

Health care providers including PTs and PTAs should participate in legal proceedings as expert witnesses to testify on behalf of patients, peers, and others to achieve justice. Being an expert witness can be considered a civic duty, similar to voting or jury duty.

Discussion Questions

1. Identify accessibility barriers in your home, school, or other public place.
2. Discuss appropriate responses to a patient who appears to be in a relationship where domestic violence is occurring.
3. The PTA is working with a patient who has called her at her home several times to ask a question and chat. The PTA feels that the situation has become more than a health care provider/patient relationship. Discuss possible respectful responses to this situation.

Learning Opportunities

1. Using the Federation of State Boards of Physical Therapy webpage (www.fsbpt.org), locate your state's licensing board and review the laws that govern PTAs in your state.
2. Use the Internet to identify the location of the closest Adult Protective Services agency. Identify what an ombudsman does and when you should contact one.
3. Create a brochure for the physical therapy profession about malpractice issues.

Summary of Part III

Part III of the text described the differences between medical ethics and medical law. Six fundamental biomedical ethical principles were discussed concentrating on confidentiality, patients' rights, cultural competence in health care and physical therapy, and informed consent as part of a patient's autonomy. HIPAA was described in regard to the privacy rule and protected health information. The general frameworks of the APTA's ethical principles for PTs and PTAs were listed. In addition, laws affecting the physical therapy profession such as the ADA, IDEA, OSHA's rules and regulations (including the bloodborne pathogens standard), VAWA (including domestic violence), licensure laws, and malpractice laws were represented.

References (Part III)

1. American Physical Therapy Association. Standards of ethical conduct for physical therapist assistants. Accessed March 2015 at: www.apta.org.
2. U.S. Department of Health and Human Services. Health information privacy. The privacy rule. Accessed December 2009 at: www.hhs.gov.
3. American Physical Therapy Association. Summary: Standards for privacy of individually identifiable health information. Accessed March 2015 at: www.apta.org.
4. American Physical Therapy Association. Access to, admission to, and patient/client rights with physical therapy services. Accessed March 2015 at: www.apta.org.
5. U.S. Department of Health and Human Services Office of Minority Health. National CLAS standards. Accessed March 2015 at: minorityhealth.hhs.gov.
6. Health Resources and Services Administration. Maternal and Child Health National Center for Cultural Competence. Accessed March 2015 at: www.mchb.hrsa.gov.
7. U.S. Census Bureau. Projection of the size and composition of the U.S. population 2014 to 2060. Accessed March 2015 at: http://www.census.gov.
8. Black, JD. Cultural competence for the physical therapy professional. *Journal of Physical Therapy Education*. April 2002; 1–14. Accessed May 2005 at: www.findarticles.com.
9. Gabard, DL, Martin, MW. *Physical Therapy Ethics*. Philadelphia, PA: F.A. Davis Company; 2003.
10. Dreeben, O. *Physical Therapy Clinical Handbook for PTAs*. Sudbury, MA: Jones & Bartlett Publishers; 2008.
11. American Physical Therapy Association. Professionalism in physical therapy: Core ethics documents. Accessed March 2015 at: www.apta.org.
12. Swisher, L, Arslanian, L, Davis, C. The realm-individual process-situation (RIPS) model of ethical decision making. *HPA Resource*. October 2005; 1–8. Accessed July 2015 at: www.apta.org.
13. American Physical Therapy Association. Value-based behaviors for the physical therapist assistant. Accessed March 2015 at: www.apta.org.
14. American Physical Therapy Association. Integrity in practice. Accessed March 2015 at: www.apta.org.
15. Title I–V American Disabilities Act of 1990. Accessed July 2015 at: http://www.eeoc.gov/.
16. U.S. Department of Education. Building the legacy: IDEA 2004. Accessed December 2009 at: http://idea.ed.gov.
17. U.S. Department of Education, Office for Civil Rights. Free appropriate public education for students with disabilities: Requirements under Section 504 of the Rehabilitation Act of 1973. Washington, DC; 2007. Accessed December 2009 at: www.ed.gov.
18. American Physical Therapy Association. Physical therapy for individuals with disabilities: Practice in educational settings. Accessed December 2009 at: www.apta.org.
19. American Physical Therapy Association. Physical therapist and physical therapist assistant licensure/regulation HOD P05-07-09-10. Accessed December 2009 at: www.apta.org.
20. American Physical Therapy Association. Physical therapist assistant licensure. Accessed March 2015 at: www.apta.org.
21. U.S. Department of Labor, Occupational Safety and Health Administration. OSHA's role. Accessed December 2009 at: www.osha.gov.
22. U.S. Department of Labor, Occupational Safety and Healthy Administration. Nursing homes and personal care facilities. OSHA standards. Accessed December 2009 at: www.osha.gov.
23. U.S. Department of Labor, Occupational Safety and Health Administration. Section 7-VII. Regulatory impact and regulatory flexibility analysis. Accessed December 2009 at: www.osha.gov.
24. Centers for Disease Control and Prevention. Understanding intimate partner violence. Accessed March 2015 at: http://usgovinfo.about.com.
25. National Guidelines Clearinghouse, Family Violence Prevention Fund. National consensus guidelines on identifying and responding to domestic violence victimization in health care settings. Accessed December 2009 at: www.guideline.gov.
26. Ron Acierno, Melba A. Hernandez, Ananda B. Amstadter, Heidi S. Resnick, Kenneth Steve, Wendy Muzzy, and Dean G. Kilpatrick. Prevalence and correlates of emotional, physical, sexual, and financial abuse and potential neglect in the United States: The National Elder Mistreatment

Study. *American Journal of Public Health*. February 2010; 100(2): 292–297.

27. U.S. Department of Justice, Office of Justice Programs. Toolkit to end violence against women from the National Advisory Council on Violence Against Women and the Violence Against Women Office. Accessed March 2015 at: www.ncjrs.gov/index.html.

28. Coker, AL. Opportunities for prevention: Addressing IPV in the health care setting. *Family Violence Prevention and Health Practice*. 2005; 1: 1–9. Accessed April 2005 at: www.endabuse.org/health/ejournal/archive/1-1/Coker.pdf.

29. American Physical Therapy Association. Excerpts from APTA's guidelines for recognizing and providing care for victims of domestic abuse. Accessed April 2005 at: www.apta.org.

30. American Physical Therapy Association. Family violence information and resources. Accessed December 2009 at: www.apta.org.

31. Durborow, N, Lizdas, K, O'Flaherty, A, Marjavi, A. Compendium of State Statutes and Policies on Domestic Violence and Health Care. 2010. Accessed July 2015 at: http://www.acf.hhs.gov/sites/default/files/fysb/state_compendium.pdf.

32. American Physical Therapy Association. Documenting domestic violence. Accessed April 2005 at: www.apta.org.

33. National Center on Elder Abuse. Public Policy. Accessed July 2015 at: http://ncea.aoa.gov.

34. Equal Employment Opportunity Commission. Laws, regulation and guidance. Accessed July 2015 at: http://www.eeoc.gov.

35. U.S. Department of Justice. Violence Against Women Act Reauthorization 2013. Accessed March 2015 at: www.justice.gov.

36. Scott, RW. *Health Care Malpractice: A Primer on Legal Issues for Professionals*. New York: McGraw-Hill; 1999.

PART IV

Communication

This part is divided into four chapters:

Part IV of this textbook, "Communication," discusses communication in health care and physical therapy and is divided into four chapters. The chapters discuss attributes of good verbal and written communication, documentation basics and components of a medical record, and discusses the PTA's role as a teacher. An additional chapter identifies issues related to reimbursement and the understanding of research articles.

PART IV

Communication

CHAPTER 8

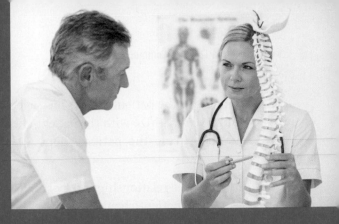

Communication Basics

OBJECTIVES

After studying this chapter, the reader will be able to:

1. Discuss the role of therapeutic communication in physical therapy.
2. Contrast empathy and sympathy.
3. Describe the significance of verbal and nonverbal communication.
4. Differentiate between verbal and nonverbal communication skills.
5. Identify the elements required to establish a therapeutic relationship with the patient.
6. Identify strategies for dealing with difficult patients.
7. Describe components of a good physical therapist/physical therapist assistant relationship.
8. Identify strategies to create trust between the physical therapist and physical therapist assistant.
9. List the eight kinds of listening skills and their importance to physical therapy.
10. Discuss effective listening skills.
11. Contrast open and closed postures.
12. Describe written communication for patients and other health care professionals.
13. Name the primary purpose of the home exercise program handout.
14. Describe the main elements of the home exercise program.

KEY TERMS

closed question
communication
empathy

open question
self-awareness
therapeutic relationship

Verbal and Nonverbal Communication

What is communication?
Communication is the most immediate tool used to interact with others.

In physical therapy, physical therapists (PTs) and physical therapist assistants (PTAs) interact with patients, clients, caregivers, and the patient/client's family. At the time of interaction, a **therapeutic relationship** is established among the PT, PTA, and patient/client. This therapeutic relationship will be highly successful if the PT and PTA convey the attitude that they:[1]

- Value the patient/client
- Are attentive to the patient/client's needs

- Acknowledge the patient/client's message
- Genuinely empathize with the patient/client
- Want to provide the patient/client with the very best care

Ideally, therapeutic relationships are partnerships among the PT, PTA, and patient/client. To achieve these partnerships and to convey positive attitudes to patients/clients, PTs and PTAs use verbal and nonverbal forms of communication.

Therapeutic Communication: Empathy Versus Sympathy

Therapeutic communication occurs when a PT or PTA interacts with a patient/client in a therapeutic or a healing manner. The communication process between the health care provider and the patient includes other elements of interaction beyond verbal and nonverbal communication factors, including the following:

- The health care provider's self-awareness, which allows communication of inner feelings, ideas, emotions, and actions between the patient and the provider
- The health care provider's total focus on the patient
- The health care provider's listening to the patient objectively without categorizing or projecting personal beliefs and values
- The health care provider's development of a trusting relationship with the patient without assuming a parental role, but conveying expertise and confidentiality

EMPATHY

The physical therapy profession can be considered a science and an art of healing. PTs and PTAs should be able to interact with patients/clients using a humanistic style of communication, placing the patient/client in a position of equality, with equal responsibility for positive outcomes in the rehabilitation process.[2] A complete therapeutic relationship between the PT/PTA and the patient/client will take place if the PT/PTA is able to understand, develop, and use the inner abilities of self-awareness and empathy in the communication process (see **FIGURE 8-1**).

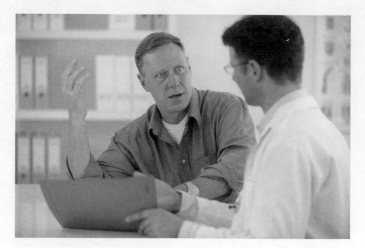

FIGURE 8-1 Interacting with the patient.
© mangostock/Shutterstock

What is empathy?

Empathy is defined as the ability to imagine oneself in another person's place and to understand the other person's feelings, ideas, desires, and actions.

As an example of empathy, it can be said that an actor or actress has empathy with the part because he or she genuinely feels and identifies with the part that is being performed. As health care providers, we genuinely feel our patient/clients' feelings, ideas, desires, and emotions. For PTs and PTAs, empathy also can be described as having the ability to understand the patient/client's health problem from within the patient/client's frame of reference.[1]

Psychologists state that to be able to feel empathy, one must have self-awareness, awareness of others, the ability to imagine, and accessible feelings, desires, ideas, and representations of actions. For example, when discussing the concept of self-awareness, the most important aspect of children's emotional development is a growing awareness of their own emotional states and the ability to discern and interpret the emotions of others. At about 2 years of age, children start becoming aware of their own emotional states, characteristics, and abilities. This phenomenon is called **self-awareness**.

The growing awareness of, and ability to recall, one's own emotional states leads to empathy, or the ability to appreciate the feelings and perceptions of others. Empathy depends not only on an individual's ability to identify someone else's emotions, but also on his or her capacity to imagine him- or herself in the other person's place and, as a result, experience an appropriate emotional response.[3]

Empathy and other forms of social awareness are important factors in the development of a person's moral sense. Moral sense or morality is an individual's personal belief about the appropriateness of what he or she does, thinks, or feels.[3] Empathy is also the result of conditioning and socialization.[3] It is possible that empathy is more important socially than it is psychologically.

The absence of empathy predisposes people to exploit and abuse others. Also, the absence of empathy means:[3]

- Emotional and cognitive immaturity
- Inability to love and truly relate to others
- Failure to respect other people's boundaries
- Inability to accept other people's needs, feelings, hopes, choices, and fears

For a health care provider, empathy depends on one's ability to put oneself in a patient's place and experience the patient's feelings of pain, anger, relief, or happiness.[3] As an example, pain can be psychologically experienced at the same time with the patient. The reason may be that the health care provider feels responsible for being there to treat the patient's condition. Thus, a learned reaction is activated and the provider experiences a form of pain as well. At that moment, this feeling is communicated to the patient and an agreement of empathy is struck between the provider and the patient.

Generally, in the relationship with patients/clients, empathy takes place in three stages:[3]

1. The cognitive stage
2. The crossing over stage
3. The coming back to own feelings stage

The first stage, the cognitive stage, involves getting into the position of the other person. This stage involves listening to the patient/client and trying to imagine what it must be like for the patient/client to experience what he or she is describing. The second stage, the crossing over stage, is the most significant because for a moment or so the PT/PTA can feel him- or herself as the patient/client, living in the patient/client's world. Then, in the third stage (coming back to own feelings stage), the PT/PTA comes back to his or her own person and feels a special alliance with the patient.

Empathy is important because it means the PT/PTA can:

- Listen better to the patient/client
- Contribute better to the patient/client's healing process
- Form therapeutic partnerships with the patient/client
- Become actively engage in the patient/client's therapeutic process
- Facilitate effective interventions by understanding the patient/client as a whole
- Involve the patient/client and his or her family/caregiver in the decision-making process
- Establish a therapeutic environment that encourages the patient/client's motivation and behavioral changes

EMPATHY VERSUS SYMPATHY

Empathy should not be considered the same as sympathy. When one has empathy for someone, they have similar feelings. When one has sympathy, they understand and have compassion for the person, but do not necessarily feel the same feelings. For example, a patient was telling me about his wife's death, which occurred 1 month earlier. As he talked about missing his wife and of his love for her, the patient's voice gradually became filled with anguish and then he burst into tears in front of me. If I felt sympathy for the patient, I would think that he was remembering his wife only with pain. I would have said to the patient, "I feel your pain." However, if I felt empathy, I would think that my patient was remembering his wife with pain and also with the joy of his love for her. I would have said to the patient, "I feel your pain and your great love for your wife."

This way of sharing the painful feelings of another person is characteristic of both sympathy and empathy. If I had only sympathy for the patient I would pay more attention to his tearful expression of pain than to the stated expression of love for his wife, whereas if I had empathy for the patient I would pay equal attention to the pain and the love. If I said to the patient, "I am sorry for your loss," this statement would convey sympathy, but not empathy. When feeling empathy I share the grieving man's emotional pain and don't just feel sorry for him. Although sympathy is also appropriate in our relationships with patients, pity is not appropriate because it is sympathy with condescension, conveying an inappropriate inequality between the patient and one's self.

The Therapeutic Relationship

The first time a PT or a PTA meets a patient, he or she has to be able to develop a rapport and a therapeutic relationship with that patient. There is no second time for making a first impression. Developing attributes of a helping professional can best be performed by imagining the behaviors that a person looks for when visiting a health care professional.

A therapeutic relationship with the patient can be established by considering the following attributes and how a PTA may behave when displaying them:

- Punctuality. It is important to be prepared for each patient and to attend to each patient in a timely fashion because it shows respect for the patient and his or her time.

- Friendliness. When initially greeting the patient, PTAs should smile and introduce themselves with their name and title. When speaking to patients, it is generally more appropriate to speak more formally. This may include calling them by their surname, rather than their first name. This formality may change after you have established a relationship, but the PTA should ask patients what they prefer to be called.

- Culturally Sensitive. In the previous chapters, cultural sensitivity was addressed and the PTA should recall how certain ethnic groups communicate in order to address the patient respectfully. For example, the PTA should be aware that some cultures differ in respect to eye contact. Many Mexican Americans and Native American Indians consider sustained eye contact when speaking directly to someone to be rude, whereas avoiding eye contact is a sign of respect.

- Communicative. The patient will expect that the PTA clearly explain in patient language the plan of care for that physical therapy session, outline the expected outcomes of the interventions, and obtain informed consent for the interventions to be performed. Informed consent involves explaining the interventions to the patient, including benefits and risks if appropriate, and receiving confirmation from the patient that the patient will participate in these interventions.

- Communication with the patient should be at the level of understanding of the individual patient. The PTA should consider the patient's age, cognitive function, and level of sensory impairment in order to explain the information appropriately. Speaking in too simplistic language may appear disrespectful to a patient whose intelligence is above that level and will be just as frustrating as the PTA speaking in medical jargon that the patient does not understand.

- Patient-Focused Behaviors. The PTA should not appear rushed or hurried while working with the patient. By focusing on the patient, the status of the patient's impairments, and the information that each member is communicating, the PTA will display respect and concern for the patient. This is an important component to building a relationship with the patient. The PTA should also remember to not become distracted. While working in a busy gym area, it may be difficult to focus energy and attention entirely on the patient, but if the PTA is constantly watching others or talking to coworkers, the relationship with the patient may suffer. The patient may believe that the PTA is not fully engaged with him or her and become distrustful or feel disrespected.

- Knowledgeable. The best way for the PTA to appear knowledgeable is to be prepared for the patient by reading the evaluation prior to interacting with the patient, asking pertinent questions of the patient, and communicating understanding of the patient's condition. The PTA should be able to answer the patient's questions. This does not mean that the PTA has to know every answer, but the PTA should always look for the answer by doing research or asking his or her supervising PT. And most importantly, the PTA must communicate his or her findings to the patient.

- Trustworthy. If the patient believes that the PTA has the patient's best interest in mind, the relationship will flourish and trust will be built. The PTA must display all of the above characteristics to develop this type of relationship.

- Helpfulness. On occasion, the PTA may be asked to perform a job or a request that is not technically part of the job. An example of this would be filling an acute care patient's water glass. Helpfulness is not forgotten by the patient. The patient remembers that the PTA went out of his or her way to do something nice for him or her and this will help to build rapport.

- Comfortable. The therapeutic relationship will develop rapidly if both the patient and PTA feel comfortable with each other. In order to develop a comfort, the PTA should be able to have a conversation with the patient. While the focus of the relationship is based on the patient's impairments, casual conversation will help to develop rapport. Talking to the patient about his or her family, occupation, or daily events in the community helps to deepen the relationship and will bring more satisfaction to both the patient and the PTA. When the PTA shows interest in the patient as a person, the PTA displays caring and compassion, which are attributes expected in a therapeutic relationship.

On occasion, the PTA may encounter patients that are not interested in forming a therapeutic relationship. The patient may sabotage the relationship by being tardy for appointments, cancelling repeatedly, or by making rude comments. While it may be human nature to return rudeness to the patient, it will do nothing for the relationship in the long run and is generally considered to be poor customer service.

Here are some strategies for dealing with difficult people. First, stay calm. When a patient or coworker becomes upset, it is easy to become upset, defensive, or reactionary. The best policy is to continue interacting in a respectful manner. The PTA should not be short or abrupt with the patient or display irritation. The PTA may need to ignore the comment or redirect the patient back to the intervention that is occurring. Secondly, focus on trying to solve the problem. The PTA should start by listening carefully to what the person is saying. In the process of listening, the PTA may come up with a strategy to alleviate the issue and even if the problem cannot be fixed, the patient usually feels better that someone at least listened

and tried to help. And lastly, try to let go of things you cannot control. Difficult people cannot always be helped, but it does not have to direct how the PTA acts or functions. For example, if the patient is continually refusing his or her treatment, the PTA should encourage the patient to participate, explain the consequences of not completing the rehab program, and inform the PT of their efforts. If the patient still refuses, then the PTA should understand that they did what they could and the patient has the right to make choices that may not seem to be in the patient's best interest.

The Physical Therapist and Physical Therapist Assistant Relationship

The relationship between the PTA and the patient is critical, but there is another relationship that requires just as much attention in order to provide effective physical therapy services. That is the relationship between the PT and the PTA. Depending upon the setting, a PTA may have one or more supervising PTs and each PT may have certain expectations and preferences for patient care. It is important that the PTA and the PT create a team that is based on understanding, trust, honesty, and effective communication (see **FIGURE 8-2**).

Each member of the team will come with varying degrees of understanding as to what his or her role is on the team. This will depend upon their education and tenure in their position. A new graduate PT may not have had an opportunity to work with a PTA previously. If the PTA has many years of experience, it is important that they learn about each other personally, but also professionally.

The following topics should be explored by the team members to help promote unity:

- Education: The first step in creating the team would be to understand the education of each member. This would include their initial physical therapy degree and should include a discussion of specific skills that are taught. Additionally, continuing education courses should be discussed to help each other understand their skill set beyond entry-level education.
- State Laws: The PT and PTA must both have the same understanding of state statutes and have a plan for the implementation of the laws and administrative rules.

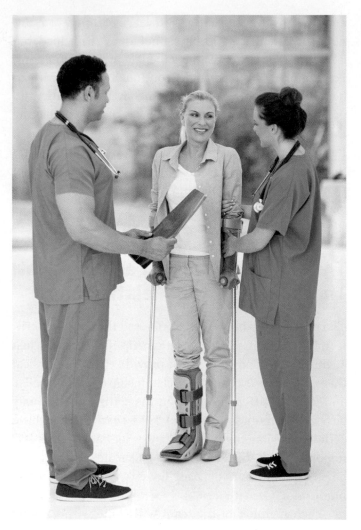

FIGURE 8-2 PT/PTA relationships require effective communication.
© michaeljung/Shutterstock

Because laws can vary from state to state, it is critical that the team abide by the current state in which they are practicing physical therapy.

- Professional and Ethical Aspects of Care: The APTA has a variety of documents that assist the PT/PTA team in understanding their role in providing quality care. The Minimum Required Skills of Physical Therapist Assistant Graduates at Entry-Level document and the Standards of Ethical Conduct for the Physical Therapist Assistant document are available from www.apta.org.[4] PTA supervision guidelines and algorithms may also assist the team in creating a plan for teamwork.
- Personal Attributes: Each member of the team will have strengths and weaknesses; it can be helpful for those to be explored and understood by each team member. An understanding of the expectations of each

member can alleviate misunderstandings and disappointment that can interfere with trust.

The APTA has recently released the Physical Therapist–Physical Therapist Assistant Team Toolkit. This electronic document is intended as a way to educate others on the importance of this relationship, but it contains valuable information that could also be utilized by a newly formed PT/PTA team.[4]

Types of Communication Forms

The two main communication forms are verbal and nonverbal.

- Verbal or oral communication uses messages conveyed orally from a sender to a receiver.
- Nonverbal communication uses messages conveyed through methods other than orally or in writing. It is divided into two groups, communication through body language and communication through facial expression including gestures and eye contact.

DEFINING VERBAL COMMUNICATION

Verbal communication is a significant part of physical therapy clinical practice, just as it is in other health care professions. The reasons for verbal communication may include:[1]

- To establish a rapport with the patient/client and/or the patient/client's family/caregiver
- To enhance the relationship among the patient/client, his or her family/caregiver, and the PT/PTA
- To obtain information concerning the patient/client's condition and progress
- To transmit pertinent information to other health care professionals and providers and supportive personnel
- To provide education and instructions to the patient/client and patient/client's family/caregiver
- To increase the patient/client's adherence to education and the continuum of care at home
- To decrease the patient/client's health risks

Cultural Diversity and Verbal Communication

From a cultural diversity perspective, problems in verbal communication may arise when the PT or the PTA and the patient/client bring two completely different world-views, languages, or backgrounds to the interactions. As the therapist interacts with patients/clients from diverse cultures, his or her individual norms of verbal communication may differ and clash with theirs. The therapist may form inappropriate judgments about the patient/client and create barriers to communication and effective patient/client care. The therapist's ethnocentrism and decreased cultural competence may cause verbal communication problems. For example, many people in the United States are uncomfortable with periods of silence and tend to associate it with a person being inarticulate or ineffectual. In contrast, African Americans often value silence and nonverbal communication. They also are often very spiritual. When in the company of strangers they can be private about their family matters.[1] Navajo Indians often appreciate long periods of silence, understanding an attentive, silent listener to be communicating interest. Asian Americans also can appreciate silence. They may verbally communicate with the therapists by agreeing with certain information in order to "save face" and not to be considered offensive.[1]

PTs and PTAs must be knowledgeable about cultural issues, especially when interacting with patients/clients and their families/caregivers who have a different cultural background and/or limited English proficiency. A patient/client's limitations in English are no reflection of the patient/client's level of intellectual functioning or his or her ability to communicate in the native language.

Familial colloquialisms, such as specific informal expressions, used by the patients/clients or their families/caregivers can also affect verbal communication in the physical therapy examination, evaluation, assessment, and interventions. Some patients/clients from other cultures prefer to use verbal communication as an alternative to written communication when receiving information about a home exercise program or certain treatment precautions. Considering linguistic cultural competence, PTs and PTAs must attempt to learn and use key words in the language of their patients/clients to be able to better communicate with them in clinical settings. Verbal communication must be presented in very different ways to be effective in different situations. In addition, consideration must be given to the patient/client's:[1]

- Health beliefs
- Health perceptions
- Attitudes
- Level of education

Health care professionals have a tendency to use family members, friends, or volunteers to communicate with patients/clients from other cultures. Doing so may present a risk of breaching patient privacy and confidentiality and not receiving necessary information from the patient/client (especially if it is sensitive). Also, filtering of information through family, friends, or volunteers can be clinically detrimental to patients/clients and can lead to malpractice problems for the PT/PTA. For example, a PT asked a patient from Russia (who was being treated for back pain), as a contraindication of treatment, if she was pregnant or trying to become pregnant. The patient stated to her American cousin in her native language: "No, no, it is impossible for me to become pregnant since I am not married." In reality the patient was more than 2 months pregnant, but she did not want her cousin to know the truth. Ultimately, this presented a negative clinical outcome for the patient and a malpractice liability for the PT. A trained medical interpreter could have circumvented such a problem. Professional interpreters are a better solution than family, friends, or volunteers.

Professional interpreters can provide culturally sensitive and high-quality language assistance services to ensure proper understanding on both sides of the medical equation. In physical therapy, the same as other areas of health care, top-quality interventions cannot be provided without effective communication. Optimal communication enhances patient satisfaction, improves outcomes, and provides greater patient/client safety. Addressing language barriers in health care must be an integral part of physical therapy efforts.

Verbal Communication Success

For health care providers, the success of verbal communication is dependent on the following factors:[5]

- The way the material is presented, including the provider's vocabulary, the clarity of voice and purpose, and the organization of the material

- The attitude of the provider
- The tone and the volume of the provider's voice
- The degree to which the patient/client listens, including the patient's mental status

During the verbal interaction, the health care provider must ensure understanding of the patient's goals immediately after meeting the patient by focusing on the patient's information and by asking questions. The material provided to the patient must be presented taking into consideration the patient's age, the presence of a language barrier, the degree of the patient's anxiety, and the level of the patient's understanding.

The health care provider's vocabulary should be precise and accurate, and contain terms understandable to the patient. For example, if the provider uses technical jargon, the technical terms can be very confusing to the patient. Also, the patient may feel that the provider is disinterested and does not empathize with him or her. The health care provider must speak clearly and concisely in a normal tone of voice. The tone and volume of voice are qualities that health care providers must be constantly aware of, especially when delivering unpleasant news to a patient. Any procedure or intervention has to be verbally explained to the patient in a logical manner, step by step, accompanied by written instructions, diagrams, or nonverbal demonstrations.

- The PTA should speak clearly in moderate tones and vary his or her tone of voice as required by the situation. PTAs should show enthusiasm, but should not be too energized as to sound or appear distractible.
- The PTA should pause in order to allow the patient to understand what the message is trying to convey. Speaking too quickly may make it difficult for the patient to comprehend the information.
- The PTA should be sensitive to the patient/client's level of understanding and cultural background.
- The PTA should explain and repeat directions as needed by the patient. Signs of irritation or frustration can be heard in the tone of voice. Responding with patience and smiling will help decrease patient anxiety and assist the patient in understanding more fully.
- The PTA should be aware that when a person feels uncomfortable or unsure, they add word fillers such as "um" or "ok." If the PTA repeatedly says the same thing to a patient, while it may be intended to be encouraging, it may sound insincere. An example is repeatedly giving praise, such as "good job" after every activity that the patient completes.

Recommendations for verbal communication:

- The PTA's verbal commands should focus on the most important aspects of the desired action for treatment.
- The PTA's instruction should remain as simple as possible and must never incorporate confusing medical terminology.
- The PTA should detail to the patient/client the general sequence of events that will occur prior to initiating treatment.
- The PTA should ask the patient/client questions before and during treatment in order to establish a rapport with the patient and to provide feedback as to the status of the current treatment.

Delivery of Verbal Communication

Verbal communication can be delivered to a patient/client through the following channels:

- Face-to-face discussions in which the PT/PTA imparts the desired meaning to the patient/client; in addition, the patient/client can ask questions. It is considered the best delivery method of verbal communication in health care.
- Telephone discussions in which the PT/PTA can interact with the patient/client; however, confidential patient/client medical information should not be discussed over the telephone.
- Group discussions in which the PT/PTA can communicate the same messages to a group of patients/clients; however, the message is not personalized because the patient/client's medical information is confidential.

Group discussion can be used in physical therapy for group exercise programs.

- Third-party discussions where the PT/PTA can communicate with the patient/client through another person (such as a family member or a caregiver). This method is limited in regard to delivering the intended meaning and by medical information confidentiality status (unless the family member is legally a personal representative of the patient/client).

EFFECTIVE AND INEFFECTIVE LISTENING AND QUESTIONING

Effective Questioning Strategies

In order to understand a patient, the PT/PTA must learn to ask questions in a way that assists in getting the information needed to perform clinical decision making. There are two types of questioning strategies: closed and open. Closed questioning asks for short factual answers. An example of a **closed question** would be: Do you have pain today? The answer could be a simple "yes" or "no." Open questioning asks the person to give a more detailed answer. An example of an **open question** would be: What types of activities are difficult because of your pain? The patient could give short answers, but the question lends itself to a more lengthy answer that will provide the PT/PTA with more clear information upon which to make clinical decisions. Many times a PT/PTA will use closed questions that lead them to more open questions that allow them to increase their understanding. The reader should be cautioned not to lead the patient in questioning, however. An example of a leading questions would be "Does that hurt?" rather than "How does that feel?" The patient may not have considered that he or she may feel pain and shouldn't be led to wonder if that was a possibility. Appropriate questioning will allow the PT/PTA to gain information that is necessary for effective patient interaction.

Effective Listening in Verbal Communication

Effective listening is meaningful in health care for a variety of reasons, including:

- To clarify information that the patient just explained to the provider
- To reflect on the patient's message and the feeling it implied

- To summarize the message the patient sent to the provider

In general, there are eight kinds of listening:[5]

- Analytical listening: Used for a specific type of information and for arranging the information in categories; an example in physical therapy would be listening to the patient's description of pain.
- Directed listening: Used for the patient's answers to specific questions; an example in physical therapy would be listening to the patient's answers about the activities and positions that increase or decrease his or her pain.
- Reflective listening: Used to clarify what the patient said; an example in physical therapy would be listening to the patient explain why a task is difficult to perform and then the PTA repeating their understanding of what they heard to clarify that they understand the patient.
- Exploratory listening: Used when a person's own interest in the subject is being discussed; an example in physical therapy would be the patient listening to the PT's recommendations of positioning techniques in sleeping to decrease the pain or the PT asking the patient specific questions about the patient's pain.
- Appreciative listening: Used for esthetic pleasure; an example would be listening to music.
- Attentive listening: Used for general information to get the overall picture of the patient; an example in physical therapy would be a PTA listening to the PT's specific recommendations for a patient's treatment.
- Courteous listening: Used when feeling obligated to listen; an example would be listening to a story the patient is describing even if it has no relevance to the patient's examination and treatment.
- Passive listening: Used when not being attentive to the matter discussed but overhearing the conversation; an example would be a patient in a hospital bed listening to the other patient's conversation in the next bed.

Generally, analytical, directed, and attentive listening can provide some relevant information about the patient to be included in the patient's documentation. Exploratory listening can provide the most relevant information about the patient (see **FIGURE 8-3**).

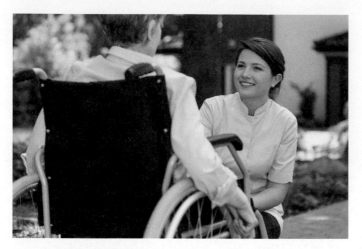

FIGURE 8-3 Listening to the patient.
© Photographee.eu/Shutterstock

The Purposes of Effective Listening

In the health care field, effective listening is the primary skill used when interacting with the patient/client. It is also a pathway for engaging in a therapeutic relationship with the patient/client, building trust, and fostering the patient/client's cooperation for treatment. In physical therapy, effective listening as a communication tool can help with the following:

- To gain better knowledge about the patient's problem(s)
- To receive better cooperation from the patient and patient's family
- To solve problems in regard to the patient's plan of care and interventions
- To encourage trust and build a therapeutic relationship between the patient and the therapist
- To improve the patient's treatment by encouraging continuous feedback from the patient

In addition, the health care provider's effective listening skills help to gain higher-quality information from the patient, save time, solve problems, and reduce and prevent medical errors. Contrarily, poor listening creates misunderstandings, wastes time, and allows for mistakes. In the health care profession, mistakes have the potential for grave effects on the lives of patients.

Methods of effective listening:

- The PT/PTA focuses his or her attention on the patient.

- The PT/PTA helps the patient to feel free to talk by smiling and looking at the patient.
- The PT/PTA pays attention to the patient's nonverbal communication such as gestures, facial expressions, tone of voice, and body posture.
- The PT/PTA asks the patient to clarify the meaning of words and the feelings involved or to enlarge the statement.
- The PT/PTA repeats the patient's message to completely understand the meaning and the content of the message. Reflective listening allows the PTA to clarify what the patient has stated and the patient can then correct any misperceptions.
- The PT/PTA takes notes as necessary to help remember or document what was said.
- The PT/PTA uses body language such as nonverbal gestures (leaning forward, nodding the head, keeping eye contact, or keeping hands at his or her side) to show involvement in the patient's message.
- The PT/PTA does not abruptly interrupt the patient and thus gives adequate time to present the full message.
- The PT/PTA empathizes with the patient.

Effective listening is a skill that can be learned and practiced by a health care provider. Effective listening requires effort, honesty, commitment, and perhaps changing one's behavior and becoming more compassionate and empathetic.

Ineffective Listening Habits

The following are ineffective listeners' habits that need to be changed, particularly when working in the health care field:

- Ineffective listeners typically listen on and off. Most people think four times faster than another person can speak, and they have too much time to think about their own affairs and concerns. To overcome listening on and off, a PT/PTA must pay attention to a patient's nonverbal communication such as gestures, eye contact, hesitation, or tone of voice.

- Ineffective listeners typically listen to words, ideas, or opinions. They prejudge the message being conveyed rather than listening to all of the information and then making a response, rather than an emotional reaction. When the PTA is effectively listening, he or she can respond calmly and with empathy.
- Ineffective listeners consider the patient boring (and not saying anything new). They may not listen if the patient is describing his or her symptoms or problems in detailed accounts. Many times a patient can express the same message over and over in regard to his or her health. This message can be significant in the patient's examination, assessment, and treatment. Also, some patients may need to explain detailed accounts of their symptoms or the effects of their treatments. To overcome wrong assumptions about the patient, a PT/PTA should listen intently to the patient's entire message (even if it was the same), and if the message is too complicated, should ask clarifying questions.
- Ineffective listeners are absorbed in their own thoughts and often daydream when another person is speaking. Daydreaming is usually a sign of tiredness and loss of concentration. To overcome daydreaming, a PT/PTA must try to take a short break from work, rest a few minutes, go back to the task, concentrate again on his or her work, and continue to listen carefully and intently to the patient.
- Ineffective listeners have favorite ideas, prejudices, and points of view that can be challenged or overturned by the patient. When that happens, the PT/PTA becomes defensive with the patient. To overcome this, the PT/PTA must respond to the patient constructively and have respect for the patient's point of view to maintain the therapeutic relationship between the PT/PTA and the patient.

Ineffective listening skills may cause ineffective treatment of the patient that can lead to fewer referrals, poor documentation that can lead to denial of payment, and poor customer satisfaction that can lead to a poor reputation of care. Appropriate listening skills must be practiced and become as important to effective care as any hands-on physical therapy skills.

DEFINING NONVERBAL COMMUNICATION

Nonverbal communication is communication through body language and facial expression including gestures and eye contact. Other types of nonverbal communication are a person's physical characteristics including clothing and grooming. In regard to physical characteristics, people sometimes inadvertently stereotype others, showing preferences for attractive people who are well dressed and well groomed. Clean clothing that fits well and good grooming can make a proper impression to a prospective employer as well as to a new patient/client. The newly hired PT should use the other employees in the department as a guide for the expectations of the employer and the patient population. The way a PTA presents him- or herself can contribute to his or her success relating to a patient/client and an employer.

The PT and the PTA should also consider that nonverbal communication varies and holds different meanings in different cultures. The receiver of nonverbal communication brings his or her own cultural understandings and expectations to the interaction. In addition, the cultural perspective complicates the interaction and opens wide the potential for miscommunication and misunderstanding.

Body Language

Body language includes a person's postures and gestures that convey messages from a sender to the receiver and from a receiver to the sender. The sender sends the message, and the receiver receives the message. Body language reveals a person's inner character and emotions. Open postures convey a person's willingness to receive a message.

Open postures can be any of the following:

- A person's standing or sitting with arms at his or her sides and legs uncrossed
- A person's standing or sitting straight
- A person's standing or sitting positioned at the same eye level with the receiver
- A person as a receiver facing the sender

Closed postures convey a person's unwillingness to receive a message (see **FIGURE 8-4**). Closed postures can be a person's standing or sitting with arms and legs crossed, being slumped over, or as a receiver turned away from the sender. Crossed arms in front of the body and crossed legs convey a closed posture that either does not allow others to send messages or that indicates superiority. Arms crossed in front of the body also display a defensive posture and that the listener is not ready to receive messages. If the receiver is turned away from the sender this shows that the receiver is avoiding communication by trying to distance her- or himself from the sender.

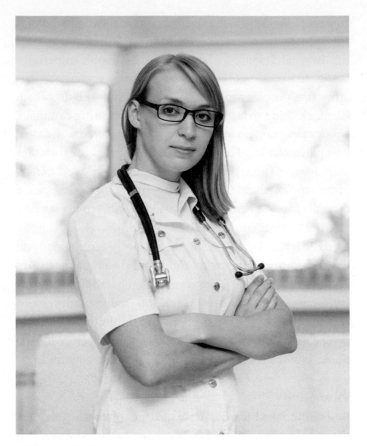

FIGURE 8-4 Closed posture.
© Ermolaev Alexander/Shutterstock

Facial expressions including gestures and eye contact can convey acceptance or rejection of thoughts and ideas presented. Acceptance of thoughts and ideas can be conveyed through a smile, by nodding, or by direct eye contact. Rejection of thoughts and ideas can be conveyed by rolling the eyes, looking up or down or away from the sender, shaking the head, or frowning.

Eye contact generally communicates a positive message. If two people want to communicate well, they will position themselves so that they can look into each other's eyes (depending on the people's culture). If a person stands while the other sits, the one who stands has subconsciously placed him- or herself in a position of authority. As health care providers, when communicating with patients, it is crucial to be at the same eye level with the patient. For example, if the patient sits in a wheelchair, the health care provider should stoop down when communicating with the patient (see **FIGURE 8-3**).

A person's body language, especially facial expressions, can communicate a genuine interest in the patient and the patient's goals, concerns, ideas, and needs. Eye contact is also significant, especially while listening to a patient/client. Looking directly in someone's eyes (without staring) can also convey honesty and decision-making capability. However, prolonged eye contact (such as staring) communicates disagreement and anger.

Health care providers may use gestures such as a comforting touch to relax a patient and to show caring and dedication to the patient. In physical therapy, touch is significant when guiding the patient in the correct performance of physical therapy activities and exercises.

Physical touch communicates a diversity of meanings across cultures. It can also be a powerful communicator of respect or disrespect and can hurt or heal. For example, a homeless patient may not have been physically touched in a long time or may have experienced harmful contact rather than a loving or respectful touch. In addition, physical touch requires special considerations across genders and diverse cultures. For example, Arab-Muslim cultures place a high value on female modesty, and it would be inappropriate for a male PT to touch the patient or even to begin an initial examination without asking permission from the patient, the patient's husband, or the patient's family. Health care providers including PTs and PTAs must remember how important nonverbal communication is, especially when interacting with patients/clients from other cultures.

DEFINING WRITTEN COMMUNICATION

Written communication represents a form of communication using messages conveyed in writing from a sender to a receiver. Written communication is used by health care providers to convey messages to patients/clients and provide information in medical records.

Written Communication Given to the Patient/Client

In physical therapy, written messages to patients/clients can reinforce verbal instructions to perform activities or exercises by including additional information, can be informed consent documents, or can be surveys to obtain data about the quality of physical therapy services rendered to the patient. Written communication allows the reader to control his or her pace of understanding the material. For patients/clients from other cultural backgrounds, all written communication must be in their language of origin.

Specific guidelines for written communication that is given to the patient/client include:[1]

- Write the information the same way you talk to the patient/client.
- Use an active voice.
- Use short sentences and common words.
- For complicated words, give examples.
- Include interaction by adding a short question and asking the patient/client to write his or her answer; this adds to the patient/client's active involvement in his or her treatment (and helps with adherence).

Examples of interaction methods for the information given to the patient/client include:[1]

- Writing a short question and asking the patient/client to write his or her answer
- Asking the patient/client to circle his or her best choice of one or two exercises from three or four pictures of exercises
- Asking the patient a few questions verbally about his or her exercises after the patient/client has read his or her written home exercise program handout

Home Exercise Program Handouts

The content of the written communication must be well organized, concise, and in layman's terms. For example, in physical therapy, written handouts for exercises or activities, called home exercise program (HEP) handouts, must be specific about the number of repetitions, the amount of exercise resistance (such as 1- or 2-pound weights), and the positions for performing the exercises or the activities. Physical therapy written handouts must have diagrams or pictures and the contact information of the PT or the PTA.

The primary mission of an HEP handout is to impart useful, actionable information to the patient/client or the patient/client's family. The words on the paper have to make complete sense to the patient. Also, the information should be consistent with the therapist's verbal explanations and demonstrations to the patient or caregiver. The handout must represent an extension of the treatment plan of care.

The HEP starts on the first day of treatment and continues to the day of discharge. If a caregiver is involved in the patient's treatment, the caregiver needs to participate early in the program to allow an easier transition when going home. The written materials should be developed in the primary language of the patient and should be short.

Technical terms and jargon must be avoided, and short sentences should be used as much as possible. For example, complex words, such as achieve, utilization, inflammation, or indication, could be replaced with simple ones, such as do, use, redness, or sign.

In relation to the written form, each sentence should present only one idea and contain no more than one three-syllable word. Lines of copy are suggested to be no more than 5 inches wide, and the type size should be 12 points or larger. To accommodate patients who may have vision deficits, the handouts should have a high contrast between the foreground and background and include large amounts of blank space on the page.

The HEP handouts should be written at the fifth-grade reading level. The exercises in the HEP handouts must be sorted in a logical manner so that the patient does not have to change positions too much, such as lying face up, then sitting in a chair, then again lying face up.

The exercises have to be simple and very clear. Writing in a conversational style implies that the material was written directly to the patient. Uncomplicated drawings may supplement the written instructions, indicating frequency, duration, number of repetitions, and the method for progressing through the exercises.

Lengthy and complicated exercise routines will discourage a patient's continuing participation. Providing the least amount of exercises needed increases the chance of a patient complying with the program. The therapist's presentation of the information constitutes another important element for the success of an HEP. For example, showing enthusiasm and interest when presenting the instructional material demonstrates concern for the patient and a degree of sensitivity to his or her needs. The element of verbal instruction and a good relationship with the patient could substantially enhance the effectiveness of a home program. A teaching aid such as the HEP handout is useless if not presented within the context of the total process of patient education and rehabilitation.

Written Communication to Health Care Professionals or Payer Sources

Written communication that is intended for other health care professionals or payer sources must be written in more formal language than that used with patients. It should avoid the use of informal language, abbreviations, slang, and should be more declarative in nature. The use of medical language is expected in this case and oversimplification of terminology should be avoided. The communication should be straightforward with its purpose clearly stated and any requests of the reader stated. If the purpose is information sharing or points are to be made, the writer should have a clear organization of the data and not embellish the communication with unnecessary information.

An example of formal written communication to another health care professional:

June 15, 2015

Dear Dr. Jones,

Your patient, John Smith, has been receiving physical therapy services for low back pain. A trial of mechanical traction has proven to benefit his pain and radiculopathy in the left lower extremity. He has been able to return to work; however, he has return of pain after 2 days. Continued use of traction will allow the patient to self-manage his pain and functional abilities. We are requesting a prescription for a home lumbar traction unit. Please contact me for any additional information.

Sincerely,

Mary Brown, PTA

Discussion Questions

1. Discuss personal experiences with health care workers and create a list of attributes or behaviors that are positive and negative.

2. Create a list of communication strengths and weaknesses that you have.

3. Create three closed questions and then convert them to open questions. Create three leading questions and then convert them to exploratory questions.

Learning Opportunities

1. Using the following skits, practice effective listening skills and reflective communication that conveys the PTA's understanding of what the patient stated.
   a. The patient is explaining how she fell down the stairs and broke her leg.
   b. The patient is describing where his pain is and what makes it better or worse.
   c. The patient is explaining the difficulty that she has taking care of her child after hurting her back.
   d. The patient describes in great detail what he did over the weekend that made his shoulder pain worse.

2. With a partner, create a paper airplane. After completing the task, analyze how you communicated during the task. Identify the attributes of a team that you displayed and if one or more partners became the leader. Compare this to how you might interact within a physical therapy team.

3. Interview a PT/PTA team and identify strategies that they employ to help them work cohesively.

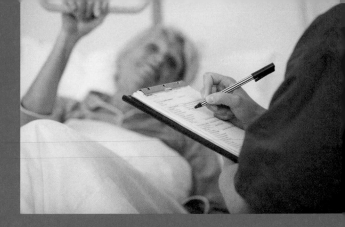

CHAPTER 9

Introduction to Documentation and the Medical Record

© racom/Shutterstock

OBJECTIVES

After studying this chapter, the reader will be able to:

1. Describe the significance and the purpose of the physical therapy medical record.
2. Identify the American Physical Therapy Association's guidelines in regard to physical therapy documentation.
3. Discuss documentation elements of the initial examination (including the patient history), visit/encounter reports, progress reports, and discharge reports.
4. Define the SOAP mnemonic and its meaning.
5. List the standardized titles and names used in physical therapy.

KEY TERMS

assessment data
functional outcome report (FOR)
objective data
problem-oriented medical record (POMR)
sign

SOAP format
source-oriented medical record (SOMR)
subjective data
symptom

Medical Records

Written communication is used by health care providers in medical records including medical documentation. In physical therapy, documentation is considered the foundation for communication between third-party payers and the providers of physical therapy services.[6]

Why do we need physical therapy documentation?

- For reimbursement
- For assurance of quality care
- For assurance of continuity of care
- For legal reasons
- For research and education
- For marketing

DOCUMENTATION FOR REIMBURSEMENT

Documentation provides the basis for coverage decisions by third-party payers. The clinical intervention must show through documentation the physical therapy clinical decision making involved, providing the necessary rationale to support the interventions.[6] To ensure reimbursement, the documentation must describe physical therapy effectiveness, showing evidence of the patient's improving functional abilities. When reading the documentation, the third-party payer is assured that physical therapy services were cost-effective and carried out by a skilled practitioner.

DOCUMENTATION FOR ASSURANCE OF QUALITY CARE

Documentation of physical therapy services provided to the patient and the patient's response to interventions is important for communicating with the physical therapy team to ensure quality care.[6] Through documentation, the members of a physical therapy team can define a patient's problems, outline the plan of care, identify barriers to recovery, and describe goals for efficient and skilled physical therapy interventions. Review of medical records can also analyze the quality of care offered to the patient (also called quality assurance).[6] Quality of care ensures a therapist's compliance, a department's efficiency and effectiveness of care, and a patient's accomplishment of functional outcomes.

DOCUMENTATION FOR CONTINUITY OF CARE

Physical therapy documentation also guides physical therapists (PTs) and physical therapist assistants (PTAs) in the intervention's outcomes and goals and establishes a communication tool among PTs, PTAs, and other health care providers who are members of the rehabilitation team. The continuity of care is reflected in physical therapy documentation through descriptions of the patient's responses to intervention and the modifications of intervention as necessary.[6]

DOCUMENTATION FOR LEGAL REASONS AND RESEARCH/EDUCATION

Legal aspects of documentation are considered in the events of lawsuits or malpractice issues by providing objective evidence of physical therapy care performed for the patient.[6] Documentation also provides useful information to researchers and educators. Accurate data from clinical practice can be objectively analyzed to determine the effectiveness of physical therapy services. Evidence-based research through clinical practice is a significant tool used in the advancement of physical therapy education as well as the progress of the physical therapy profession.

DOCUMENTATION FOR MARKETING

Documentation can also be an important marketing tool because it includes descriptions of successful functional outcomes achieved by the patient and the skilled and efficient quality of care offered to the patient.

THE AMERICAN PHYSICAL THERAPY ASSOCIATION'S DOCUMENTATION GUIDELINES

The following are the American Physical Therapy Association's (APTA) documentation guidelines:[2]

- The documentation must be consistent with the APTA's Standards of Practice and all jurisdictional and regulatory requirements.
- Every visit/encounter requires documentation.
- All documentation must be legible and use medically approved abbreviations or symbols.
- All documentation must be written in black or blue ink, and the mistakes must be crossed out with a single line through the error, initialed, and dated by the PTA.
- When utilizing electronic health records, security measures to ensure patient confidentiality must be utilized.
- Each intervention session must be documented; the patient's name and identification number must be on each page of the documentation record.
- Informed consent for the interventions must be signed by a competent adult. If the adult is not

competent, the consent must be signed by the patient/client's legal guardian. If the patient is a minor, the consent must be signed by the parent or an appointed guardian.

■ Each document must be dated and signed by the PT/PTA using their first and last names and their professional designation. Professional license number may be included, but it is optional.

■ All communications with other health care providers or health care professionals must be recorded.

■ PT students' notes should be co-signed by the PTs.

■ PTA students' notes should be co-signed by the PTs and/or PTAs.

■ Nonlicensed personnel notes should be co-signed by the PT.

■ Documentation of referral sources or self-referral should occur within the initial documentation.

■ Cancellations and no-shows should be documented.

Data from American Physical Therapy Association. APTA Governance. Terminology. Accessed February 2006, at: www. apta.org.

Types of Medical Records

Physical therapy documentation can be written using different types of medical records. The most-used include POMR and SOMR.

PROBLEM-ORIENTED MEDICAL RECORDS

Physical therapy documentation uses a **problem-oriented medical record (POMR)**, which was introduced in health care in the 1970s by Dr. Lawrence Weed. POMR is a method of establishing and maintaining the patient's medical record so that problems are clearly listed in order of importance, and a rational plan for dealing with them is stated.[6]

The sections of the POMR may include the following:

■ Data

■ Problem list

■ Intervention plan

■ Progress notes

■ Discharge notes

Each section contains the appropriate information from each discipline. The data included in the POMR are kept at the front of the chart and are evaluated as frequently as indicated with respect to recording changes in the patient's status as well as progress made in solving the problems. Using the POMR, health care facilities can create comprehensive medical records containing information from each discipline. This method enhances communication between health care providers, ultimately helping with the patient's care.

The advantages of POMR include provision of organization and structure of the medical information, chronological description of interventions, a specific plan for managing the patient's problems, and the improvement of communication between health care providers.

SOURCE-ORIENTED MEDICAL RECORDS

The **source-oriented medical record (SOMR)** is another type of organization method for medical records. An SOMR is arranged in accordance with the medical services offered in the clinical facility.[6] Some hospitals use SOMRs by labeling a section in the chart for each discipline with a tab marker. The first section of the SOMR is the physician's section, followed by sections for nursing, pharmacy, dietary, social services, physical therapy, occupational therapy, speech and language pathology, and test results.[6] The health care providers from each discipline document their content in the section designated for their discipline. The SOMR format is criticized by some health care providers because it is difficult to read through each section for information.

SOAP RECORDS

Medical records written in the **SOAP format** were also created by Dr. Weed as a component of the POMR.[6] SOAP is an acronym for an organized structure to keep the progress notes in the chart. Each entry contains the date, patient's identification number, and the title of the patient's particular problem followed by the SOAP headings.

The SOAP headings represent the following:

■ *Subjective findings:* Information provided by the patient or patient's family/caregiver

(continues)

- *Objective findings:* Results of tests, measurements, and interventions
- *Assessment:* Overall response to interventions and the effects of interventions, changes in patient status, and the health care provider's opinion about the patient's progress
- *Plan:* The plan for further diagnostic or therapeutic action or for the next intervention session

The beginning of a SOAP organized note can identify the discipline's diagnosis or problem and should be placed in the problem list section of the POMR.

Types of Physical Therapy Documentation Reports

Physical therapy uses four types of documentation reports:

- Initial evaluation report
- Visit/encounter treatment notes
- Progress reports
- Discharge reports

INITIAL EXAMINATION/EVALUATION REPORT

The initial examination and evaluation report constitutes the foundation of all other reports that follow, such as visit/encounter notes, progress reports, and discharge reports.[6] Through the initial evaluation report, the PT establishes the primary purpose for intervention and outlines the expectations for progress.

The initial examination and evaluation report can be written in the SOAP format, a narrative format, or another format. Because the POMR format does not focus on the patient's functional limitations but mostly on the patient's impairments, some PTs prefer to use a different type of format called the **functional outcome report (FOR)** in the initial examination report.

The FOR format follows a sequence of information different from the SOAP format. The FOR format is more appropriate in an initial examination report because it includes such elements as the reason for referral, the patient's functional limitations, physical therapy assessment, therapy problems, functional outcome goals, and intervention plan and rationale.[6] The FOR format is becoming popular in physical therapy because it can easily demonstrate the effect of impairments on functional limitations, and it is relatively uncomplicated for reviewers.

Initial Examination and Evaluation Report Elements

The initial examination and evaluation report may contain the following elements:[6]

- Referral, including the reason for referral and the specific treatment requested by the referral source
- Data accompanying the referral, including the primary diagnosis (or onset date), secondary diagnoses, medical history, medications, and other complications or precautions
- Physical therapy history, including the patient's date of birth, age, gender, start of care, and the primary complaint
- Referral diagnosis, including the mechanism of injury and the prior diagnostic imaging (or testing)
- Prior therapy history
- Evaluation data, including the patient's cognition, vision, hearing, vital signs, vascular signs, sensation and proprioception, coordination, balance, posture, pain, edema, active range of motion (AROM) and passive range of motion (PROM), strength, bed mobility, transfers, ambulation (level and stairs), wheelchair uses, orthotic/prosthetic devices, durable medical equipment used or needed, activity tolerance, special tests, architectural considerations, requirements to return to prior activity level (including work, school, or home), outcome measures data, and wound description (for wound care, including the incision status)
- Prior level of function, including mobility at home and in the community, employment, or school
- Treatment diagnosis
- Assessment, including the reason for skilled care
- Problems
- Plan of care, including specific intervention strategies, frequency, duration, patient instruction/home

program, caregiver training, short-term goals and dates of achievement, long-term goals and dates of achievement, and patient's rehabilitation potential

Patient History

Patient history is part of the initial examination and evaluation. As described in the examination and evaluation section in Chapter 4, patient history refers to a complete medical history of the patient's chief complaints, present illness, past history, allergies, current medications, lifestyle and habits, social history, vocational and economic history, and family history. The history is taken in an orderly sequence, keeping the patient focused while discouraging irrelevant information (see **FIGURE 9-1**). Patient history can include the following documentation elements:[6]

- Personal information, including patient's age, gender, and occupation
- Medical diagnosis and any precautions related to physical therapy
- Patient's chief complaint, including the patient's description of his or her condition, the reason for seeking assistance, and identification of the patient's primary problem
- Patient's present illness, including the symptoms associated with the patient's primary problem such as location of the problem (may use a body chart), severity, nature (such as aching, burning, or tingling), persistence (constant versus intermittent), and aggravated by activity versus relieved by rest
- Onset of the patient's primary problem including mechanism of injury (if traumatic), sequence and progression of symptoms, date of the initial onset and status up to the current visit, prior treatments and results, and associated disability
- Patient's past history, including prior episodes of the same problem; prior treatments and responses; other affected areas (or body parts); familial, developmental, and congenital disorders; general health status; medications; and x-rays or other pertinent tests
- Patient's lifestyle, including the patient's profession or occupation, assistance from family or friends, occupational and family demands (spouse, children, job expectations), activities of daily living (hobbies, sports), and the patient's concept of the impact of functional (including cosmetic) and socioeconomic factors

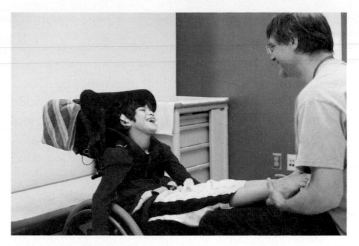

FIGURE 9-1 Child with PT.
© Jaren Jai Wicklund/Shutterfly

TREATMENT NOTES

Treatment notes (written by the PTs and/or PTAs) are generally short, depending on the format and frequency of the report, the practice setting, the patient type, and the payer involved. As is done with the initial evaluation report, the treatment notes must include the patient's full name, date of birth, medical records number, and room number. The information in the treatment notes can be written as SOAP notes or as narrative format notes.

The SOAP notes also follow the sequence of data organization corresponding to subjective, objective, assessment, and plan. The narrative format notes vary. However, the narrative format notes must be organized properly and have consistency in describing comparisons between treatments. The SOAP notes are used the most in physical therapy for treatment notes.

PROGRESS REPORTS

Progress reports are written by the PTs and provide documentation of the continuum of care to justify the skilled physical therapy services rendered.[6] The focus of progress reports is on reevaluation of problems identified in the initial evaluation or any other new problem that developed since the last formal reevaluation. The progress reports need documentation describing the skilled interventions, the complicating factors that affected the duration of skilled care, and the comparative data from the initial evaluation or the last reevaluation. The format of a progress report varies; however, it must contain the following general elements:[6]

- Attendance
- Current baseline data, including patient's cognition, vision, hearing, vital signs, vascular signs, sensation and proprioception, coordination, balance (sit and stand), posture, pain, edema, AROM and PROM, strength, bed mobility, transfers, ambulation (level and stairs), wheelchair utilization, orthotic/prosthetic devices, durable medical equipment used or needed, activity tolerance, special tests, architectural considerations, requirements to return to prior activity level (including work, school, or home), and wound description (for wound care and including the incision status)
- Treatment diagnosis
- Assessment, including the reason for skilled care
- Problems
- Plan of care, including specific treatment strategies, frequency of treatment, duration of treatment, patient instruction/home program, caregiver training, short-term goals and dates of achievement, long-term goals and dates of achievement, and the patient's rehabilitation potential

DISCHARGE REPORTS

Discharge reports are the last of the four types of reports used in physical therapy. Per APTA requirements, they are written by the PT and describe the success of physical therapy services provided.[6] The essential elements of a discharge report include the following:

- Attendance
- Current baseline data, including patient's cognition, vision, hearing, vital signs, vascular signs, sensation and proprioception, coordination, balance (sit and stand), posture, pain, edema, AROM and PROM, strength, bed mobility, transfers, ambulation (level and stairs), wheelchair use, orthotic/prosthetic devices, durable medical equipment used or needed, activity tolerance, special tests, architectural considerations, requirements to return to prior activity level (including work, school, or home), outcome measures data, and wound description (for wound care, including the incision status)
- Treatment diagnosis

- Assessment, including the reason for skilled care
- Problems
- Plan of care, including specific intervention strategies, frequency of treatment, duration of treatment, patient instruction/home program, caregiver training, short-term goals and dates of achievement, long-term goals and dates of achievement, and discharge prognosis

SOAP Writing Format

The SOAP-format reports are used the most in physical therapy practice. They can be written daily or weekly.

VISIT/ENCOUNTER SOAP-FORMAT REPORTS

The daily or weekly SOAP-format reports can be written by the PT or the PTA.

The SOAP format data can be used as follows:

- By the PT to write the initial examination and evaluation reports
- By the PT to write the reexamination and reevaluation progress reports
- By the PT and the PTA to write their visit/encounter progress notes

---

The SOAP initial examination and evaluation reports are written by the PT during the initial examination and evaluation. The SOAP reexamination and reevaluation reports, called progress reports, are written by the PT periodically throughout the time the patient is receiving physical therapy. The visit/encounter SOAP progress notes are written by the PT or the PTA on a daily basis. The PT is also responsible for the discharge examination and the discharge evaluation reports, which are the patient/client's final examination and evaluation. The APTA considers the establishment of the discharge plan and documentation of the discharge summary/status the responsibility of the PT, and not the PTA. However, the laws in various states may differ. The PTA can write a SOAP note (called a discharge summary) summarizing the care a patient received in his or her last physical therapy intervention, without any reexamination and reevaluation (interpretation of the data), as well as write the post-discharge plan of care.

SUBJECTIVE DATA IN SOAP-FORMAT REPORTS

As stated earlier, the SOAP mnemonic stands for **s**ubjective, **o**bjective, **a**ssessment, and **p**lan. The S section at the beginning of the SOAP note contains the **subjective data**, and includes information provided by the patient or the patient's family. The subjective data also include any pertinent information regarding physical therapy that the patient's family and the patient's caregiver offer. Every time the patient is seen in physical therapy, he or she is interviewed about his or her chief complaint(s). The complaints causing the patient to seek medical help are called symptoms and are included in the subjective part of the SOAP note.

Patient's Symptoms

- A **symptom** is any change in the body or its functions perceived by the patient.

- A symptom represents the subjective experience of a disease. Some frequent examples of patients' symptoms in physical therapy are pain, stiffness, weakness, numbness, and loss of equilibrium.

- Elements of the patient's symptoms (in the SOAP note) may include the date when the symptoms occurred, the location of the symptoms, the manner in which they occurred, aggravating or relieving factors, the severity, and any associated symptoms.

PHYSICAL THERAPY DIAGNOSIS VERSUS MEDICAL DIAGNOSIS

When using the POMR format, the patient's problems are listed (and numbered in certain facilities) prior to the subjective section of the SOAP note. The patient's medical diagnosis is different from his or her physical therapy diagnosis.

The patient's medical diagnosis is the identification of the cause of the patient's illness or discomfort. A medical diagnosis is determined by a physician's evaluation and

diagnostic tests. The medical diagnosis is equivalent to the patient's pathology.

As per the *Guide to Physical Therapist Practice*, physical therapy diagnosis is the clinical classification by a PT of a patient's impairments, functional limitations, and disabilities.[7] As per the International Classification of Impairments, Disability, and Handicaps (ICIDH) developed by the World Health Organization, physical therapy diagnosis also represents the data obtained by physical therapy examination and other relevant information to determine the cause and nature of a patient's impairments, functional limitations, and disabilities.[7] For example, for a musculoskeletal problem, a patient's medical diagnosis could be "right hip fracture." The physical therapy diagnosis, in contrast, could be "transfer and gait dependency." A patient's difficulties with transfers and a patient's dependency on assistive devices while walking represent the patient's impairments and functional limitations. For a neurologic problem, a medical diagnosis could be "multiple sclerosis." The physical therapy diagnosis could be "ataxic gait and frequent falling." A patient's difficulties, such as lack of muscular coordination while walking and frequent falling, represent patient impairments and functional limitations.

SUBJECTIVE DATA IN PROGRESS SOAP-FORMAT NOTES

The subjective data in the progress SOAP note include information about the patient and the patient's condition that is described to the PT or the PTA by the patient or a representative of the patient. Subjective information must be relevant to the patient's physical therapy diagnosis and treatment plan. As a result, the subjective information must not include all the patient's complaints but just the condition(s) relevant to the physical therapy diagnosis/ prognosis and intervention plan.

To include relevant information in the subjective section, the PTA needs to use active, directed, attentive, and exploratory listening. For example, to write about the subjective data, the PTA can use verbs such as states, reports, and says. Also, the patient can be directly quoted, especially in regard to a patient's attitude about physical therapy or descriptions of activities that the patient can or cannot perform. When the subjective information is provided by someone other than the patient, the PTA must document the name of the person who provided the information and the person's relationship to the patient.

Pain information can be located in the subjective or objective part of the SOAP note. As the patient describes the pain to the PT/PTA it would be reported in the S section. If a standardized tool such as the McGill Pain Questionnaire is used, the information may be more appropriately documented in the O section. The documentation location should be consistent within the practice so that all personnel working can locate the information easily. The description of pain must be illustrated by the patient. It can be depicted in some form of a pain profile using pain scales, a checklist of descriptive words, or body drawings.

The subjective data may include the following:[6]

- Patient's complaints of pain
- Patient's response to the previous intervention
- Patient's description of functional improvements, such as being able to do activities of daily living (ADLs)
- Patient's lifestyle situation, such as being able to go out to dinner or entertain friends like he or she used to do before this condition
- Patient's goals, such as to be able to drive his or her car in 2 to 3 weeks
- Patient's compliance or difficulties with the home exercise program (HEP)

The SOAP examination note written by the PT in the initial examination and evaluation (or reexamination) is much more detailed than the visit/encounter progress SOAP note written by the PT and the PTA during physical therapy interventions. The initial examination SOAP note includes, in addition to the patient's complaints, information about the patient's medical history, environment, emotions and attitudes, level of functioning, and goals.

An example of a subjective part of the progress SOAP note for a patient who had a right total knee replacement 4 weeks ago might be:

S. Patient reports that for the past weekend she was able to walk (using the cane) in her home up and down five stairs, three times/day without her right knee buckling.

Other examples of subjective information in the progress note may include:

- Patient described having numbness and tingling in the back of her left leg down to her calf.
- She said that she was diagnosed with herniated disc of her back last year.
- Patient rates his pain in his right arm and shoulder at 6 with movement and 2 without movement.
- She said: "I need to get better fast and be able to go to work as a secretary."
- He denies any discomfort in his back while sitting at his desk.
- Patient stated that he had the car accident on February 15, 2015.

OBJECTIVE DATA IN SOAP-FORMAT NOTES

The O section of the SOAP note contains the objective data. The **objective data** are information that can be reproduced or confirmed by another health care provider with the same training as the one gathering the objective information.

Patient's Signs

The health care provider includes in the objective section of the SOAP note the signs of the patient's disease or dysfunction. A **sign** is objective evidence or a manifestation of an illness or disordered function of the body.[6] Signs are apparent to observers whereas symptoms may be obvious only to the patient/client.[6]

A sign can be seen, heard, measured, or felt by the diagnostician. Finding of such signs can be used to confirm or deny the diagnostician's impressions of the disease suspected of being present. An example of a sign in physical therapy would be the patient's gait pattern such as flexed posture and shuffling gait (as in Parkinson's disease).

In physical therapy, the objective part of the SOAP note also contains the patient's treatment session.

OBJECTIVE DATA IN PROGRESS SOAP-FORMAT NOTES

The PTA should write the objective data of the progress SOAP note considering that another PTA may need to reproduce or continue the intervention, and that a reader untrained in physical therapy (such as an insurance representative or a lawyer) may determine the effectiveness of the treatment session.

> The objective section in the progress SOAP note may contain the following:[6]
>
> - The results of the physical therapy measurements and tests, such as manual muscle testing, goniometry, gait assessment, and specific neurologic assessments (such as balance, sensation, or proprioception)
> - The description of the interventions provided to the patient, such as physical agents and modalities, therapeutic exercises, wound care, functional training (such as gait using assistive devices), patient education/instruction (such as postsurgery precautions), and discussion and coordination with other disciplines (such as occupational therapy practitioners who want to give the patient a shoehorn to be able to put his or her shoes on)
> - The description of the patient's function, such as performing transfers, gait (with or without assistive devices, on even or uneven surfaces and stairs), or bed mobility (such as turning from supine to side-lying to sitting)
> - The PTA's objective observations of the patient during interventions (such as the increase in the number of exercise repetitions), tests and measurements (such as compensating for muscular weakness), and patient education/instruction (such as understanding the HEP on the first performance)

Data about visual or tactile observations such as posture or palpation reassessments performed by the PT or the PTA are also included in the objective part of the SOAP note. Additionally, other data such as written copies of the home exercise program (HEP) are found in the objective section of the SOAP note.

The objective information of the progress SOAP note must include the following:[6]

- Description of the reason(s) for intervention and the intervention provided to the patient. These data must include enough detail that another PT or PTA could read the description and replicate the intervention. Documentation should not be repetitive of the previous treatment note, but should include rationale for changing the intervention. For example, descriptions of why therapeutic exercise was progressed, a modality was discontinued, or observable changes in functional status of the patient will indicate patient progress.
- Description of the patient's response to each intervention. These data are important for the PT/PTA to be able to replicate or change the intervention to obtain the most effective patient response. The PT/PTA should not write what he or she did regarding the intervention (such as "Applied moist hot pack to the patient's lower back"). Instead, the PT/PTA should write the patient's response to the moist hot pack (such as "Patient had decreased muscular spasm of right erector spinae at L2–L4 level after application of moist hot pack to the muscles for 20 minutes while the patient was in prone position").
- Description of tests/measurements after interventions. These data are significant because by repeating tests and measurements that were performed in the initial examination, the PT/PTA can describe the results by relating them with the initial examination findings. Outcome measures are standardized assessments that identify functional outcomes and help to establish the progress toward the outcomes that were established during the evaluation. Periodic assessment of the patient's progress will help to determine if the physical therapy is successful.
- Medicare also requires specific reporting under the Physician Quality Reporting System (PQRS). This reporting requirement is for payment of specific interventions and varies by diagnosis. The APTA website has updated information for current guidelines that usually change annually.[8]
- Utilization of words that describe the patient performing a function. Descriptions of the quality of a patient's movement define the patient's true ability to complete

functional tasks and develop the reader's visualization of the patient's functional status.

■ Logical organization of information. These data can give the reader a clear image of the patient's interventions and progress.

■ Utilization of words that portray skilled physical therapy services. Documentation should include specific decision-making rationale that relates the impairment and functional limitation to the intervention that no one other than the PT or PTA could provide.

■ Inclusion of copies of any additional written information (such as exercises and/or patient education material) that was given to the patient for home use.

The objective data of the initial examination and evaluation (or reexamination) SOAP note (written by the PT) are more complex than the objective information of the progress SOAP note (written by the PT and the PTA). The data in the initial examination SOAP note may contain the following information:[6]

■ Patient's cognitive status, communication, and judgment

■ Patient's musculoskeletal findings, such as range of motion, strength, or posture

■ Patient's neurologic findings, such as pain, reflexes, or sensation

■ Patient's cardiovascular findings, such as blood pressure, pulse, respiration, or endurance

■ Patient's functional status, such as transfers, mobility, ADLs, or work/school activities

■ Patient's outcome measure data

Example of Objective Information in Progress SOAP Notes

An example of an objective part of the progress SOAP note for a patient who had a right total knee replacement 4 weeks ago might be:

O. Patient performed: 10 minutes stationary bicycle; closed kinetic chain (CKC) strengthening exercises standing at the wall and bending right knee 10 times, 3 sets with 1-minute rest between sets; sitting in a chair, strengthening exercises for right knee extension, using 3-pound weight around right ankle,

10 repetitions, 3 sets with 1-minute rest between the sets; standing and holding onto the back of the chair, strengthening exercises for right knee flexion, using 3-pound weight around right ankle, 10 repetitions, 3 sets with 1-minute rest between the sets; long sitting ice pack for 10 minutes to right knee; patient sitting reassessed for right quadriceps strength using manual muscle test (MMT): is 4/5.

Other examples of objective information in the progress note may include the following:

■ Patient transferred partial weight bearing (PWB) on right lower extremity (RLE) from bed to w/c and back with maximum assist of one for strength and balance, and with verbal cuing for PWB status.

■ Blood pressure (BP) 140/90; pulse 95 beats per minute (BPM), irregular.

■ Active range of motion (AROM) of right shoulder flexion 0° to 115°.

■ Patient performed self-stretching exercises, three repetitions, to increase right shoulder flexion and abduction with elevation, sitting, and sliding the right arm on the table.

■ The diameter of the wound from the right to the left outer edge is 5 cm today compared to 6.2 cm on 9-27-15.

ASSESSMENT DATA IN SOAP-FORMAT NOTES

The A section of the SOAP note contains the **assessment data**, which represent a summary of the information from the subjective and objective sections of the SOAP note. The assessment is one of the most important sections of the SOAP note because it tells the reader whether physical therapy is helping the patient.

In the assessment section, the PTA discusses the patient's response to intervention and the effectiveness of the intervention, and also comments about the patient's progress/lack of progress toward the goals established by the PT in the initial examination and evaluation. Also in the assessment section, the PTA remarks about the patient's progress toward the patient's own goals as expressed by the patient in the subjective section of the SOAP note. (These goals are tied in with the intervention and the reassessment data from the objective section of the SOAP note.)

All comments in the assessment section of the progress SOAP note must be supported by evidence from the subjective and objective sections' data. During the interventions, the patient's reassessments are conducted by the PT or the PTA on a regular basis and are documented in the objective assessment section of the SOAP note to determine the effectiveness or lack of effectiveness of the interventions.

The assessment section may contain the following:[6]

- Patient's overall response to intervention, such as decreased pain, improved range of motion, or improved gait pattern
- Patient's progress toward short- and long-term goals (from the PT's initial evaluation)
- Explanations as to why the interventions are necessary
- Effects of interventions on the patient's impairments and functional limitations
- Comparison of patient's abilities from previous date to current date

---

When interpreting the data in the assessment section of the SOAP report, the PTA (or the PT) should avoid the following documentation errors:

- Making undetermined general comments about the patient's condition or progress, such as "patient is walking better today" or "patient tolerated treatment well."
- Describing the patient's progress without showing evidence in the subjective and objective sections of the SOAP note.
- Overlooking meeting the patient's short- and long-term goals (from the initial examination and evaluation).

The assessment data of the initial examination and evaluation (or reexamination) SOAP notes (written by the PT) are more complex than the assessment information

in the progress SOAP note. The data may contain the following:[6]

- Analysis of the problems and plan of action (including summary of impairments, functional limitations, and disabilities)
- Short-term goals that can be accomplished in 2 to 3 weeks from the start of the intervention
- Long-term goals that are functional goals (written in functional terms) that can be accomplished in 4 to 5 weeks (or longer) from the start of the intervention

Example of Assessment Information in Progress SOAP Notes

An example of the assessment part of the progress SOAP note tying in information from the subjective and the objective sections of the SOAP note for a patient who had a right total knee replacement 4 weeks ago might be:

S. Patient reports that for the past weekend she was able to walk (using the cane) in her home up and down five stairs, three times/day without her right knee buckling.

O. Patient performed: 10 minutes stationary bicycle; closed kinetic chain (CKC) strengthening exercises standing at the wall and bending right knee 10 times, 3 sets with 1-minute rest between sets; sitting in a chair, strengthening exercises for right knee extension, using 3-pound weight around right ankle, 10 repetitions, 3 sets with 1-minute rest between the sets; standing and holding onto the back of the chair, strengthening exercises for right knee flexion, using 3-pound weight around right ankle, 10 repetitions, 3 sets with 1-minute rest between the sets; long sitting ice pack for 10 minutes to right knee; patient sitting, reassessed for right quadriceps strength using manual muscle test (MMT): is 4/5.

A. Patient is progressing in physical therapy: tolerated increased weight to 3 pounds with strengthening exercises; patient met short-term goal #1 to ascend and descend five steps independently; right knee scar is red and healing.

Other examples of assessment information in the progress note may include:

- Strengthening exercises were effective in increasing patient's strength by 1/2 of MMT grade. Patient met his short-term goal #1 to transfer from sit to stand independently.
- Patient was consistently using proper body mechanics and using the leg muscles while lifting.
- Patient needed frequent verbal cues for total hip replacement (THR) precautions to maintain right lower extremity (RLE) in abduction while transferring from bed to w/c.
- Patient is not progressing toward goal of independence in ambulation for 50 feet with standard walker (SW).

All of these data need to be supported by the subjective and objective information in the note.

PLAN DATA OF SOAP-FORMAT NOTES

The P section of the SOAP note contains the plan. The plan data of the progress SOAP note contain information that the PTA may need to apply regarding the patient's interventions before and during the treatment session(s) or between the sessions. They also indicate when the next session will take place or how many sessions are to be scheduled. The plan section of the progress SOAP note uses verbs in the future tense. PTAs should avoid meaningless and nonspecific documentation, such as "continue with current plan of care."

The plan section may contain the following:[6]

- Plan for next treatment session, including justification for continued care
- Plan for consultation with another discipline
- Frequency of the treatment
- Plan for reevaluation or discharge by the PT
- Plan to discuss with the PT changes in the patient's condition, introduction of new exercises, or specific patient goals or complaints

The plan data of the initial examination and evaluation (or reexamination) SOAP note written by the PT are more complex than the plan information in the progress SOAP note written by the PT and the PTA. The examination SOAP note contains information about the specific intervention plan for the patient's identified problem(s) and the frequency and duration of the interventions.

An example of a plan part of the progress SOAP note for a patient who had a right total knee replacement 4 weeks ago could be:

P. Will continue with therapeutic exercise and increase repetitions and weights next session to improve patient's ability to independently transfer in and out of his bed; will start neuromuscular reeducation using proprioception exercises next session to improve balance during transfers.

Other examples of plan information in the progress note may include the following:

- Will discuss with the PT the possibility of adding self-stretching exercises as an HEP.
- The PT will see the patient next visit for reassessment.
- Will order a rolling walker to be available for next treatment session on 10-25-15.
- Will do gait training on stairs next visit to allow patient to return home.
- Next visit will increase the weights to 5 pounds in PRE-strengthening exercises to allow patient to lift objects above his head at work.

Legal Issues in Documentation

In physical therapy, documentation guidelines should specifically comply with the jurisdictional requirements, regulatory requirements, and insurance company (including Medicare/Medicaid) requirements.

General guidelines applying to physical therapy documentation are:[6]

- The patient's right to privacy should be respected regarding written information in the SOAP examination and evaluation, reexamination and reevaluation, and the SOAP note.

- The release of the medical information, including written physical therapy documentation, must be authorized by the patient in writing.

- All inquiries for medical information to the PTA should be directed to the supervising PT.

- Written physical therapy records should be kept in a safe and secure place for 7 years.

In physical therapy documentation, verbal communication is used in telephone conversations regarding the following:

- Verbal referrals for physical therapy treatment from other health care providers
- Receiving information about the patient from the patient (or the patient's representative)
- Receiving inquiries about the patient's medical condition or treatment from different persons

When a PTA verbally takes a telephone referral from another health care provider, the PTA needs to document in writing the following:[6]

- The date and time of the call
- The name of the person calling and the name of the health care provider who referred the patient
- The name of the PTA who took the referral
- The name of the patient and all other details in regard to the referral
- The date when a written copy of the referral will be sent to the physical therapy office/ department
- The name of the PT who will be responsible for the referred patient

In addition, PTAs may receive calls about changes in a patient's condition. These calls also need to be documented in writing regarding the date and time of the call, the name of the person calling, the name of the PTA taking the call, and a summary of the conversation. If it is an emergency situation, the PTA should direct the caller to call 911 or the nearest hospital's emergency department.

Standardized Titles and Names Used in Physical Therapy

The physical therapy profession has created a standardized terminology for consistency in titles identifying professionals' areas of expertise.[2] This terminology is recognized by the APTA. The following paragraphs define the uniform terminology that should be used for physical therapy:[2]

- When the acronym APTA is used in public relations and marketing, it should be used in conjunction with the title American Physical Therapy Association.
- The APTA supports the use of PT as the regulatory designation of a physical therapist. Other letter designations such as RPT, LPT, or academic and professional degrees should not be substituted for the regulatory designation of PT. PTA is the preferred regulatory designation of a physical therapist assistant.
- The APTA supports the recognition of the regulatory designation of a PT or a PTA as taking precedence over other credentials or letter designations. To promote consistent communication of the presentation of credentials and letter designations, the APTA recognizes the following preferred order:
  - PT/PTA
  - Highest earned physical therapy–related degree
  - Other earned academic degree(s)
  - Specialist certification credentials in alphabetical order (specific to the American Board of Physical Therapy specialties)
  - Other credentials external to the APTA
  - Other certification or professional honors (e.g., FAPTA)
- The APTA supports the designations SPT and SPTA for PT students and PTA students, respectively, up to the time of graduation. Following graduation and prior to licensure, graduates should be designated in

accordance with state law. If state law does not stipulate a specific designation, graduates should be designated in a way that clearly identifies that they are not licensed PTs or licensed or regulated PTAs.

- The APTA is committed to promoting the PT as the professional practitioner of physical therapy and promoting the PTA as the only individual who assists the PT in the provision of selected physical therapy interventions. The PT is responsible for the patient and patient/client management. The PTA makes changes in selected interventions only to progress the patient as directed by the PT and to promote patient safety and comfort. The APTA is further committed to incorporating this concept into all Association policies, positions, and program activities, wherever applicable.
- The term *professional*, when used in reference to physical therapy services, denotes the PT. The practice of physical therapy is conducted by the PT.
- The PTA is a technically educated health care provider who assists the PT in the provision of physical therapy.
- The PTA is an educated individual who works under the direction and at least general supervision of the PT. The PTA is the only individual who assists the PT, in accordance with the APTA's policies and positions in the delivery of selected physical therapy interventions. The PTA is a graduate of a PTA education program accredited by the Commission on Accreditation in Physical Therapy Education (CAPTE).
- The APTA uses the term *physical therapist professional education* to refer to the basic education of the PT to qualify him or her to practice physical therapy, and the term *physical therapist post-professional education* to refer to the advanced physical therapy educational studies undertaken by a PT to enhance his or her professional skills and/or knowledge. The term *professional*, when it is used in reference to physical therapy services, denotes the PT.
- Only PTs may use or include the initials PT or DPT, and only PTAs may use or include the initials PTA in their technical or regulatory designation. Additionally, the APTA supports the inclusion of language to protect the exclusive use of these terms, titles, and designations in statutes and regulations.

Defensible Documentation

PTs and PTAs should be aware that defensible documentation is an intrinsic part of contemporary physical therapy clinical practice. PTs have been continuously seeking to integrate the latest evidence into their practices. The evidence can include better tests and measures, new and improved equipment, new theories of disease pathology, and more efficient interventions.[9] Consequently, the evidence-based practice needs to be documented using researched clinical guidelines and approved physical therapy protocols. Third-party payers, other health care providers, and consumers expect this form of documentation from physical therapy providers.[9]

PTs have a large role in creating effective defensible documentation. They should include documentation that:[9]

- Reflects the PT's decision-making process
- Indicates evidence of the PT's unique body of knowledge and skill
- Provides the PT's verification of his or her professional judgment

PTAs should work closely with PTs to help facilitate the patient/client's functional outcomes using evidence-based interventions. This can be accomplished by evaluating and discussing with the PTs current research from journal articles and reviews regarding evidence-based interventions. The APTA's website, PT Now Article Search, Hooked on Evidence, and the Physical Therapy Outcomes Registry provide literature review for evidence-based interventions.

The APTA recommends the following tips for documentation that reflects evidence-based care:[9]

- PTs should incorporate valid and reliable tests and measures as appropriate.
- PTs and PTAs should keep up to date with current research through journal articles and reviews, and the APTA's PT Now and Hooked on Evidence website.
- PTs should include standardized tests and measures in the clinical documentation.
- PTs and PTAs should review and incorporate evidence-based interventions into clinical physical therapy.

Computerized Documentation

Computer-based documentation is rapidly becoming the norm in physical therapy facilities. While not compelled to utilize electronic health records (EHRs), regulations are changing that may require physical therapy to utilize computerized systems in the next few years. Documentation systems can run on desktop computers, notebook or laptop computers, touchscreen computers, and personal digital assistants (PDAs) see **FIGURE 9-2**. Notebook computers and PDAs both allow the PT/PTA to enter information while performing examinations/evaluations, assessments, or interventions with the patient. Wireless communication also allows the PT/PTA to instantly retrieve the patient's record electronically. The benefits of computerized documentation include the following:

- Submitting information to insurance companies electronically
- Monitoring the clinician's productivity

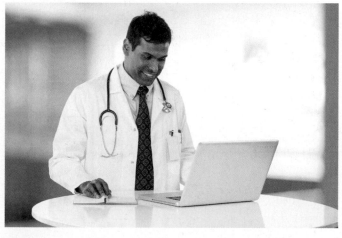

FIGURE 9-2 Electronic records are becoming commonplace in health care.
©Stuart Jenner; Shutterstock, Inc.

- Tracking patients' visits
- Easing patient scheduling
- Minimizing documentation paperwork
- Integrating billing
- Maximizing efficiency
- Increasing reimbursement
- Improved communication between health care teams[10]

Discussion Questions

1. Describe the six reasons that documentation is required and discuss how those reasons are related.
2. Utilizing the APTA website, locate the *Defensible Documentation for Patient/Client Management* webpage. Discuss the components of appropriate documentation and the common errors made that can lead to payment issues.
3. Watch a classmate complete a functional task, such as picking up an object from the floor or putting on his or her coat. Write a descriptive paragraph of the activity. Within a group, analyze how effectively the information would fit into the observation section of a SOAP note.

Learning Opportunities

1. Create a reference sheet for what information goes into each section of the SOAP note.
2. Create a list of pros and cons of electronic medical records.
3. Interview a PTA in clinical practice about the challenges of documentation in today's reimbursement environment.

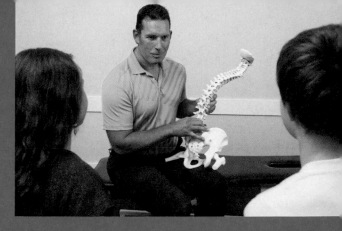

CHAPTER 10

Teaching and Learning

OBJECTIVES

After studying this chapter, the reader will be able to:

1. Discuss the teaching and learning aspects of physical therapy.
2. Describe patient education methods for people who have difficulty reading, for patients who are older adults, for patients who have visual and hearing impairments, for patients who cannot speak English, and for patients from other cultures.

KEY TERMS

learning
teaching

Communication Methods for Teaching and Learning

Teaching and learning are important patient education processes that take place during physical therapy interventions. Patient education or patient instruction is considered an essential aspect of health care delivery. Physical therapists (PTs) and physical therapist assistants (PTAs) must be able to assess the patient/client as the learner, understand his or her learning needs, and also provide a suitable teaching and learning environment. **Teaching** involves planning the process of imparting information and then implementing the plan. **Learning** involves a change in the learner that creates understanding of information, changes in behavior and attitude, and the desire to utilize the information to help make life decisions.

TEACHING

In general, teaching means explaining and supplying information to the learner. Teaching also involves building the learning environment to help make it conducive to learning.

PTs and PTAs may be involved with academic teaching at colleges, universities, and other technical institutions, as well as clinical teaching. Clinical teaching or clinical instructional activities can take place with patients/clients and the patient/clients' family and caregivers, and PT/PTA students. Teaching opportunities involving health care teaching are important to provide communities with information on specific conditions and interventions or health prevention topics. Examples might include speaking about appropriate exercise to members of a local Multiple Sclerosis Society or providing a training session for Certified Nursing Assistants on appropriate patient transfers to protect their backs.

In order for learning to occur, good teaching attributes should be present. First, the teacher should be enthusiastic about the topic. Teaching and learning should be fun so it is important that the teacher show that he or she enjoys talking about the topic. Secondly, the teacher should have the knowledge of his or her topic. For clinical instruction, PTs and PTAs generally know the information well enough that they do not need to prepare; however, when creating in-services for other health care providers or presentations for the public, it is best to perform research to organize and present the information well. Lastly, the teacher should employ appropriate feedback and cueing to the learner. In the beginning, the teacher should encourage the learner with appropriate praise, such as "You're doing great!" or "Keep going, you're getting it!" While the PT/PTA often acts as the patient's cheerleader at this stage, it is important to be aware that not every patient action requires praise, and repeating the same phrase over and over loses its motivating power. Likewise, if the teacher is attempting to cue a mistake or refinement of movement, he or she should use words that encourage as well as correct. An example of this would be, "If you contract your trunk muscles before you squat, you will get better control of your leg movements." Or "Look in the mirror as you are lifting your arm in the air, what do you see?" These types of statements don't focus on the patient being wrong, but the statements do allow them to correctly move and assist the patient in self-awareness and self-correction (see **FIGURE 10-1**).

Clinical Instructional Activities

In physical therapy, PTs and PTAs teach patients/clients:

- Information to help improve the patient/client's ability to manage acute and chronic conditions
- Information for prevention, wellness, and opportunities for healthier lifestyles
- Material regarding exercises for reducing the effects of impairments/functional limitations
- Methods for active involvement in the patient/client's physical therapy plan of care

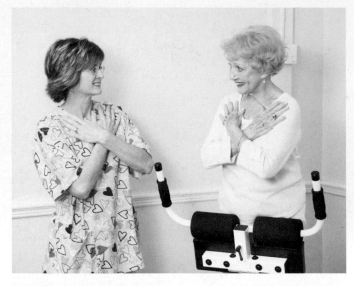

FIGURE 10-1 Teaching proper form.
© Lisa F. Young/Shutterstock

- Material regarding adherence with home exercise, activities, and/or wellness programs
- Methods to maximize and promote independence in patient/clients' activities of daily living and continuity of care

In addition, the clinical instructional activities must provide information to increase the patient/client's understanding of his or her diagnosis and the specific rationales for interventions. The patient/client can use the information to manage his or her condition and to adapt to the home or work environment.

The clinical instructional activities are also directed at the patient/clients' family and caregivers. Family and caregiver instructional activities may include training in specific techniques that increase, promote, and produce the identified patient/client outcomes. Most of the instruction focuses on the safety of the patient/client and the patient/client's family and caregivers.

While teaching generally means that the professional is imparting information to the patient, it is important to recognize that the goal is really that the patient will learn new attitudes and behaviors that will improve his or her health and well-being.[11]

Prior to teaching a patient, it is important that the PT or PTA assess the learner to find out his or her current understanding and personal needs. Patient-centered teaching involves learning who the patient is and tailoring the teaching experience to the patient. Ask the patient how they learn best—via demonstration, written information, video, or auditory. People can learn in multiple ways and varying the teaching style may help the patient remain engaged in the learning process. Most patient teaching occurs over a number of treatment sessions, so developing a rapport of trust and understanding will help the practitioner create a teaching plan that the patient will be more likely to embrace.[11]

Clinical instruction modes for patients/clients can take the following formats:

- Discussions
- Demonstrations
- Presentations
- Lectures
- Audiovisual materials or web-based learning methods
- Return demonstrations
- Illustrations of written information

When making demonstrations or presentations, the PTA should demonstrate or present the most important information first, keep the content brief and concise, emphasize the most important points, and be specific. The demonstrations and presentations should be presented at the level of the learner. The PTA should avoid technical terms when patients/clients are involved, and limit extraneous information that may distract the learner.

When delivering lectures to the patient/client (and family/caregiver), the PTA should be very concise, building on the information the learner has already processed and adding visual aids such as illustrations, diagrams, or models. For example, before displaying audiovisual materials, the PTA should review the information, explaining any technical terms used or identifying any equipment or intervention the patient/client may need. The PTA should also stop the video at appropriate times to explain critical aspects of performance the patient/client may have to perform. After viewing the video, return demonstrations allow the PTA to assess how well the patient/client grasped the concepts presented. The PTA should observe

the patient/client's performance of the task, critique it, praise it, or help to refine it.

Clinical instruction activities require that the clinician teacher provide the following things for the learner:[11]

- Respect for the patient's values, preferences, and expressed needs
- An overview of the objectives and purpose of the learning activity
- A description of how the learning activity fits with the patient's personal goals
- An environment that is quiet and appropriate for learning
- Reduction of conditions that have a negative impact on learning such as pain or discomfort, anxiety, fear, frustration, feelings of failure, humiliation, embarrassment, boredom, or time pressures
- A teaching plan that is logical and sequential, using patient-friendly language and understandable for the patient given his or her own personal traits (e.g., culture, age, intellect and educational levels)
- Ample time for practice and answering questions
- Specific instructions to ensure that the clinician and patient have the same perceptions
- Appropriate assessment of learning immediately following the teaching and in subsequent treatment sessions
- Involvement of family members or friends to provide a support system for the patient

Other types of clinical instructional activities are clinical in-service and clinical education. Clinical in-service are activities in which PTs, PTAs, or PT/PTA students prepare short educational programs designed to impart specific aspects of knowledge to peers. This tool can be an excellent way to teach others about topics from continuing education courses that the professionals have attended. Presentation skills and organization of the topic will help the learner absorb and assimilate information quickly. Whenever possible, engage the learners by asking open-ended questions or having them participate in an activity (see **FIGURE 10-2**). When reviewing hands-on skills that the learner may already know, it may be useful to have the participants perform peer assessment. This will actively engage them in the learning process and tap into the skills that they already have. An example where this may be appropriate could be a review of safe transfer training with certified nursing assistants in a skilled nursing facility.

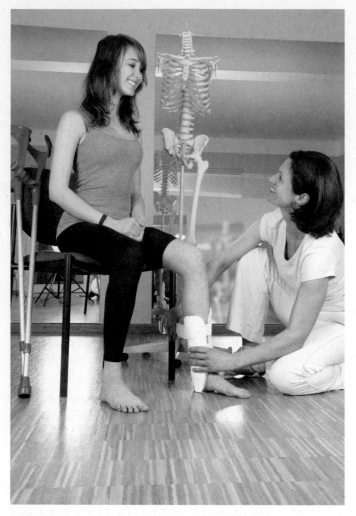

FIGURE 10-2 Teaching patients about their injury and how to use crutches.
© RioPatuca/Shutterstock

Clinical education involves activities in which the PT or PTA participates in guiding the learning experiences of a student in the clinical environment. The American Physical Therapy Association (APTA) has a program to help clinical instructors learn strategies for teaching students—the Credentialed Clinical Instructor Courses. These courses help with organization, development, and implementation of teaching within the clinical environment.

Communication Methods for Patient Education

PTAs should be aware of the communication skills used to deliver patient education. Each patient/client is different and has various learning requirements. As a result, communication modes may need to be adjusted to match each patient/client's learning needs.

PATIENT EDUCATION

Patient education constitutes a significant form of intervention in physical therapy clinical practice. The PT and the PTA must assess the patient/client's abilities and learning styles and identify obstacles to learning. The instructional method of patient education needs to be adapted to the patient/client, especially for a patient/client who may have cognitive deficits or learning disabilities.

During patient education, the PT or PTA's communication skills are critical. The therapist should communicate clearly and simply by using everyday words, rephrasing as necessary, and explaining new words. To ensure the message gets to the patient, besides speaking and writing, the therapist can use other materials such as audiotapes, videotapes/DVDs, support groups, hotlines, and websites for online information. In addition, the patient's understanding of information can be verified by asking open-ended questions and asking the patient to demonstrate how he or she will accomplish the instructions.

Barriers to Learning

In some cases, PTs and PTAs will need to adjust their teaching methods to accommodate a patient's ability to learn. Patients who have learning impairments, visual or auditory impairments, who lack concentration or who lack motivation to learn will need other accommodations in order for learning to occur.

The following ideas may help to reduce barriers to learning:

- By adjusting the teaching method, therapists can adjust to a patient's learning style and special needs. This also can be done by finding out the patient's preference for learning, such as reading, listening, watching, or doing.
- The teacher should focus on the patient's concerns and relate the importance of the topic being taught to those concerns. Avoid using fear tactics to gain the patient's attention. Instead, focus on the positive importance of learning and using the learned information. Especially when teaching a patient who appears unmotivated, it

is important to utilize a factor that is important to the patient as motivation.

- The patient should be encouraged to bring a family member or a friend to the teaching session for support and to reinforce and clarify information.
- The teacher should break up information into logical "bits of information" so that the patient has time to process what is being taught.
- Allow for practice. Many learners learn best kinesthetically so practicing "hands on" will improve learning. For more didactic learning, do not rely on closed questioning to verify learning. "Do you understand?" or "Do you have any questions?" may be answered "yes" or "no" without ever allowing the teacher to substantiate understanding of the material taught.
- For those who have difficulty reading, make sure the materials are written in plain language, consistently using the same words. When using new terms, define them and use repetition to reinforce the information. Sentences should be short and simple, and each should be marked with a bullet point. Only five or six bullet points should be on each list. Attention can be drawn to essential information by making circles or arrows or adding dividers or tabs to the material.
- For individuals who are older adults, the therapist needs to assess how and when the patient is ready to learn by finding out the patient's interest, determining his or her level of motivation to learn, and tying new information to past experiences. The learning process can be enhanced by an environment conducive to learning such as a quiet place, sitting near the patient, speaking clearly, and teaching in brief sessions (instead of long ones). Instructions can be taught one step at a time by demonstrating and describing the procedure and encouraging the patient to practice each step.
- For patients who have visual impairments, therapists can introduce themselves and other people present in the room, asking if the patient wants assistance and providing directions. When writing for a patient who has visual impairments, the best method is to write the material in large print size (16 points), to use simple fonts, to avoid italics, and to write clearly and concisely (or to print information in Braille).
- When speaking with patients who have hearing impairments, the therapist can move a chair closer to face the patient, get the patient's attention by touching him or her, and speaking clearly and distinctly (not

loudly). Pronunciation does not need to be exaggerated; however, distracting and interfering sounds need to be reduced. The light in the room has to be adequate because many patients with hearing impairments read lip movements and look at gestures, expressions, and pantomime actions.

- For patients who cannot speak English, the therapist can use certified interpreters to communicate key information to the patient. The patient must be comfortable with the interpreter, especially when discussing potentially embarrassing topics. Patients who cannot speak English will be very happy to be greeted in their native language, and to have their names pronounced correctly. The therapist should speak clearly and concentrate on the most important message(s) for each patient.
- For patients from other cultures, the therapist needs to understand the patient's values and beliefs and to pay attention to nonverbal communication such as voice volume, postures, gestures, and eye contact. Working with the family decision maker, who may be different from the patient, is essential for the success of intervention. The treatment has to be creative and may involve a spiritual advisor.

PTs and PTAs are teachers who need to recognize their own strengths and weaknesses as teachers and pay close attention to their learners' needs. By utilizing knowledge, enthusiasm, and encouragement, the PT/PTA will be effective in teaching and improving the status of the patient.

Discussion Questions

1. The PTA is teaching a patient about good posture. Describe specific strategies that could be used to perform this task.

2. A patient with osteoporosis of the knee has come to physical therapy to manage his pain and in hopes of prolonging the need for a total knee replacement. The patient is morbidly obese and does not exercise regularly. The PTA recognizes that the patient's weight is part of the issue in resolving the knee pain and achieving the patient's goal of delaying surgery. Discuss methods of teaching this patient about his condition while respectfully understanding his personal obstacles.

3. Discuss the pros and cons of the different types of instructional modes (discussions, demonstrations, presentations, lectures, audiovisual material, web-based materials, return demonstrations, and illustrations of written information).

Learning Opportunities

1. Utilizing one of the teaching strategies (demonstration, written communication, lecture, or discussion), prepare a plan to teach a patient how to move from supine to sit.

2. Create an educational brochure about a topic that would be relevant to physical therapy that could be used as a learning tool. An example might be safety in the home.

3. Explore the Internet to find technology to assist in teaching patients who are hearing or visually impaired.

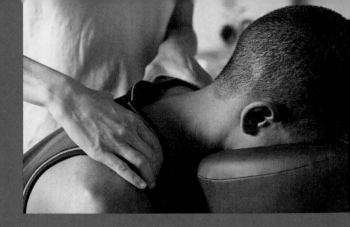

CHAPTER 11

Reimbursement and Research

OBJECTIVES

After studying this chapter, the reader will be able to:

1. Define commonly used terminology in reimbursement.
2. Describe reimbursement for Medicare, Medicaid, private insurance companies, and health maintenance organizations.
3. Compare and contrast the value of the different types of research to provide evidence for clinical physical therapy practice.
4. Describe the value of validity and reliability in research.
5. Discuss the main elements of a research study.
6. Describe how to write a research report.

KEY TERMS

experimental research
health maintenance organization (HMO)
Medicaid
Medicare

nonexperimental research
preferred provider organization (PPO)
research

Reimbursement Issues in Physical Therapy

Reimbursement is the payment of funds by a patient or an insurer to a health care provider for services rendered. As future employees, physical therapist assistant (PTA) students need to be familiar with insurance and reimbursement concepts and terminology.

REIMBURSEMENT TERMINOLOGY

Reimbursement terminology is significant in physical therapy clinical practice:

- The patient is considered the first party. The physical therapist (PT), as the health care professional delivering physical therapy services, is considered the second party. The insurer is the third party.
- The insurer is also considered the payer that makes payment for services under the insurance coverage policy.
- The term capitation means a reimbursement method that pays the provider a set fee each month, based on the number of patients enrolled in the insurance plan. A capitated payment is a form of reimbursement for health care services in which a health care provider is paid a predetermined (fixed) amount for each patient enrolled in his

or her care. Capitation and capitated payment are terms used mostly by managed care organizations (MCOs).

- Fee-for-service payment is a payment for specific health care services that were provided to a patient. The payment can be made by the patient or by an insurance carrier. As opposed to the capitated payment, a fee-for-service payment means that when a procedure was performed, a fee was charged, and the fee was paid by the insurance company. In the past, PTs were reimbursed for 100 percent of the billed procedures. The current health care market has caused insurance companies to reimburse only a percentage of the total bill.

- Managed care means a variety of methods of financing and organizing the delivery of health care in which costs are contained by controlling the provision of benefits and services. Physicians, hospitals, and other health care agencies contract with the managed care system to accept a predetermined monthly payment for providing services to patients enrolled in a managed care plan. The enrollee's access to health care is limited to the physicians and other health care providers who are affiliated with the plan. Clinical decision making is influenced by a variety of administrative incentives and constraints (specific rules and regulations).

- A **health maintenance organization (HMO)** is a prepaid health care program of group practice that provides comprehensive medical care, especially preventive care, whose main goal is to control health care expenditures. A **preferred provider organization (PPO)** is similar to an HMO; however, it will allow patients to choose out-of-network providers, but will not pay 100 percent of those charges.[12]

- Copayment is a monetary amount to be paid by the patient to health care professionals each time a service is provided. Deductibles are portions of health care costs that the patient must pay prior to getting benefits from the insurance company. For example, a deductible of $1,000 means that the patient will pay the first $1,000 of health care costs and the insurance company will then begin assisting with health care bills.

- Health care professionals dislike the term *denial* because it means refusal by an insurer to reimburse for services that have been rendered.

- Eligibility is the process of determining whether a patient qualifies for benefits, based on factors such as enrollment date, preexisting conditions, and valid referrals.

- Prior authorization is a procedure required by some health care insurers that requires that the patient or health care provider contact them to approve procedures or health care. Examples of activities that require preauthorization are surgical procedures or physical therapy services. In addition, some insurers limit the number of visits that can be provided in a calendar year or per diagnosis.[12]

- The term *CPT 2014* stands for Current Procedural Terminology 2014. The CPT is a list of descriptive terms that contains five-character, numeric codes assigned to nearly every health care service. When billing occurs, health care providers must choose a CPT code that identifies the services provided.[13] Some examples of CPT codes are 97530, which represents therapeutic activities, or 97110, which represents therapeutic exercise.

- ICD-10-CM refers to the *International Classification of Diseases, tenth revision, Clinical Modification*. These codes create a standardized classification of diagnoses across all health care settings and providers. Health care insurers require that ICD-10 codes be identified during billing. ICD-10 codes are also used to report diagnoses, symptoms, and inpatient procedures.[14]

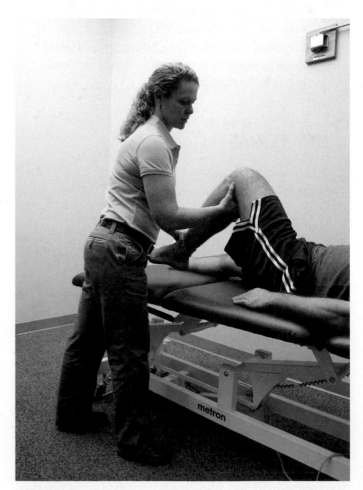

REIMBURSEMENT ORGANIZATIONS

Physical therapy services can be reimbursed by Medicare, Medicaid, private health insurance companies, and health maintenance organizations (HMOs).

Medicare

Medicare is the largest provider of health care services in the United States. Medicare was established in 1965 by the U.S. Congress as Title XVIII of the Social Security Act to provide medical coverage and health care services to individuals age 65 years old or older.

Medicare is a health insurance program for:[15]

- People age 65 or older
- People under age 65 with certain disabilities
- People of all ages with end-stage renal disease (permanent kidney failure requiring dialysis or a kidney transplant)

The Centers for Medicare and Medicaid Services (CMS) administers the Medicare program and, in partnership with the states, the Medicaid program. CMS central and regional offices share seven key objectives outlined in the CMS Strategic Plan 2013–2017:[16]

1. Improve quality care
2. Improve preventive health benefits
3. Strengthen consumer protections
4. Expand coverage
5. Strengthen program integrity
6. Improve payment models
7. Transform business operations

Medicare has four parts: Part A, hospital insurance; Part B, medical insurance; Part C, Medicare Advantage; and Part D, Medicare Prescription Drug Coverage. Most people don't pay a premium for Part A because they or a spouse already paid for it through their payroll taxes while working.[15] However, most people pay a monthly premium for Part B. Part C, Medicare Advantage includes health plans offered by private companies and approved by Medicare.[15] Medicare Advantage plans require individuals who are on Medicare to pay additional monthly premiums. Part D, Medicare Prescription Drug Coverage is typically available to everyone with Medicare,[15] but also involves additional cost.

Medicare payments for physical therapy services vary based on where the services are provided.[12]

Medicare Part A (hospital insurance) helps cover:[15]

- Inpatient care in hospitals, including critical access hospitals, and skilled nursing facilities (not custodial or long-term care)
- Hospice care and some home health care (beneficiaries must meet certain conditions to get these benefits)

Medicare Part B (medical insurance) helps cover:[15]

- Doctors' services and outpatient care.
- Medically necessary services to diagnose or treat a medical condition.
- Part A claims for patients whose claim limit has been exhausted or has been denied due to ineligibility of claims. An example of this is when a patient does not meet the qualifications for a hospital stay but is placed in the hospital for observation.
- Some other medical services that Part A doesn't cover, such as some of the services of physical and occupational therapists, and some home health care. Part B helps pay for these covered services and supplies when they are medically necessary.

- The prospective payment system (PPS) is a fixed payment that is matched to diagnosis classifications known as diagnosis related groups (DRGs) in the acute care setting. PPS is also utilized in inpatient rehabilitation hospitals, skilled nursing facilities, long-term care hospitals, home health care, hospice, hospital outpatient departments, and inpatient psychiatric facilities.
- Within the skilled nursing facility (SNF), Medicare pays for therapy via Part A or Part B. Each patient entering the SNF receives an assessment known as the minimum data set (MDS), which looks at functional skills, hearing, vision, cognitive skills, and so on. This information is used to determine the amount of skilled care that the resident will require from the staff (nursing, PT, OT, SLP). The resource utilization group (RUG) classification will determine what

amount of reimbursement that Medicare will pay for the resident. RUG levels are determined by adding up the amount of nursing care and the number of minutes a patient receives physical therapy, occupational therapy, and speech-language therapy. Examples of levels include: ultra, very high, high, medium, and low. The American Physical Therapy Association (APTA) provides updates when CMS mandates changes to the system. This complex process requires conscientious education of changing regulations and documentation to support the need for physical therapy to avoid denial of payment.

- When a patient enters an inpatient rehabilitation facility, a system similar to that in a skilled nursing facility is utilized. Patients are assessed using the Functional Independence Measure (FIM). These scores are utilized in the inpatient rehabilitation facility patient assessment instrument (IRF PAI) to classify the patient and identify the predetermined payment amount.
- The Outcome and Assessment Information Set (OASIS) is the assessment tool utilized for home health care. This tool shows patient improvement over time and is also used to classify the patient for payment groups.

In addition to the predetermined groupings to determine payment, Medicare does allow health care providers to identify when services are being provided to patients with multiple health problems and also adjusts the amount of payment based on geographic location.

As of July 2015, another restriction placed on physical therapy by Medicare is a capped payment of $1,940 per year for the combined costs for physical therapy and speech-language pathology services paid under the Part B program. Patients may qualify for an exception to the therapy cap if the treatments are medically reasonable and necessary.

Medicaid

Medicaid was enacted in 1965 as a jointly funded program in which the federal government matched state spending to provide medical and health-related services. Medicaid was originally established by the U.S. Congress as Title XIX of the Social Security Act. Although there are specific federal requirements for Medicaid concerning eligibility, benefits, and provider payments, states have a wide degree of flexibility to design their programs. Medicaid services are designed for children, non-elderly low-income

parents, other caretaker relatives, pregnant women, non-elderly individuals with disabilities, and low-income elderly people. CMS requires that states provide the following services:[16]

- Inpatient hospital services
- Outpatient hospital services
- EPSDT: Early and Periodic Screening, Diagnostic, and Treatment Services
- Nursing facility services
- Home health services
- Physician services
- Rural health clinic services
- Federally qualified health center services
- Laboratory and x-ray services
- Family planning services
- Nurse midwife services
- Certified pediatric and family nurse practitioner services
- Freestanding birth center services (when licensed or otherwise recognized by the state)
- Transportation to medical care
- Tobacco cessation counseling for pregnant women

Other services are considered optional and are determined on a state-by-state basis. This may include physical therapy services.

Additionally, some states have regulations that do not allow PTAs to provide services to Medicaid patients in an attempt to contain costs. Other notable state regulations may include a small premium or a copayment for services that must be paid by the Medicaid enrollee.

The Affordable Care Act requires that states expand the services of Medicaid to provide coverage to non-elderly, non-disabled adults with incomes at or below 138 percent of the federal poverty level.[17] The health plans must cover the following benefits: (1) ambulatory patient services; (2) emergency services; (3) hospitalization; (4) maternity and newborn care; (5) mental health and substance use disorder services, including behavioral health treatment; (6) prescription drugs; (7) rehabilitative and habilitative services and devices; (8) laboratory services; (9) preventative and wellness services and chronic disease management; and (10) pediatric services, including oral and vision care. A Supreme Court ruling determined that states have the right to choose or decline the Medicaid expansion. States that choose to expand receive federal government subsidies from 2014 through 2020.[17] States that choose not to expand retain the right to create a variety of optional benefit services. It is critical that PTs and PTAs are aware of the regulations within their state. The Medicaid.gov website and the APTA website offer up-to-date information and webpage links that can provide valuable information about regulations and requirements for providing care to patients with Medicaid coverage.

For up-to-date information about Medicare and Medicaid, its rules, and current application, students should refer to the Medicare website at www.cms.gov.

Private Insurance

Private insurance companies, such as Blue Cross Blue Shield, Humana, and Coventry, provide insurance to individuals and employees through employer provided plans. Each plan purchased may have a variety of benefits, require copayments, and may require authorization for services. It is important for the patient and the health care provider to understand the requirements for the physical therapy episode. The APTA has developed the Physical Therapy Model Benefit Plan Design as a resource to help insurance companies understand the purpose and benefits of physical therapy to their policyholders.[19]

In 2010, Congress passed the Affordable Care Act (ACA). The law requires that uninsured Americans gain access to insurance and that Centers for Medicare and Medicaid Services and states create Health Insurance Marketplaces, expand Medicaid, and regulate private health insurance plans.[16] The goal of the ACA is to improve health care access and move to an outcome-based health care system.

Workers' compensation is an employer purchased insurance to cover medical costs when an employee is injured while performing his or her job. This insurance is purchased from the state; employers in almost every state are required to purchase this for their employees. Just as with the other insurances, there are a variety of requirements and cost-containment practices that must be known in order to provide cost-effective physical therapy.

Health Maintenance Organizations

A health maintenance organization (HMO) is a form of managed care. Managed care provides health care services by a limited number of health care professionals for a fixed prepaid fee. A managed care company is a third-party payer that directs patients to specific providers that have contracted with the managed care company. Managed care monitors health care services to the patient to avoid excessive and inappropriate treatment. The goals of managed care are to ensure favorable patient outcomes and to contain medical expenses. For example, in managed care services, a patient has access first to the primary care physician (PCP). The patient cannot see a specialist before the PCP determines whether the patient needs to see the specialist. The PCP also determines if an outpatient (less costly) intervention is necessary instead of an inpatient (more costly) intervention. Also, patients in need of health care are required to have an office visit first instead of an emergency department visit, and use less expensive (older) medications instead of more expensive (newer) medications. As a general rule, the treatments or the procedures may not be paid by the managed care system if they are found to be outside of managed care guidelines.

An HMO is a form of managed care that requires enrollees to visit only providers within the HMO network. Managed care and HMOs were originally created to curb the enormous expense of health care costs that arose in the 1960s and 1970s. The initial role of HMOs was to decrease health care costs by providing preventative health care. Instead of treating individuals as they become ill, an HMO's purpose is to keep these individuals healthy by providing preventative medicine. Health care providers who are members of an HMO receive a fixed annual fee for each member. In general, HMOs and managed care organizations are under financial pressure to limit the spending on each and every patient. This demand, in many situations, may cause (from the health care providers' perspectives) inequitable health care decisions in regard to patients' interventions.

HMOs can be divided into four distinct groups:[20]

- Staff HMOs, in which the health care providers are employees of the HMO, providing care only for HMO members
- Group HMOs, in which the health care is provided by a separate group of physicians (not employees of the HMO) having contracts with the HMO to treat only members of the HMO
- Individual practice associations (IPAs), in which there are contracts between the HMO and the individual physicians stipulating that the physicians can use their own offices to treat HMO and non-HMO patients
- Network HMOs, similar to IPA HMOs, except that instead of contracts with individual physicians, the HMO has contracts with a number of large physicians' groups who treat HMO as well as non-HMO patients

There are also different types of HMO plans: the prepaid group plan (PGP), preferred provider organization (PPO), and individual practice association (IPA). Typically, an employer contracts for managed care or HMO services as a benefit to its employees. Employees may have to pay a small fee for each visit as a copayment.

In general, the primary care physician (PCP) is the gatekeeper that authorizes other medical services such as diagnostic testing or rehabilitation services. In managed care, the gatekeeper or the PCP refers the patient to the provider being designated as the one who directs an individual patient's care. In practical terms, the gatekeeper or the PCP is the one who refers patients to specialists or subspecialists for care.

PTs must obtain a provider number to treat patients within a specific HMO. Also, HMOs require authorization of physical therapy services even if the PCP made the referral. The HMO may deny physical therapy payment for services in spite of the fact that the authorization for physical therapy was granted. PTAs may not be authorized to treat HMO patients in outpatient or home care settings.

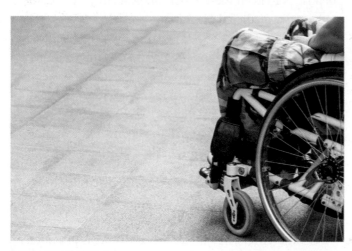

© panumas nikhomkhai/Shutterstock

Tricare and the Veterans Health Administration System

Tricare is a health program for members of the armed services and their families. It acts as an insurance company providing services to these eligible candidates only. Just as with private insurance, benefits, copayments, and authorization for services will vary with the plan that the member chooses.

The Veterans Health Administration is the health care system for active and retired active military personnel who qualify. Services are available at inpatient hospitals and outpatient clinics and include preventative care, diagnostic, and treatment services.

Basic Research Elements

Research is described as a creative process by which professionals (such as PTs) systematically challenge their everyday practice.[20]

THE SIGNIFICANCE OF PHYSICAL THERAPY RESEARCH

The APTA supports PTs' role in practicing evidence-based physical therapy by accessing and applying clinical research to patients/clients. Research determines the effectiveness or lack of effectiveness of various physical therapy services for patients/clients. The evidence that emerges from physical therapy research can be used as a guide in clinical practice. Sometimes, the results of research may support current clinical practice. Other times, research results may point to areas of clinical practice that need to be modified.

> Why physical therapy research is necessary:[20]
>
> - To establish a body of knowledge for physical therapy
> - To determine the efficacy of physical therapy treatments
> - To improve patient care in physical therapy

The body of knowledge rationale for physical therapy research has to do with characteristics of the physical therapy profession such as identity and performance. Because physical therapy, as with other applied medical professions, encompasses in its body of knowledge a combination of arts and sciences, its identity and performance can be discovered and enhanced only through research. The efficacy of physical therapy in health care can also be demonstrated through research by augmenting established interventions and perhaps discovering new ones. However, the most important reason for research in physical therapy as well as in health care in general is improving patient care. Through clinical research, PTs and PTAs (under the supervision of PTs) are able to apply the obtained information to their patients. This is why PTAs, as members of the physical therapy clinical team, need at least a basic knowledge of research elements to understand and evaluate physical therapy research literature.

In 2008, the APTA began developing Clinical Practice Guidelines (CPGs) utilizing research evidence to improve the effectiveness, safety, outcomes, and efficiency of health care. In 2014, the APTA had approved seven diagnosis-specific CPGs and was working on further submitted proposals. To further the initiative of research in 2015, the APTA will begin compiling data on patient outcomes via the Physical Therapy Outcomes Registry. These two initiatives are only possible through the work of everyday clinicians becoming involved in evidence-based research.[21]

TYPES OF RESEARCH

There are two main types of research: experimental and nonexperimental. **Experimental research** is research in which at least one independent variable is subjected to controlled manipulation by the researcher. On the contrary, **nonexperimental research** does not manipulate the independent variable. Variables are certain characteristics that take different forms in a research study. Examples of variables include physical therapy treatments such as electrical stimulation, gait training, or ultrasound. Other variables can be patients' signs and symptoms such as pain, tingling, weakness, strength, or range of motion (see **FIGURE 11-1**).

Independent and Dependent Variables

The independent variable is a research variable that is manipulated by the researcher. The independent variable is believed to cause a change in the dependent variable. The effects of the independent variable can be seen and measured in the dependent variable. Dependent variables are variables that are only measured or registered. The dependent variable also determines the outcome that is being evaluated. For example, in a research article titled "The Effects of Electrical Stimulation in the Treatment of Low Back Pain," the independent variable is electrical stimulation and the dependent variable is low back pain. The researcher manipulates electrical stimulation to see its effects in the patient's level of low back pain.

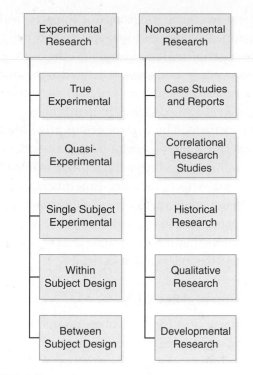

FIGURE 11-1 Types of research.

The term *independent variable* applies mostly to experimental research in which the variable is manipulated or observed by the researcher so that its value can be related to that of the dependent variable. Although the independent variable is often manipulated by the researcher, it can also be a classification where subjects are assigned to groups. In a study where one variable causes the other, the independent variable is the cause. In a study in which groups are being compared, the independent variable is the group classification. It can be said that in a research study, the independent variable defines a principal focus of research interest, and the dependent variable is the outcome of the research. In an experiment, the dependent variable may be what was caused or what changed as a result of the study. In a comparison of groups, the dependent variable is what the groups differ on.

Experimental Research

There are different types (or designs) of experimental research such as true experimental, quasi-experimental, single-subject experimental, within-subject design, and between-subjects design. For example, the difference between true experimental and quasi-experimental research is the researcher's level of control in the experiment. In the true experimental design, the researcher uses at least two separate groups of subjects, with random assignment of subjects to groups. In these two groups, one is the experimental group and the other is the control group. The experimental group is defined as the group that receives a new treatment that is under investigation. The control group is defined as the group that does not receive the new treatment. The control group provides a baseline for interpretation of results. The quasi-experimental design, in contrast, uses only a single group without having a control group. Also, in the quasi-experimental design the subjects are not randomly assigned to the group. Both true and quasi-experimental research studies are clinically significant because they maintain some level of control when manipulating the independent variable.

Nonexperimental Research

Nonexperimental research involves no manipulation of an independent variable. The researcher examines records of past phenomena, documents existing phenomena, or observes new phenomena. Examples of types of nonexperimental research are case reports (case studies), correlational research studies, developmental research, historical research, and qualitative research. Case reports (or case studies) are very popular among physical therapy research articles because they contain an in-depth investigation of an individual, a group, or an institution. An example of a case report is a description of implementation of a cycling training program as an exercise for two patients who had strokes. Usually clinicians reading case studies may be able to try to implement the treatments (or activities) in their clinical practices. Many physical therapy clinicians doing research feel that case reports (case studies) can help them share clinical experiences, develop new hypotheses for new research, identify problem-solving skills, and in the long run, develop practice guidelines.

Another type of nonexperimental study is the correlational research study, which attempts to determine whether a relationship exists between two or more quantifiable variables, and if so, the degree of that relationship. Although correlational studies describe and predict relationships between variables, they do not actively manipulate the variables. Examples of correlational studies are retrospective, descriptive, or predictive. Developmental research studies are also a type of nonexperimental study. These are most often found as articles describing behaviors differentiating individuals at different levels of age, growth, or maturation. An example can be a study describing the development of kicking movements in preterm and full-term infants by videotaping them and analyzing the infants' kicking frequency. Research data might have been collected for these infants at different ages such as 6 weeks, 12 weeks, and 18 weeks. In such an example, the infants were described at more than one point in time to document the effects of the passage of time. Another type of nonexperimental study is a longitudinal study, which is designed to collect data over time for the purpose of describing developmental changes in a particular group. Contrary to longitudinal research, cross-sectional nonexperimental research is based on observations of different age or developmental groups at one point in time, providing the basis for inferring trends over time.[20]

Historical research involves investigation of a variety of data sources and determining relationships based on analyses and inferences. Historical studies investigate the authenticity of the data, and evaluate the value of the data. Historical research uses primary and secondary sources of data. The primary sources are original documents, eyewitness accounts, or direct recordings of events. The secondary sources are descriptions of events by those other than eyewitnesses, summaries of information from textbooks, or newspaper accounts.

Qualitative studies seek facts about or causes of social phenomena and complex human behavior. Using inductive reasoning (from a set of specific facts to a general conclusion), qualitative studies develop concepts, insights, and understanding from patterns within the data. Qualitative research involves the use of qualitative data to understand and explain social phenomena. Qualitative data sources include observation and participant observation (fieldwork), interviews and questionnaires, documents and texts, and the researcher's impressions and reactions. Some examples of qualitative research methods are action research, case study research, and ethnography. Qualitative research was not very popular in earlier physical therapy studies, perhaps because of its holistic approach to people and settings. However, considering advanced current physical therapy social phenomena, the role of qualitative research in physical therapy science—and in research generally—has been dramatically changed.

SIGNIFICANT ELEMENTS OF RESEARCH

Some significant elements of a research article, besides the variables, are the research question, hypothesis, reliability, validity, scales of measurement, and subjects.

Research Question

Researchers typically address questions that contribute to scientific knowledge. The purpose of a research study is to examine a specific research question. Generally, the research question must be answerable and feasible. Questions involving judgments or philosophical questions are very difficult to study. Also, the experiment may be too expensive or unrealistic as far as the time or the resources needed to be able to answer the question. The researcher should determine the study's risks and benefits and be able to justify the demands placed on the subjects during data collection.

Hypothesis

Once the research question is formulated and variables are defined, the researcher proposes an educated guess about the outcome of the study. This guess is called a hypothesis. A study's hypothesis is defined as a statement of the expected relationship between variables. A hypothesis can be either a null hypothesis, stating that no relationship exists between the variables, or a research hypothesis, stating that there is a relationship between the variables. A null hypothesis is also a statistical hypothesis. The research hypothesis states the researcher's true expectation of the results.

Reliability

Research articles also must have reliability to see the degree of consistency with which an instrument measured a variable. Intrarater reliability is the degree to which one rater can obtain the same rating on multiple occasions of measuring the same variable. For example, an experienced PTA performs a clinical experiment applying a "special" stretch to see if it increases a patient's elbow flexion range of motion. After 10 experimental treatments applying the special stretch, the PTA uses a goniometer to measure the patient's elbow flexion range of motion three times. Each goniometric measurement was taken at a different time. After each measurement, the PTA records the degrees and observes that each of the three measurements recorded 110 degrees. In this example the PTA obtained intrarater reliability of his or her experiment. Then the PTA asked two experienced PTs to also measure the patient's range of motion three times after 10 treatments of the special stretch. Each goniometric measurement was taken by the PTs at three different times. If the PTs also found that each measurement was 110 degrees, then the PTA obtained

interrater reliability of his or her experiment. Interrater reliability is the degree to which two or more raters can obtain the same ratings for a given variable.

Validity

Validity means how meaningful test scores are as they are used for specific purposes. In other words, it means the degree to which an instrument measures what it is intended to measure. For example, the validity of the "special" stretch that the PTA performed on the patient to increase the patient's elbow flexion range of motion can be questioned in regard to the position of the stretch, the type of stretch, and the PTA's experiences performing the stretch. In this example, the special stretch is the independent variable that may or may not cause a change in the dependent variable, the patient's elbow flexion range of motion. The experiment can be evaluated looking at internal validity or external validity. Internal validity is the degree to which the observed differences on the dependent variable are the direct result of manipulation of the independent variable, and not some other variable. In the example, to establish internal validity for this study, it would have to be proven that the special stretch, and not other variables, caused improvements in the patient's elbow flexion range of motion. To achieve internal validity the relationship between the independent and dependent variable must be free from the effects of extraneous factors. External validity is the degree to which the results are generalizable to individuals (the general population) outside the experimental study. To achieve external validity is almost an impossible task, because it is dependent on the experiment interaction with the specific type of subjects tested, the specific setting in which the experiment was carried out, or the time in history when the study was performed.

Scales of Measurement

Researchers use measurement as a way of understanding, evaluating, and differentiating characteristics of people and objects. The researcher classifies physical or behavioral characteristics of variables or scores on scales such as nominal, ordinal, interval, or ratio. These scales help the researcher communicate information in objective terms and not in vague interpretations.

The nominal scale classifies variables or scores into two or more mutually exclusive categories based on a common set of characteristics. For example, the subjects can be classified by gender (male or female), by clinical diagnosis, or by nationality. The ordinal scale classifies and ranks variables or scores in terms of the degree to which they have a common characteristic. In the ordinal scale the intervals between the ranks are not equal. For example, manual muscle grading (testing) in physical therapy, using choices such as normal, good, fair, poor, trace, and zero, uses an ordinal scale of ranking. Other examples of an ordinal scale can be patients' functional status or pain.

The interval scale classifies and ranks variables or scores based on predetermined equal intervals. The interval scale does not have a true zero point and does not represent an absolute quantity. Examples of interval ranking are students' scores ranging from 0 to 100, or temperature scales in Fahrenheit and Celsius. The ratio scale classifies and ranks variables or scores based on equal intervals and a true zero point. The ratio scale is the highest and the most precise level of measurement used in research. Examples of ratio ranking are scales for height, weight, distance, age, time, or goniometric measurements.

Subjects

Researchers utilize subjects for experimental purposes. Researchers need informed consent documents to be able to include human subjects in their studies. Typically, an informed consent document consists of disclosure of information about the study, the subject's comprehension of that information, and the consent elements, such as:[22]

- The purpose of the research project, explaining clearly the reason for doing the research and for selecting this particular subject
- The research procedures, explaining in detail what will be done to the subject
- The risks and discomforts of the research study, stating the risks that may result and the discomfort that can be expected
- The research benefits, describing the potential benefits to the subject as the participant, to general knowledge, or to the future administration of health care
- The alternatives to participation, describing reasonable alternative procedures that might be used in the treatment of this subject when a treatment is being studied
- The confidentiality statement of the procedures, used to ensure the anonymity of the subject in collecting,

storing, and reporting information and the persons or agencies that have access to the information
- The request for more information, stating that the subject may ask questions about or discuss participation in the study at any time
- The right to refuse to participate or to discontinue participation at any time
- The injury statement, describing the measures to be taken if injury occurs as a direct result of the research activity
- The consent statement, confirming that the subject consents to participate in the research project
- The signatures of the subject, a parent or guardian (for minors), and a witness

The consent must be voluntary, and special consideration is given to subjects who are "vulnerable" such as patients who have mental illness, diminished mental capacity, or developmental disabilities. The subjects can withdraw the consent at any time before or during an experiment, or even after data collection when a subject might request that his or her data be discarded.

EVALUATING A RESEARCH ARTICLE

When evaluating a research article, the PTA can consider the following questions:

- What problems are the researchers solving? Why are these problems important?
- What did they really do (as opposed to what the researchers said or implied they did)?

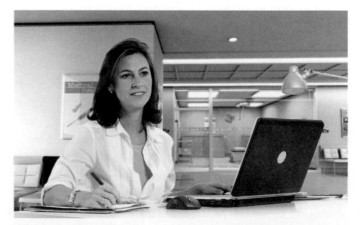

FIGURE 11-2 Evidence-based practice requires PTs and PTAs to critically read research.
© Monkey Business Images/Shutterstock

- What methods are they using?
- What is the contribution of their work (such as what is interesting or new in their work)?
- Would you as a researcher solve the problem differently?
- What were the results? Did the researchers do what they set out to do?
- Are the results reliable and valid?
- Do all the pieces of the researchers' work fit together logically?

Elements of a research study:
- Title and abstract
- Introduction
- Methods
- Results
- Discussion and conclusion

Title and Abstract

The title of a research article should be informative so that the reader is able to learn enough about the research content. After reading the title, if the reader is interested in the topic, he or she reads the abstract. Abstracts of research articles must contain specific information about the purpose, method, results, and major conclusions of the presented work. The information reported in the abstract must be consistent with the information reported in the research article.

Introduction

The purpose of the introduction is to acquaint the reader with the rationale behind the work, with the intention of defending it. The introduction places the work in a theoretical context, and enables the reader to understand and appreciate the objectives. The introduction should allow the reader to distinguish between previous research and the current study. From the introduction, the reader can find out the type of study, the hypothesis, the specific purposes of the study, if the research literature is pertinent, and if the references are appropriate and comprehensive.

The following questions are the central points for the evaluation of the introduction section of a research article:[22]

- Is the problem important? Has the problem been clearly stated?
- Did the researcher provide a theoretical context for the research study?
- Did the researcher utilize the research literature for the framework of his or her study?
- Did the researcher utilize the references appropriately and comprehensively?
- Is the type of study design clear (such as experimental or nonexperimental)?
- Are the purposes of the study and the hypothesis (or guiding questions) stated clearly?

Methods

The methods section of a research article contains essential information to evaluate the validity of the study. The methods section includes information about the subjects, the study design (if experimental or nonexperimental), the instrumentation or the equipment used in the study, the research procedures reporting data collection, operational definitions, issues of validity, and the data analysis describing how the data were analyzed. The reader of the methods section can find out who the subjects were, what inclusion or exclusion criteria were used for these subjects, and how the subjects were selected. The type of research design specified in the methods section can tell the reader about control groups, the number of independent or dependent variables, and/or how often the treatments or measurements were applied. The instrumentation subsection of the methods section documents the reliability and validity of the instruments used in the study, and the data analysis subsection discusses statistical analysis or other appropriate procedures to analyze the data. The methods section gives the reader a clear picture of what was done in the study at each step.

The following questions are the central points for the evaluation of the methods section of a research article:[22]

- How were the subjects selected, and how many subjects were researched?
- Was the design of the research study identified, and is it appropriate for the study?
- Was randomization used when the subjects were included in groups?
- Was a control group used?
- How many independent variables were used?
- How often were physical therapy treatments and measurements applied?

- Was the instrumentation described in enough detail?
- Were the reliability and validity of the instruments documented?
- Were data collection procedures described clearly and in enough detail to be replicated?
- Were operational definitions for all independent and dependent variables provided?
- Were statistical analyses appropriate? Did the researcher explain the reason for using the stated statistical analyses?
- Did the researcher address each research question in the data analysis?
- What was the alpha level?

Alpha level is the probability of concluding that the null hypothesis is false (when in fact it is true). The alpha level is set by the researcher before data analysis and is usually contrasted with the probability level, which is generated by the data analysis. The statistical result using the acceptable alpha level (which is 0.05) can allow rejection of the null hypothesis and acceptance of the research hypothesis. The alpha level as a probability can be set typically between 0.05 and 0.01. The lower the alpha level, the better the experiment. If the statistical alpha level is equal or lower than the alpha level set by the researcher before data analysis, the results show that the expected difference is due to chance. The statistical results of an experiment due to chance typically indicate that there are true differences in the measured dependent variable. For example, an alpha level at 0.05 means that the statistical results of the experiment can happen 5 times out of every 100.

Results

The purpose of the results section of a research article is to present and illustrate the research findings. These findings should be presented objectively without interpretation or commentary. In this section, the reader can evaluate what the major finding of the study was, if the results were presented clearly, if tables and figures were presented accurately, if the hypothesis was addressed, and if the results were statistically significant.

The following questions are the central points for the evaluation of the results section of a research article:[22]

- Did the researcher present the results clearly?
- Did the researcher present the figures and tables accurately?
- Are the results statistically significant?

Discussion and Conclusion

The discussion and conclusion section of the research article provides an interpretation of the study's results and supports the conclusions using evidence from the experiment and from generally accepted knowledge. The reader should be able to agree with the conclusions drawn from the data, examine if the conclusions were overgeneralized, and look for factors that could have influenced or accounted for the results.

The following questions are the central points for the evaluation of the discussion and conclusion section of a research article:[22]

- How did the researcher interpret the results?
- Did the researcher clarify if the hypotheses were rejected or accepted?
- Did the researcher consider alternative explanations for the obtained findings?
- Are the discussions of the results supported by the research literature?
- Does the researcher provide the limitations of the study?
- Are the results of the study clinically important?
- Does the researcher mention how the results apply to clinical practice?
- Does the researcher provide suggestions for further study?
- Do the research conclusions flow logically from the obtained results?

Finally, at the end of the evaluation of the research article, the PTA as the reader can reflect on the study by concentrating on particular questions and deciding whether the researcher's answers were true, appropriate, and justified. The PTA can use the same approach to evaluate oral and poster presentations.

SUGGESTIONS FOR READING A RESEARCH PAPER

Some readers prefer to read a research paper sequentially from the beginning to the end; however, some readers prefer a different sequence, such as the following:

- Read the title. What is the paper about?
- Read the abstract. It should give you a concise overview of the paper.
- Read the introduction. Look for motivations, relation to other work, and a more detailed overview.
- Read the structure of the paper. What do the remaining sections address? How do they fit together?

- Read the previous/related work section. How does this work relate? What is new or different about this work?
- Read the conclusions. What were the results?
- Read the body of the paper. Some people may want to skip the statistical analyses the first time through.

The references will be important for the reader only if the topic is important. The references can point the reader to related research as well as research upon which the current study builds.

HOW TO WRITE A RESEARCH REPORT

After reading a research article, a PTA student may want to write a research report about the published research literature. The written research report should have two main components:

- A concise summary of the research article, providing an overview of what the researcher did (and why), what methods the researcher used, and what the results were
- A brief critique of the research article, giving a technical (physical therapy) evaluation of the work, explaining what things were unclear or not addressed, and describing the merits of the work

The following are guidelines for writing a research report:

- The research article should be read critically and not superficially.
- The PTA student should use his or her understanding of the research article to write a cohesive summary, not a play-by-play account of the article.
- The PTA student should be concise but include some technical physical therapy details.
- The PTA student should understand the key points of the research article.
- The PTA student should not copy choice phrases from the research article.

Discussion Questions

1. Utilizing the Internet, discuss the issues surrounding the capitation of physical therapy services at $1,940 per year for Medicare patients.
2. Describe the differences between Medicare and Medicaid.
3. Identify what the following acronyms stand for and their relationship to reimbursement.
   a. CMS
   b. DRG
   c. PPS
   d. ACA
   e. CPT
   f. ICD-9-CM
   g. HMO
   h. SNF
   i. RUG

Learning Opportunities

1. Research the tenets of the Affordable Care Act and describe how it affects physical therapy.
2. The PTA is working with a PT to develop an evidence-based assessment tool for new patients who have total knee arthroplasty. Develop a plan for obtaining research that would help you with this task.
3. The PTA is presenting an in-service for the physical therapy department in which he is interning. He is utilizing case studies for his evidence. Describe the value of case studies and list the value of other types of research that may assist him with his presentation.

Summary of Part IV

Part IV of this text described the significance of verbal and nonverbal communication and identified the concept of the therapeutic relationship in physical therapy. Types and modes of listening skills and written communication were discussed. Teaching and learning skills were discussed. The elements of the HEP and the APTA's guidelines for physical therapy documentation were listed. The SOAP progress notes, written daily or weekly, were depicted as the PTA's main documentation responsibility. Patient education and the role of the therapeutic relationship were included, as well as the distinction between empathy and sympathy. This part concluded with reimbursement topics in physical therapy, and the basic elements of physical therapy research.

References (Part IV)

1. Dreeben, O. *Patient Education in Rehabilitation*. Sudbury, MA: Jones & Bartlett Publishers; 2010.
2. American Physical Therapy Association. APTA governance. Terminology. Accessed February 2006 at: www.apta.org.
3. Davis, CM. *Patient Practitioner Interaction: An Experiential Manual for Developing the Art of Health Care*. Thorofare, NJ: SLACK Incorporated; 1994.
4. American Physical Therapy Association. PTA patient care and supervision. Accessed April 2015 at: www.apta.org.
5. Purtilo, R, Haddad, A. *Health Professional and Patient Interaction*. Philadelphia, PA: W.B. Saunders Company; 1996.
6. Bircher, WD. *Lukan's Documentation for Physical Therapist Assistants*. 3rd ed. Philadelphia, PA: F.A. Davis Company; 2007.
7. American Physical Therapy Association. *Guide to Physical Therapist Practice*. Alexandria, VA: APTA; 2014.
8. American Physical Therapy Association. Medicare physician quality reporting system. Accessed April 2015 at: www.apta.org.
9. American Physical Therapy Association. APTA's defensible documentation for patient/client management. Accessed January 2010 at: www.apta.org.
10. American Physical Therapy Association. Get connected with APTA Connect! Accessed January 2010 at: www.apta.org.
11. Falvo, DR. *Effective Patient Education. A Guide to Increased Adherence*. 4th ed. Sudbury, MA: Jones & Bartlett Publishers; 2011.
12. Erickson, ML, McKnight, R. *Documentation Basics. A Guide for the Physical Therapist Assistant*. Thorofare, NJ: SLACK Incorporated; 2012.
13. Green, MA, Rowell, JC. *Understanding Health Insurance. A Guide to Billing and Reimbursement*. 9th ed. Clifton Park, NY: Delmar Cengage Learning; 2008.
14. American Physical Therapy Association. ICD-10. Accessed August 2014 at: www.apta.org.
15. Centers for Medicare and Medicaid Services. Your Medicare coverage. Accessed July 2015 at: www.medicare.gov.
16. Centers for Medicare and Medicaid Services. CMS Strategy: The Road Forward 2013–2017. Accessed August 2014 at: www.cms.gov.
17. American Physical Therapy Association. Making sense of health care reform. Accessed August 2014 at: www.apta.org.
18. Drafke, MW. *Working in Health Care: What You Need to Know to Succeed*. Philadelphia, PA: F.A. Davis Company; 2002.
19. American Physical Therapy Association. Private insurance. Accessed August 2014 at: www.apta.org.
20. Domholdt, E. *Physical Therapy Research: Principles and Applications*. Philadelphia, PA: W.B. Saunders; 2000.
21. American Physical Therapy Association. Practice and patient care. Accessed August 2014 at: www.apta.org.
22. Gross, PL, Watkins, MP. *Foundations of Clinical Research: Applications to Practice*. 3rd ed. Upper Saddle River, NJ: Prentice Hall/Pearson Education Company; 2008.

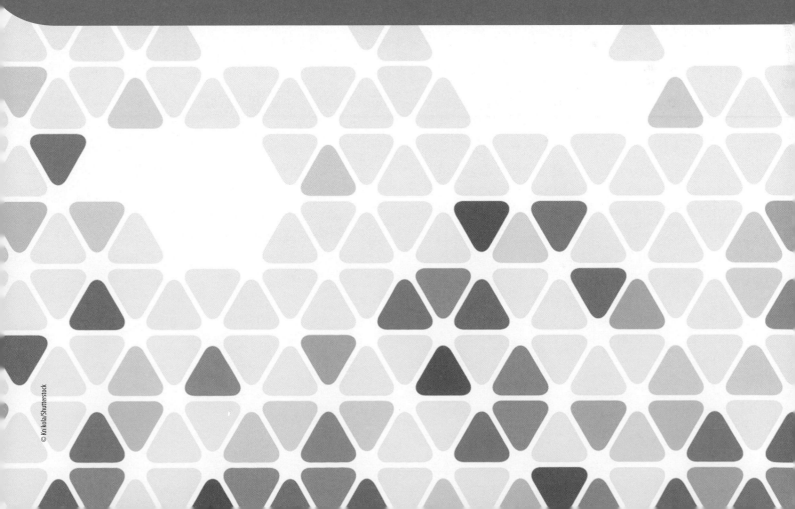

PART V

Planning for Success

This part is divided into two chapters:

- CHAPTER 12: Student Learning Success
- CHAPTER 13: Lifelong Success

This part discusses the steps students can take to be successful in physical therapist assistant school and when beginning their careers. These two chapters allow students to examine their own learning, provide knowledge about learning approaches, and help students create plans and strategies to achieve their goals. Utilizing the last chapter in the text allows the future physical therapist assistant to begin the program with an understanding of future opportunities, a plan for personal success, and a path to developing their career as a PTA.

CHAPTER 12

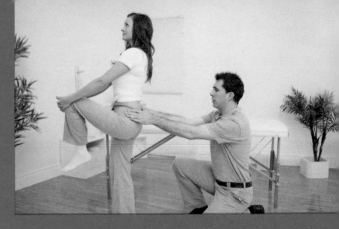

Student Learning Success

OBJECTIVES

After studying this chapter, the reader will be able to:

1. Identify rules for learning.
2. Describe learning styles.
3. Discuss learning resources and strategies.
4. List learning and test-taking strategies.
5. Create a lifelong learning plan.

KEY TERM

SQ3R

Becoming a Physical Therapist Assistant Student

Physical therapist assistant (PTA) students can come from a variety of life experiences. Some are new to college, some are nontraditional students, some have college degrees or on-the-job experience, but one thing that they all have in common is that they must become focused in a short-lived and fast-paced learning experience. Students are generally enthusiastic and excited to begin learning, but often find that the pace of learning and the amount of material to be learned can be overwhelming. This chapter will explain some strategies for learning and examination that will assist the PTA student during school and eventually in preparing for the National Physical Therapy Examination (NPTE).

Learning

There are basic understandings of learning and researchers are constantly studying how we learn in an attempt to assist students in the process. There are several principles that help us understand learning.

1. The brain can adapt. The brain is constantly processing all of the information coming in to make sense of it. A person's thoughts, processing of sensory information, emotions, and imagination all influence how someone perceives what is occurring to, or around, him or her.[1] Students should be aware that their perception is different from the person presenting the information and the others in the room.
2. The brain is social. Innately within each of us is the need to interact with others. To feel like we belong is

hardwired. So it is important for students to make connections to one another as they learn.[1]

3. The brain looks for patterns.[1] As we learn, the brain is searching for ways to make sense of the information. One way to do this is to look for similarities in what we already know. This allows the learner to connect the information to the pattern that they already know and understand. This is learned at a very early age, when children sort things into like colors or objects.

4. Emotions are important.[1] If a person thinks back to an early childhood memory, it almost always is of an event that evoked great emotion; a birthday party that was exciting, a tragic moment that was frightening, or an angry altercation. Memories that are attached to strong emotion are memories that can be recalled with greater clarity. When students are learning material, if they can create excitement in their learning, they will be much more likely to remember it long term.

5. The brain will work as one unit.[1] Students are often asked to learn bits of information, such as the names of anatomical parts. However, for long-term retention of such information, the brain prefers to think in context of not just the parts, but as the whole. In physical therapy, this occurs frequently. While teaching a patient to move from sit to stand, the physical therapist (PT) may break the process into parts and practice each section. In order to be functional and cement the learning of this movement, the PT must put the action back together and have the patient complete the entire movement as one.

6. What is going on around you matters.[1] Students often believe that their cell phone, music, television, or friends are not distracting them while they are studying. But brain research shows us that the brain really cannot multitask. Distractions will take away the ability to truly concentrate. Even daydreaming in one's own mind is a form of distraction. To truly learn, students must set themselves up for success by limiting their distractions.

7. In order to learn, the student must think about the learning.[1] Processing information requires that the student consider what it is that has been presented and make sense of it. And then more importantly, use the ideas, skills, or experiences to cement the learning. By manipulating the information, the brain can create meaning of the learning and store it in memory.

8. The brain can always create new learning connections.[1] The brain is infinite in its ability to learn and it does this by creating new neuronal connections. While learning may be easier for children as the brain is developing, age is not a limitation to learning. Anyone, of any age, who is motivated, can learn something that matters to them.

9. Intelligence is not fixed and learning occurs only through challenge.[1] Some of the most successful people did not find success just because they were intelligent, but rather because they did not give up. Research by Allison Lee Duckworth at the University of Pennsylvania has focused on this exact hypothesis. In her research, she has found that developing "grit" or the ability to stick with a task even though it is difficult is a primary skill needed for success in school and work. When students care about something, they will give more effort, even if it is difficult.[5] Duckworth and her colleagues have also focused their research on self-control. Self-control or the ability to delay gratification in order to achieve a more long-term goal has also been noted as a trait of successful people.[2] Consider the story of the tortoise and the hare as a lesson in the grit, self-control, and perseverance of the tortoise. Success in life and PTA school will be determined by many traits and opportunities, but it appears that development of grit, self-control, and perseverance could serve the student well.

LEARNING STYLES

Learning styles are defined as particular methods to gain, process, and store information (see **FIGURE 12-1**). Research on personality and brain function (especially related to the differences in left and right hemispheric functions) indicates that each person gains, stores, and communicates information in a preferred way. Each person has a predominant learning style. Some people use a combination of learning styles, but most people have at least one preferred learning style.

There is not a best learning style, but some styles tend to exchange information more effectively than others. Teachers are always striving, especially in the sciences, to identify and adapt their teaching styles to their students' preferred learning styles. As students and clinicians, PTs and PTAs are also making efforts to identify their own learning styles and their patients' learning styles to be able to adapt these to the learning and teaching processes.

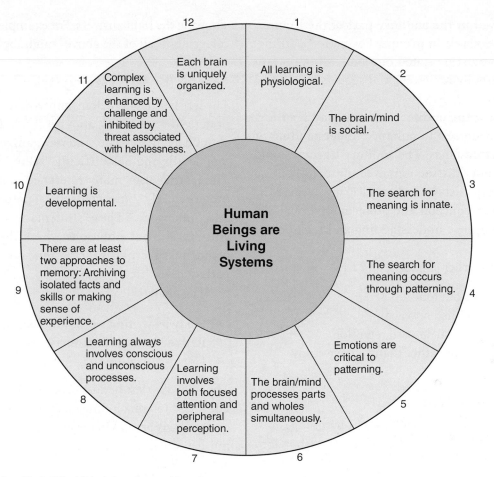

FIGURE 12-1 The Caines' Brain/Mind Principles of natural learning.
http://www.cainelearning.com/brain-mind-principles/; 12 Brain/Mind Learning Principles in Action: Developing Executive Functions of the Human Brain, 2nd Edition, 2008, Corwin, p. 255.

Understanding one's own preferred learning style can make a person an effective learner and problem solver. However, learning occurs in a variety of ways—visual, auditory, via movement, and so on—and students should not limit the way that they learn to only their preferred style.

Visual Learning Style

The visual learner prefers seeing the information. The learner prefers symbols, charts, diagrams, pictures (including motion such as in videos), and colors. Sometimes the learner may be easily distracted by images and may not concentrate on the lecture. Highlighting the information; organizing the material as acronyms or mnemonics; and using CD-ROMs, videotapes, or photographs may be helpful.[3]

The visual learner should utilize mind mapping to study, use graphic organizers by replacing words with symbols, turn phrases into images, and reconstruct images in different ways. For the visual learner, the written words will have less significance without visual aids. As study aids, the visual learner can utilize visual aids by:

- Drawing diagrams/pictures, graphs, and symbols
- Creating flashcards to identify concepts
- Practicing imaging techniques (by turning visual images into words or concepts)
- Recollecting mental pictures of his or her notes
- Utilizing the learning objectives to identify the learning task

Auditory Learning Style

The auditory learner prefers to hear lectures and is eager (if not shy) to discuss any topic. The learner prefers to use a tape recorder instead of taking notes because he or she is too involved in the auditory part of the lectures. The learner works well in groups. For better learning, the information must be stated out loud, all important facts must be verbally reviewed, and sequences must be written out.[3]

As study aids, the auditory learner may read text aloud to him- or herself to enhance understanding or may listen to lecture tapes. The auditory learner should study where auditory distractions are minimal. Working with a partner can assist the auditory learner because the student can explain concepts and problem solve out loud, which helps to improve understanding and retention of information.

The auditory learner should:

- Explain concepts out loud
- Record lectures to listen to again
- Utilize repetition to help with retention
- Utilize study groups rather than solitary study

Kinesthetic Learning Style

The kinesthetic learner prefers to learn by doing, most often using trial and error. The learner prefers laboratory work, field/clinical activities, and manipulating objects or things. The learner prefers to read the instructions as the last resort. He or she prefers not to listen to lectures, take notes, or read the material. The learner prefers "hands-on" experience. Also, the learning process can be reinforced by using gestures or certain movements.[3] The learner should be cautious when learning procedures, as it is difficult to "unlearn" an incorrect technique.

The kinesthetic learner should:

- Use illustrations and note taking during lectures to stay focused
- Talk or study with another kinesthetic learner
- Role-play the case studies (or scenarios)
- Write practice answers
- Utilize a motion when learning, such as counting on fingers to learn a list of symptoms
- Study in shorter blocks of time rather than marathon study sessions

The kinesthetic learner should read all the material (including the introduction and the summary). During tests, the kinesthetic learner should not make hasty decisions when choosing the right answers. For example, answer A may be correct, but "all of the above" might be better.

Analytic (Linear) Learning Style

The left-hemisphere dominant analytic (linear) learner prefers to read, think about it, reread, organize, think about it again, rewrite, and reorganize. The learner prefers details and has difficulty seeing the "big picture." The learner uses many reference materials. He or she prefers clearly stated goals, lists, patterns, practice sets, and homework.[3] These students will have more difficulty in clinical situations where they must be aware of not just factual information, but social aspects of patient care.

The analytic learner should:

- Study by writing words and lists over and over
- Rewrite ideas in different ways
- Use organization charts

The analytic (left-hemisphere dominant) learner should not spend too much time studying unnecessary concepts or details. When taking tests, the analytic learner should not get stuck on one question, but should continue to answer all questions.

Spatial Learning Style

The right-hemisphere dominant spatial learner prefers to learn by recognizing sequencing of symbols, objects, and events. The learner sees the "big picture" first before the details. Learning is typically informal, spontaneous, and creative.[3]

The spatial (right-hemisphere dominant) learner should:[3]

- Study by processing the information from whole to parts
- Use additional study time
- Work with others
- Learn to apply the new material

The spatial (right-hemisphere dominant) learner should first look at the similarities of the information and form a total picture of the material before evaluating the details. Also allowing more time to assimilate the new ideas and writing them down can be very helpful for this learner.

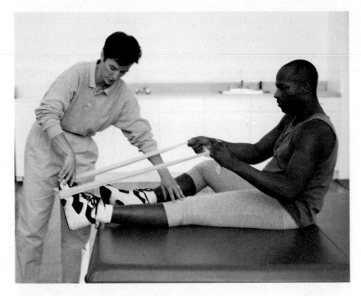

© wavebreakmedia/Shutterstock

Learning Resources

TEXTBOOKS

Textbooks are intended to be a primary resource for student learning. The advent of electronic versions can make finding information very easy and the organization of notes can be done with the click of a button. Learning how to use a textbook is important and can make the process of learning easier.

One technique that has been utilized for years is the **SQ3R**. This stands for Survey, Question, Read, Recite, and Review. Students should begin by surveying the chapter to be read. Looking at the way the author has outlined the chapter and the objectives that are intended to be met helps the reader to be prepared for the reading process. Secondly, the student should think about questions that can be answered by the reading. This is an important step that many students skip, but makes the difference between reading and understanding. In order to understand and learn something, the student must connect the information to something that he or she already knows. In preparation of this process, students should consider what they already know and what questions they might have about the subject. Finally, the student is ready to actually read the chapter. Students should consider if their questions are being answered as they read. Looking at the pictures and figures can help bring clarity to the reading. At the end of each passage, the student should recite what he or she has learned from the reading. This helps to organize the information in the student's mind and will lead to memory retention. Additionally, if the student does not understand a passage, he or she should reread the section, discuss it with classmates, and ask questions of the instructor. Taking notes during this activity can assist the student in reviewing the material later. Students should plan to review their notes on a daily basis to make sure that they are remembering the material. A student can quiz him- or herself by covering up the material and using the headings to recite the important concepts in that section of the chapter.[4]

THE INTERNET

The Internet has changed the way that we live our lives and how we learn. It has been said that you can find anything on the Web; however, just because you find it doesn't mean that it is true. Students must learn how to identify credible websites that can be trusted to give accurate information. The first thing to do is to identify who is putting the information on the website. Credible sources can include universities and colleges (.edu), government webpages (.gov), medical organizations (.org), or hospital related sites (.org). The website should have clearly identified authors with expertise or should provide a bibliography for the information provided. Students should be leery of websites that are commercialized, endorse products, or sell products from the website. Students should also look for information that is current by identifying when the webpage was last updated.

THE LIBRARY

Every university and college and many cities have libraries. And more importantly, they have librarians. Librarians are excellent resources to help students find materials that are relevant and useful in answering their questions. They can assist with selecting the correct database to perform research in and can make suggestions about relevant words and terminology to use when performing research queries. This can save valuable time by helping to limit the available data to those which are most relevant to the project the student is working on. Librarians can also assist the student in ordering materials that may not be located in that library or on the Internet.

STUDENT SERVICES

Every university or college has a student service center that is intended to assist students to be successful. One common offering is tutoring. This sometimes comes in the form of group tutoring, review sessions with a graduate student, or can be individual tutoring. The center usually offers study skill instruction and can assist students in test-taking skills. Students should not overlook those offerings. Students should not wait until they are failing a class to seek assistance either. Learning these skills early in a student's academic career can save the student anxiety and money.

INSTRUCTOR ASSISTANCE

Go early, go often. Instructors have office hours for students to come and get further assistance in the learning process. Students should go to the instructor with specific questions, not vague statements of not understanding. When students explain to the instructor what they do understand and what does not make sense, the instructor is better able to focus the answers on the specific topic. Students who have been reading the assigned material and attending class will be more successful with this learning strategy than those who expect the instructor to explain all of the material again.

SCHEDULES AND CALENDARS

As a general rule, students underestimate the amount of time that instructors expect students to spend on studying outside of class. Students may be used to instructors handing them the material to learn, they memorize it for the exam, and end of story. Application and problem solving require more than memorization. Manipulating the information in your mind, using it to solve problems, and formulating a rationale for choices are much better strategies. They prepare the student for comprehensive exams, clinical work, and the NPTE.

Students in PTA school often are juggling school, jobs, and families. This requires them to be very organized and to develop efficient use of their time. By utilizing a calendar, students can identify upcoming examinations and assignments so that they have adequate time to prepare. Additionally, students may need to utilize a calendar that helps them plan out each day more specifically so that they can schedule study time, time for relaxation, time

for exercise, and time for work, school, or chores. Busy schedules can be overwhelming when they are not planned out. Decreasing the anxiety by being aware and prepared allows the student to feel calmer and to feel in control of his or her daily life.

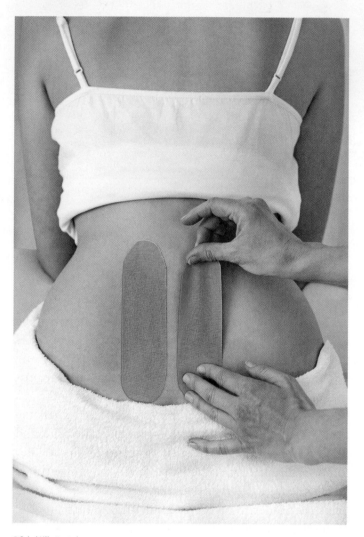

© Bulushi/Shutterstock

Strategies for Success in PTA School

Students will find that they are most successful when they consider not just their own learning style, but when they reflect on their learning as a whole. How successful have their strategies been? How organized is their studying? How committed have they been to learning the information, applying the information, and problem solving? When students identify their motivation, effort, and strategies, they are better able to choose new strategies that will help them improve their learning skills.

LEARNING STRATEGIES

- Create a preferred learning environment. Students should consider the time of day, the type of lighting, surrounding sounds, temperature, type of seating, and snacks/drinks needed. Students who pay attention to these preferences will create a setting that improves their learning abilities by removing distractions and creating comfort.

- Read with purpose and recognize the value of note taking. Taking notes from reading or lectures helps to organize the information from the student's perspective. This will help the student to understand the information better. Students who do not have good note-taking skills should devise a shorthand to help them become faster at note taking. Utilize the lecture's organization to create an outline for the notes.

- Create mnemonics to help remember lists of information. Creating rhymes or putting information to music can also assist the mind in long-term recall.

- Develop supportive relationships; this is the easiest way to improve learning skills. Students who feel isolated in a classroom are less likely to be successful than those who make connections with other students.[5]

- Recognize the personal learning style's strengths and build on them; at the same time, value other learning styles.

- Do not solve problems alone; learning power can be increased when working with others. In addition, working with people with opposite learning styles can add more to the learning process.

- Relate classwork to clearly defined long-range goals. Students who are motivated and have clear goals will see their learning as a stepping stone to reach their goal of becoming a PTA. The motivated student recognizes that effort is important and that setbacks are part of the process.[6]

- PTA school and clinical practice require a strategy and thought process different from those that students may have encountered before. Because every patient is different, students will need to appreciate that not every answer is black and white. In reality, students will be expected not only to show competency in skills but the ability to rationalize when it is appropriate to deviate from the norm. And students should learn to use research evidence to justify their reasoning.

- Recognize the need for active learning strategies. Memorization of information typically does not lead to long-term recall of the data unless the student creates some personal meaning of the information. In order to learn and truly know the necessary information, students should practice skills and review material repeatedly. Secondly, students should understand the information well enough to be able to explain it to others. Students should be able to provide examples to relate the information to the "bigger picture." And lastly, students should use the information to solve a problem, make a recommendation, or explain the rationale for a selected choice.

- Utilize review questions that come with the textbook to deepen learning and test understanding. This could be done in a group setting to allow for discussion of the answers or individually to test the student's preparedness for an exam. This can be a valuable way to identify errors or omissions in understanding and can generate questions that the student can discuss with the instructor.

TEST-TAKING SKILLS

PTA students who do not learn good test-taking skills are working with an unseen disadvantage. In almost every objective test (such as in physical therapy), these students give up points needlessly because of undisciplined testing behaviors, irrational responses to test items, or a variety of other bad habits. As in other sciences, successful test taking in physical therapy involves applying critical reading and thinking skills to the test to avoid making careless mistakes. These careless mistakes can be any of the following:

- Not reading the directions carefully; students should not be in a great hurry to start the test, but should read the instructions first.

- Not monitoring the test time; students should monitor their progress periodically to make sure that they don't get caught in a time crunch.

- Changing the original answers due to second-guessing; students should keep their original answers—research shows that the first intuition is more likely to be correct. Students should change their answers only when they strongly feel that the original answer was incorrect.

- Not allowing enough time to go through the test so that at the end no items are left blank or are misread by a computerized grading program.
- Not clearly identifying what the question is asking. Students should underline or highlight important words that help to answer the question or help to provide context to the question.

The three phases of test-taking strategies for PTA students are:

- In the first phase, the student should go through the test and answer only those items that he or she is confident about; the other questions can be skipped momentarily. This strategy builds up confidence and assures that the student will get credit for what he or she knows if running low on time.
- In the second phase, the student should go through the test and focus on items he or she skipped in the first phase. The student should identify and eliminate incorrect answers by eliminating choices that are definitely wrong or unlikely.
- In the third phase, the student should think critically by doing the following:
  - Being cautious of items that contain absolute terms such as always, never, invariably, none, all, every, and must
  - Substituting a qualified term such as frequently or typically, for an absolute term, such as always or most, to see if the statement is more or less valid than the original one
- When taking multiple-choice tests, a good strategy is to read only the "stem" of the question and not the multiple choices, to see if the correct answer can be determined without having to be prompted by the choices. If no answer can be found that way, the student can read each multiple-choice answer separately and consider whether it is a "true" or "false" choice. The answer that sounds most valid or most true should be the final choice. Sometimes, teachers are limited in their supply of decoy answers, and as a result will make up terms to use for that purpose. For a student who missed classes or has not studied, the decoy is hard to detect; however, if the student has been attending classes regularly and has done a good job of preparing for the test, the student will not choose an answer that sounds totally new.

- When taking a test with true–false items, students generally have a difficult time reading and considering the choices carefully. A slight alteration in the phrasing of the item can make a big difference. The basic ground rule for answering true–false items is that if any part of the statement is not true, the student should select false as the answer. At the same time, true–false items can be overanalyzed to the point that the student goes beyond the scope of the question, looking to find an extreme exception to what the question is testing or the "trick" suspected to be somewhere in the phrasing. The student should read the question carefully, but judge what the question is actually saying.

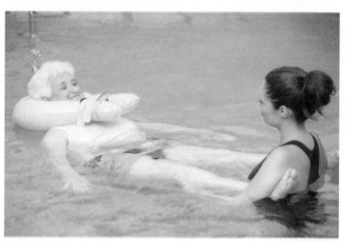

© Monkey Business Images/Shutterstock

Lifelong Learning

While it may be difficult for a student to think about lifelong learning activities at the beginning of his or her career, it is imperative that the student appreciate that learning does not end at graduation. Because of the ever-changing nature of health care, conscientious professionals will always be curious and interested in learning new developments in the field. In beginning the process, students should consider all of the different aspects of this textbook that have suggested resources, introduced topics of learning, or piqued their interest. Making a list of topics that you find interesting and locating resources for learning can help you create a lifelong learning plan. As your career develops, physical therapy practice changes and health care evolves, and so too will your lifelong learning plan.

Discussion Questions

1. With your classmates, discuss learning strategies that have helped you in the past. Explain whether this varies by the type of learning task.
2. Complete an online learning inventory using the sources below. Share your results with your classmates.
   a. Education.com
   b. Multiple Intelligences Assessment (http://www.edutopia.org/multiple-intelligences-assessment)
   c. The Vark Questionnaire (http://vark-learn.com/the-vark-questionnaire/)
3. Discuss learning services available on your campus.

Learning Opportunities

1. Utilizing your course syllabi and schedule, create a daily/monthly calendar that includes school, work, and family/social obligations. Identify when completing homework and studying will fit into the schedule.
2. Utilize the SQ3R strategy to read a chapter in a textbook.
3. List activities that will be part of a lifelong learning plan.

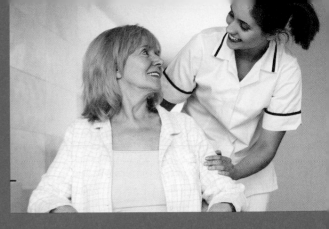

CHAPTER 13

Lifelong Success

OBJECTIVES

After studying this chapter, the reader will be able to:
1. Identify attributes that lead to successful careers.
2. Describe strategies for developing a satisfying career.
3. Create a career plan.

KEY TERMS

competence
initiative
networking

As students enter a new professional program, it may be difficult to imagine career success and project future happiness in the job and life. If one stops to think about life's journey, however, it may be very helpful to consider developing skills and a mind-set that can lead to just those things. Developing skills and enhancing personality traits may make the difference in a job that is satisfying and one that just pays the bills.

Attributes of Successful People

John Maxwell, in his book *The 21 Indispensable Qualities of a Leader,*[7] outlines attributes that leaders have and how to grow those attributes in one's self. These attributes can also lead to success in the workplace and may hold some answers to happiness in life. Those that lead to success include optimism, commitment, passion, competence, initiative, flexibility, generosity, and relationships.[7]

OPTIMISM

There has been quite a bit of research showing that developing the skill of "looking on the bright side" will lead a person to becoming happier and more satisfied with life. To become an optimist, it may be best to spend less time with the perpetual complainers in the workplace. It is easy to fall into the trap of always looking for what is wrong in a situation or complaining over that which you have no control. Optimists try to see what is of value in every situation and expect to succeed. They focus on what is within their influence and what works with their own personal strengths. The power of a positive attitude, resilience in the face of adversity, and recognizing that mistakes create learning opportunities are all part of an optimistic outlook.[8]

COMMITMENT

No one sets out to do a job poorly. Boredom, feeling of being unappreciated, or pressure to do more work can cause a person to cut corners or give up caring about providing the best care. A person who is truly committed to his or her job will make decisions that benefit the whole company, not just him- or herself. Good work performance and doing the right thing are important in physical therapy because they lead the person to develop character. When one has good character, others will come to depend upon that person. Additionally, employers will come to see that the employee is trustworthy and will reward this effort in the long run. This is particularly important for the physical therapist assistant (PTA) who works closely with the physical therapist (PT) to provide patient care. Showing commitment to the patient will help develop the bond of trust necessary in the PT/PTA relationship.

PASSION

When PTA students are asked why they want to become a PTA, a frequent response is because they want to help people. That is a great answer, but typically wouldn't sustain anyone throughout a whole career. Instead, they must come to feel passion about physical therapy. Feelings of excitement, joy, wonder, and awe are what sustain people throughout their work careers. This passion for physical therapy can be contagious, so it is helpful to surround yourself with people who are also passionate about what they are doing.

COMPETENCE

Competence is a cornerstone principle in physical therapy education. The assessment of skills and knowledge is completed by showing competence through skill checks, practical exams, and clinical internship evaluations. All of this leads to completing the National Physical Therapy Examination to show minimum competency. However, no one remains competent in physical therapy without retaining curiosity and initiative to keep learning. Health care research constantly forces a professional to continue to learn and to look for ways to improve. This drive toward excellence prevents PTAs from becoming bored with their jobs and pushes them to remain competent in the field. Lifelong learning is an important component and will help the PTA become more successful in patient care.

INITIATIVE

Initiative is doing more than what is expected of you. Recently, a PTA was honored for doing more than what was expected of her. Her patient was having difficulty with swelling in her arm due to cancer treatments. This patient did not have health care insurance that would assist her in paying for a compression garment, which was critical to controlling the swelling. So, the PTA made one for her using her sewing machine at home. This PTA took the initiative to do more for her patient, not because she had to, but because she wanted to. When people do more for others (their patients, their employers, their coworkers), they end up feeling more happiness and eventually reap rewards that they had no idea could happen.

FLEXIBILITY

Flexibility helps a person recognize change will occur and one must learn to adapt. This is a critical attribute for anyone in health care. Health care laws and payment for health care services are constantly changing. It is imperative that the PTA be aware of the changes and adapt to them. Being flexible and thinking creatively can help the PT/PTA team to look for new ways to provide care for their communities and to show value in the care that they provide. As the population of the United States ages and becomes more culturally diverse, physical therapy must learn to adapt and be proactive in creating opportunities. Flexibility and becoming an agent of change will help the PTA feel more in control and will prevent anxiety that often comes with change.

GENEROSITY

Part of developing gratitude and feeling satisfaction in life is appreciating what one has. The act of being generous to others takes the focus off of one's self. Monetary generosity is only part of the equation. People have many talents and often generosity has more to do with sharing one's talents and time. Generosity shows others a spirit of compassion and caring that connects a community together. And all people have a drive to be connected to others. PTAs will be offered many opportunities to share their talents such as pro bono clinics, community education, events to assist elderly residents in the community, opportunities to bring awareness to diseases through research funding activities, and assisting those less fortunate.

RELATIONSHIPS

It may seem like a foregone conclusion that PTs and PTAs enjoy working with people. Students should not underestimate the value of developing relationships. Work becomes more enjoyable when a person has a good relationship with those he or she works with and this creates more job satisfaction. A work relationship should have trust, good communication, and mutual respect to allow for productivity. This should be extended to the PTA's relationship with the supervising PT and with the patients.

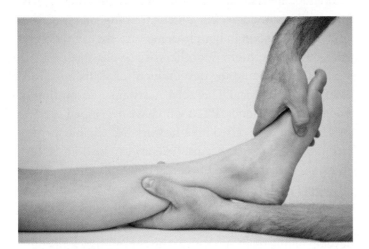

© Image Point Fr/Shutterstock

Developing a PTA Career

NETWORKING

As a student, it may be helpful to identify working members of the profession who might act as mentors. Mentors can assist students in navigating the transition from classroom to clinic to the first job. Mentors may be found through joining national, state, and college physical therapy organizations, via alumni of the college the student is attending or through hometown physical therapy community members. Creating a relationship with a mentor can help a student understand the expectations and behaviors that will lead him or her to job opportunities and career success. The American Physical Therapy Association (APTA) offers a mentoring program for new graduates that connects them to more seasoned professionals who can answer questions and help guide their early career decisions.

The APTA has many opportunities for students to network, starting with the student assembly. The student assembly was created to help students understand the APTA, to connect with current leadership and members, and to connect with other students across the United States and the world. Leaders communicate with students via Twitter, Facebook, and Skype. Student leaders have created a newsletter called *The Loop* and have developed a network of core ambassadors to help communicate opportunities and information to all students. Students have opportunities to attend the National Student Conclave, the Next Conference, Combined Sections, and the House of Delegates and National Assembly meeting of PTA leaders. At the state chapter level, student special interest groups exist to help connect students from area colleges and universities together and allow networking with the state chapter. All of these opportunities allow for networking and learning within the physical therapy community that will help the student find his or her niche.

CAREER DEVELOPMENT

Before beginning a job search, students should start by identifying their career goals. This will help new graduates clearly identify if the company meets their career values, how they will best fit within the company, and will assist them in identifying their attributes that will benefit the company. Skill surveys are available online that can assist graduates in identifying career goals, creating a list of skills that can highlight their interests and strengths; personality assessments can identify values and personality traits. Graduates can utilize these assessments to create resumes and to evaluate job opportunities. Career-Intelligence.com and iSeek.org are two websites that feature these assessments.

The APTA has created a document, *Considerations for Practice Opportunities and Professional Development*, to assist graduates in assessing whether or not certain job openings would meet their professional goals.[9]

> Some questions graduates should ask themselves include:[9]
>
> **Financial Considerations**
>
> - How is the management of the facility set up?
> - What opportunities are available for advancement?
> - What are the wages and benefits?
>
> *(continues)*

Professional Development Considerations

- Does the facility provide opportunities for continuing education?
- Does the facility have a mentoring program?
- Does the facility have a plan for growth and sustainability?

Ethical and Legal Considerations

- How does the business handle its financial operations?
- Do PTs control patient care decisions?
- What is the role of PTAs and physical therapy aides?

Quality of Care Considerations

- What is the job description of the PT and PTA?
- What input do the employees have into the practice of physical therapy, policies and procedures, and quality improvement practices?
- What are the policies for providing quality care and concern for patient outcomes?

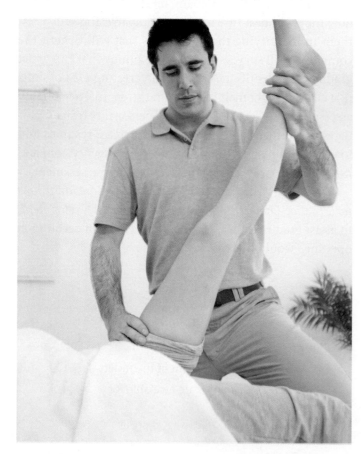

© wavebreakmedia/Shutterstock

CONTINUING COMPETENCE

During the identification of career goals, new graduates should consider what areas or topics of physical therapy that they found most interesting in school. Because physical therapist assistant education prepares graduates to work with entry-level skills, students can utilize their interest areas to develop a continuing education plan. This plan will help graduates to further develop skills that may set them apart from others in the workforce. This can be a valuable tool when applying for jobs or it can create opportunities for specialization. Some students find that returning to college for degrees in athletic training, massage therapy, or certification in lymphedema care, for example, can open doors that might not otherwise be possible.

Another avenue for development of skills and leadership is the Physical Therapist Assistant Recognition of Advanced Proficiency. PTAs who have developed specific skills within a specified area of work are eligible for this recognition. The advance proficiency can be done in several specialized areas: acute care, aquatic, cardiovascular/pulmonary, education, geriatric, integumentary, musculoskeletal, neuromuscular, oncology, and/or pediatric physical therapy. The advanced recognition can be utilized to develop public relations within the community and could be used as an identification of advanced skills when applying for a new job.

As students advance through their PTA program, they are immersed in reading research and identifying evidence-based practice. This practice should continue after graduation and can lead graduates to identify areas of practice that they find interesting. Creating journal reading groups with other professionals can help to facilitate learning and collegiality between practitioners. Learning through journal readings and continuing education courses will help to develop a deeper understanding of physical therapy questions. This may even lead graduates to research of their own.

An additional component of continuing competency is that many states require continuing education as a requirement of relicensure. The purpose of this requirement is to increase knowledge, increase clinical competence, increase enthusiasm and contentment in professional work, and improve benefits to business. The number of hours vary by state, but research shows that PTs in states that require continuing education hours actually complete more hours than those in states that do not require any continuing education.[10]

LEADERSHIP DEVELOPMENT

In addition to the discussion of career development and continuing education, membership in the national professional organization can lead PTs and PTAs to leadership roles in the association, the community, or places of employment. The APTA has programs developed through the student assembly to help students develop leadership skills. The APTA also has a professional development program available for members through the learning center. The Health Policy and Administration Section of the APTA has developed a leadership certificate called LAMP (Leadership, Administration, Management, and Professionalism). This program requires a series of courses, projects, and mentoring to help the person develop these skills.

Every year the Association recognizes members, who are graduates with 5 years or less experience who have stepped into leadership roles in the APTA, with the Emerging Leader award. Members have the opportunity to become leaders in the PTA Caucus, at the chapter level or within sections.

Leadership within the workplace can also be a gratifying endeavor. PTAs can become leaders within their teams, may be employed in supervisory positions such as MDS coordinators or rehabilitation team leaders in skilled nursing facilities, or may become clinical instructors for PTA programs. Some PTAs may also choose to continue their careers as instructors within PTA programs. In addition, success within the workplace may also take the form of ownership in physical therapy clinics.

Discussion Questions

1. Describe a person that you feel is successful and list the attributes that make you feel this way.
2. Discuss what your career goals are in 5 years, 10 years, 15 years, and so on.

Learning Opportunities

1. Create a plan to develop the attributes of successful people.
2. Develop a timeline of career goals and connect them to activities to assist you in achieving them.

Summary of Part V

Part V provides students with an opportunity to plan for success in both their academic career and their clinical career. A discussion of learning styles and learning strategies provides insight into study strategies that can assist in becoming successful. Learning resources are also explored. In Chapter 13, the text explored attributes of leaders and opportunities to become leaders in physical therapy. Development of a career starts with identifying career goals and understanding what options for development are available.

References (Part V)

1. Caine, G, Caine, R. Brain mind principles. Accessed April 2015 at: http://www.cainelearning.com/brain-mind-principles/.
2. Duckworth, AL, Yeager, DS. (in press). Measurement matters: Assessing personal qualities other than cognitive ability for educational purposes. *Educational Researcher*. Accessed April 2015 at: https://sites.sas.upenn.edu/duckworth/pages/research.
3. Dreeben, O. *Patient Education in Rehabilitation*. Sudbury, MA: Jones & Bartlett Publishers; 2010.
4. Study Guides and Strategies. SQ3R reading method. Accessed April 2015 at: http://www.studygs.net/texred2.htm.
5. Erickson, B, Peters, C, Strommer, D. *Teaching First-Year College Students*. San Francisco, CA: Jossey-Bass; 2006.
6. Pink, D. *Drive, the Surprising Truth about What Motivates Us*. New York City, NY: Riverhead Trade; 2011.
7. Maxwell, JC. *The 21 Indispensable Qualities of a Leader*. Nashville, TN: Thomas Nelson; 1999.
8. Sigelman, M. *Learned Optimism: How to Change Your Mind and Your Life*. New York City, NY: Vintage Books; 2006.
9. American Physical Therapy Association. Considerations for practice opportunities and professional development. Accessed May 2015 at: www.apta.org.
10. Landers, MR, McWhorter, JW, Krum, LL, Glovinsky, D. Mandatory continuing education in physical therapy: Survey of physical therapists in states with and states without a mandate. *Physical Therapy Journal*. September 2005; 85(9): 861–871.

APPENDIX A

Hippocratic Oath

I swear by Apollo the physician, and Aesculapius, and Health, and All-heal, and all the gods and goddesses, that, according to my ability and judgment, I will keep this Oath and this stipulation: to reckon him who taught me this Art equally dear to me as my parents, to share my substance with him, and relieve his necessities if required; to look upon his offspring in the same footing as my own brothers, and to teach them this art, if they shall wish to learn it, without fee or stipulation; and that by precept, lecture, and every other mode of instruction, I will impart a knowledge of the Art to my own sons, and those of my teachers, and to disciples bound by a stipulation and oath according to the law of medicine, but to none others.

I will follow that system of regimen which, according to my ability and judgment, I consider for the benefit of my patients, and abstain from whatever is deleterious and mischievous.

I will give no deadly medicine to any one if asked, nor suggest any such counsel; and in like manner I will not give to a woman a pessary to produce abortion. With purity and with holiness I will pass my life and practice my Art. I will not cut persons laboring under the stone, but will leave this to be done by men who are practitioners of this work.

Into whatever houses I enter, I will go into them for the benefit of the sick, and will abstain from every voluntary act of mischief and corruption; and, further from the seduction of females or males, of free men and slaves.

Whatever, in connection with my professional practice or not, in connection with it, I see or hear, in the life of men, which ought not to be spoken of abroad, I will not divulge, as reckoning that all such should be kept secret.

While I continue to keep this Oath unviolated, may it be granted to me to enjoy life and the practice of the art, respected by all men, in all times! But should I trespass and violate this Oath, may the reverse be my lot!

APPENDIX B

Patient's Bill of Rights

1. The patient has the right to considerate and respectful care.
2. The patient has the right to obtain, from their certified provider, complete current information regarding their diagnosis, treatment, and prognosis in terms the patient can reasonably be expected to understand. When it is not advisable to give such information to the patient, the information should be made available to an appropriate person on their behalf.
3. The patient has the right to receive from their certified provider information to make informed consent prior to the start of any procedure or treatment. This shall include such information as the medically significant risks involved with any procedure and probable duration of incapacitation. Where medically appropriate, alternatives for care or treatment should be explained to the patient.
4. The patient has the right to refuse any and all treatment to the extent permitted by law and to be informed of any of the medical consequences of their action.
5. The patient has the right to every consideration of privacy concerning their own medical care program limited only by state statutes, rules, regulations, or imminent danger to the individual or others.

6. The patient has the right to be advised if the clinician, hospital, clinic, or others propose to engage in or perform human experimentation affecting their care or treatment. The patient has the right to refuse to participate in such research projects.
7. The patient has the privilege to examine and receive an explanation of the bill.
8. Insurance companies may not discriminate against children who have preexisting conditions.
9. Insurance companies may not cancel coverage based upon prior illness or errors in application for insurance. Additionally, coverage may not be limited based upon total lifetime coverage limits.
10. Insurance companies may not limit the consumer's choice of health care providers including which emergency room location a patient may access.
11. Patients may appeal denied services to an independent third party.
12. Young adults may remain on their parent's insurance until age 26.
13. Patients will receive preventative care without cost such as mammograms, immunizations, and prenatal and new baby care.

Data from: Advisory Commission on Consumer Protection and Quality in the Health Care Industry. Patients' Rights and Responsibilties. Found at: http://www.hcqualitycommission.gov/final/append_a.html. Accessed March 17, 2010.

APPENDIX C

American Physical Therapy Association's Code of Ethics for Physical Therapists

HOD S06-09-07-12 [Amended HOD S06-00-12-23; HOD 06-91-05-05; HOD 06-87-11-17; HOD 06-81-06-18; HOD 06-78-06-08; HOD 06-78-06-07; HOD 06-77-18-30; HOD 06-77-17-27; Initial HOD 06-73-13-24] [Standard]

Preamble

The Code of Ethics for the Physical Therapist (Code of Ethics) delineates the ethical obligations of all physical therapists as determined by the House of Delegates of the American Physical Therapy Association (APTA). The purposes of this Code of Ethics are to:

1. Define the ethical principles that form the foundation of physical therapist practice in patient/client management, consultation, education, research, and administration.
2. Provide standards of behavior and performance that form the basis of professional accountability to the public.
3. Provide guidance for physical therapists facing ethical challenges, regardless of their professional roles and responsibilities.
4. Educate physical therapists, students, other health care professionals, regulators, and the public regarding the core values, ethical principles, and standards that guide the professional conduct of the physical therapist.
5. Establish the standards by which the American Physical Therapy Association can determine if a physical therapist has engaged in unethical conduct.

No code of ethics is exhaustive nor can it address every situation. Physical therapists are encouraged to seek additional advice or consultation in instances where the guidance of the Code of Ethics may not be definitive.

This Code of Ethics is built upon the five roles of the physical therapist (management of patients/clients, consultation, education, research, and administration), the core values of the profession, and the multiple realms of ethical action (individual, organizational, and societal). Physical therapist practice is guided by a set of seven core values: accountability, altruism, compassion/caring, excellence, integrity, professional duty, and social responsibility. Throughout the document the primary core values that support specific principles are indicated in parentheses. Unless a specific role is indicated in the principle, the duties and obligations being delineated pertain to the five roles of the physical therapist. Fundamental to the Code of Ethics is the special obligation of physical therapists to empower, educate, and enable those with impairments, activity limitations, participation restrictions, and disabilities to facilitate greater independence, health, wellness, and enhanced quality of life.

Principle #1

Physical therapists shall respect the inherent dignity and rights of all individuals.

(Core Values: Compassion/Caring, Integrity)

1A. Physical therapists shall act in a respectful manner toward each person regardless of age, gender, race, nationality, religion, ethnicity, social or economic status, sexual orientation, health condition, or disability.

1B. Physical therapists shall recognize their personal biases and shall not discriminate against others in physical therapist practice, consultation, education, research, and administration.

Principle #2

Physical therapists shall be trustworthy and compassionate in addressing the rights and needs of patients/clients.

(Core Values: Altruism, Compassion/Caring, Professional Duty)

2A. Physical therapists shall adhere to the core values of the profession and shall act in the best interests of patients/clients over the interests of the physical therapist.

2B. Physical therapists shall provide physical therapy services with compassionate and caring behaviors that incorporate the individual and cultural differences of patients/clients.

2C. Physical therapists shall provide the information necessary to allow patients or their surrogates to make informed decisions about physical therapy care or participation in clinical research.

2D. Physical therapists shall collaborate with patients/clients to empower them in decisions about their health care.

2E. Physical therapists shall protect confidential patient/client information and may disclose confidential information to appropriate authorities only when allowed or as required by law.

Principle #3

Physical therapists shall be accountable for making sound professional judgments.

(Core Values: Excellence, Integrity)

3A. Physical therapists shall demonstrate independent and objective professional judgment in the patient/client's best interest in all practice settings.

3B. Physical therapists shall demonstrate professional judgment informed by professional standards, evidence (including current literature and established best practice), practitioner experience, and patient/client values.

3C. Physical therapists shall make judgments within their scope of practice and level of expertise and shall communicate with, collaborate with, or refer to peers or other health care professionals when necessary.

3D. Physical therapists shall not engage in conflicts of interest that interfere with professional judgment.

3E. Physical therapists shall provide appropriate direction of and communication with physical therapist assistants and support personnel.

Principle #4

Physical therapists shall demonstrate integrity in their relationships with patients/clients, families, colleagues, students, research participants, other health care providers, employers, payers, and the public.

(Core Value: Integrity)

4A. Physical therapists shall provide truthful, accurate, and relevant information and shall not make misleading representations.

4B. Physical therapists shall not exploit persons over whom they have supervisory, evaluative, or other authority (e.g., patients/clients, students, supervisees, research participants, or employees).

4C. Physical therapists shall discourage misconduct by health care professionals and report illegal or unethical acts to the relevant authority, when appropriate.

4D. Physical therapists shall report suspected cases of abuse involving children or vulnerable adults to the appropriate authority, subject to law.

4E. Physical therapists shall not engage in any sexual relationship with any of their patients/clients, supervisees, or students.

4F. Physical therapists shall not harass anyone verbally, physically, emotionally, or sexually.

Principle #5

Physical therapists shall fulfill their legal and professional obligations.

(Core Values: Professional Duty, Accountability)

5A. Physical therapists shall comply with applicable local, state, and federal laws and regulations.

5B. Physical therapists shall have primary responsibility for supervision of physical therapist assistants and support personnel.

5C. Physical therapists involved in research shall abide by accepted standards governing protection of research participants.

5D. Physical therapists shall encourage colleagues with physical, psychological, or substance-related impairments that may adversely impact their professional responsibilities to seek assistance or counsel.

5E. Physical therapists who have knowledge that a colleague is unable to perform their professional responsibilities with reasonable skill and safety shall report this information to the appropriate authority.

5F. Physical therapists shall provide notice and information about alternatives for obtaining care in the event the physical therapist terminates the provider relationship while the patient/client continues to need physical therapy services.

Principle #6

Physical therapists shall enhance their expertise through the lifelong acquisition and refinement of knowledge, skills, abilities, and professional behaviors.

(Core Value: Excellence)

6A. Physical therapists shall achieve and maintain professional competence.

6B. Physical therapists shall take responsibility for their professional development based on critical self-assessment and reflection on changes in physical therapist practice, education, health care delivery, and technology.

6C. Physical therapists shall evaluate the strength of evidence and applicability of content presented during professional development activities before integrating the content or techniques into practice.

6D. Physical therapists shall cultivate practice environments that support professional development, lifelong learning, and excellence.

Principle #7

Physical therapists shall promote organizational behaviors and business practices that benefit patients/clients and society.

(Core Values: Integrity, Accountability)

7A. Physical therapists shall promote practice environments that support autonomous and accountable professional judgments.

7B. Physical therapists shall seek remuneration as is deserved and reasonable for physical therapist services.

7C. Physical therapists shall not accept gifts or other considerations that influence or give an appearance of influencing their professional judgment.

7D. Physical therapists shall fully disclose any financial interest they have in products or services that they recommend to patients/clients.

7E. Physical therapists shall be aware of charges and shall ensure that documentation and coding for physical therapy services accurately reflect the nature and extent of the services provided.

7F. Physical therapists shall refrain from employment arrangements, or other arrangements, that prevent physical therapists from fulfilling professional obligations to patients/ clients.

Principle #8

Physical therapists shall participate in efforts to meet the health needs of people locally, nationally, or globally.

(Core Value: Social Responsibility)

8A. Physical therapists shall provide pro bono physical therapy services or support organizations that meet the health needs of people who are economically disadvantaged, uninsured, and underinsured.

8B. Physical therapists shall advocate to reduce health disparities and health care inequities, improve access to health care services, and address the health, wellness, and preventive health care needs of people.

8C. Physical therapists shall be responsible stewards of health care resources and shall avoid overutilization or underutilization of physical therapy services.

8D. Physical therapists shall educate members of the public about the benefits of physical therapy and the unique role of the physical therapist.

APPENDIX D

American Physical Therapy Association's Standards of Ethical Conduct for Physical Therapist Assistants

STANDARDS OF ETHICAL CONDUCT FOR THE PHYSICAL THERAPIST ASSISTANT HOD S06-00-13-24 [Amended HOD 06-91-06-07; Initial HOD 06-82-04-08] [Standard]

Preamble

This document of the American Physical Therapy Association sets forth standards for the ethical conduct of the physical therapist assistant. All physical therapist assistants are responsible for maintaining high standards of conduct while assisting physical therapists. The physical therapist assistant shall act in the best interest of the patient/client. These standards of conduct shall be binding on all physical therapist assistants.

Standard 1 A physical therapist assistant shall respect the rights and dignity of all individuals and shall provide compassionate care.

Standard 2 A physical therapist assistant shall act in a trustworthy manner towards patients/clients.

Standard 3 A physical therapist assistant shall provide selected physical therapy interventions only under the supervision and direction of a physical therapist.

Standard 4 A physical therapist assistant shall comply with laws and regulations governing physical therapy.

Standard 5 A physical therapist assistant shall achieve and maintain competence in the provision of selected physical therapy interventions.

Standard 6 A physical therapist assistant shall make judgments that are commensurate with their educational and legal qualifications as a physical therapist assistant.

Standard 7 A physical therapist assistant shall protect the public and the profession from unethical, incompetent, and illegal acts.

(See also Ethics and Judicial Committee document *Guide for Conduct of the Physical Therapist Assistant*)

Relationship to Vision 2020: Professionalism; (General Counsel, ext. 3252)

[Document updated: 12/14/2009]

Explanation of Reference Numbers: *BOD P00-00-00-00* stands for Board of Directors/month/year/page/vote in the Board of Directors Minutes; the "P" indicates that it is a position (see below). For example, BOD P11-97-06-18 means that this position can be found in the November 1997 Board of Directors minutes on Page 6 and that it was Vote 18.

P: Position | S: Standard | G: Guideline | Y: Policy | R: Procedure

Visit www.apta.org for complete and up-to-date standards.

APPENDIX E

Problem-Solving Algorithm Utilized by PTAs in Patient/Client Intervention

This algorithm, developed by the American Physical Therapy Association's Departments of Education, Accreditation, and Practice, is intended to reflect current policies and positions on the problem-solving processes utilized by physical therapist assistants in the provision of selected interventions. The controlling assumptions are essential to understanding and applying this algorithm (see **FIGURE E-1**). (This document can be found in *A Normative Model of Physical Therapist Assistant Education: Version 2007.*)

- The physical therapist integrates the five elements of patient/client management—examination, evaluation, diagnosis, prognosis, and intervention—in a manner designed to optimize outcomes. Responsibility for completion of the examination, evaluation, diagnosis, and prognosis is borne solely by the physical therapist.

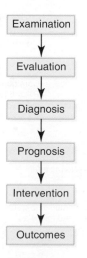

FIGURE E-1 Controlling assumptions.

The physical therapist's plan of care may involve the physical therapist assistant to assist with selected interventions. This algorithm represents the decision making of the physical therapist assistant within the intervention element.

- The physical therapist will direct and supervise the physical therapist assistant consistent with the APTA House of Delegates positions, including Direction and Supervision of the Physical Therapist Assistant (HOD P06-05-18-26); APTA core documents, including Standards of Ethical Conduct for the PTA; federal and state legal practice standards; and institutional regulations.
- All selected interventions are directed and supervised by the physical therapist. Additionally, the physical therapist remains responsible for the physical therapy services provided when the physical therapist's plan of care involves the physical therapist assistant to assist with selected interventions.
- Selected intervention(s) includes the procedural intervention, associated data collection, and communication, including written documentation associated with the safe, effective, and efficient completion of the task.
- The algorithm may represent the thought processes involved in a patient/client interaction or episode of care. Entry into the algorithm will depend on the point at which the physical therapist assistant is directed by the physical therapist to provide selected interventions.
- Communication between the physical therapist and physical therapist assistant regarding patient/client care is ongoing. The algorithm does not intend to imply a limitation or restriction on communication between the physical therapist and physical therapist assistant (see **FIGURE E-2**).

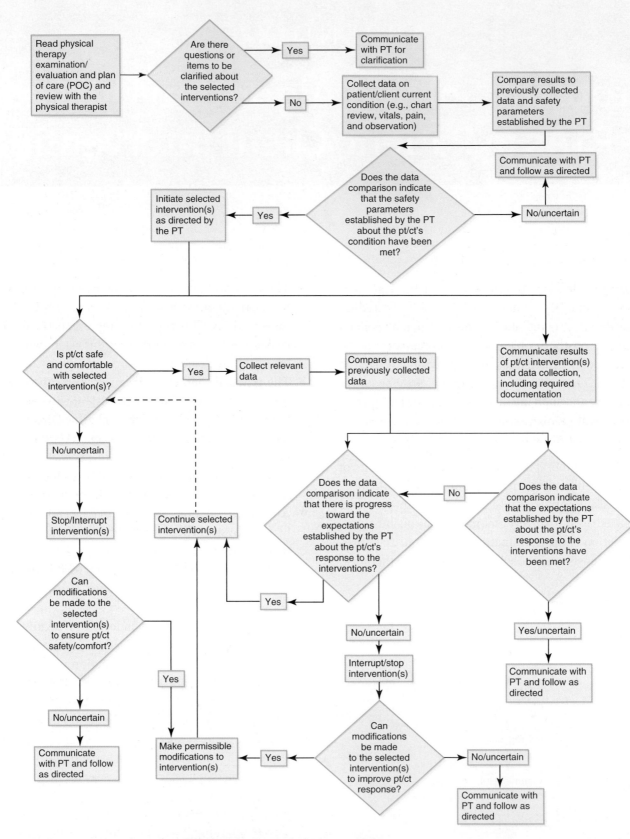

FIGURE E-2 Problem-solving algorithm utilized by PTAs in patient/client intervention.

Issued by Advisory Panel of Physical Therapist Assistant and adopted by the American Physical Therapy Association Board of Directors, January 2011. Available at www.apta.org, Accessed July 2015, with permission of the American Physical Therapy Association. This material is copyrighted, and any further reproduction or distribution is prohibited.

* See controlling assumptions

Glossary

American Physical Therapy Association (APTA): The American Physical Therapy Association (APTA) is an individual membership professional organization representing member physical therapists (PTs), physical therapist assistants (PTAs), and students of physical therapy.

Americans with Disabilities Act (ADA): The Americans with Disabilities Act of 1990 (ADA) prohibits discrimination and ensures equal opportunity for persons with disabilities in employment, state and local government services, public accommodations, commercial facilities, and transportation.

APGAR screening: A system of evaluating an infant's physical condition at birth, created by Virginia Apgar, an American anesthesiologist; the infant's heart rate, respiration, muscle tone, response to stimuli, and color are rated at 1 minute, and again at 5 minutes after birth.

Assessment data: Data that include an appraisal or evaluation of a patient's condition based on clinical and laboratory data, medical history, and the patient's accounts of symptoms; data included in the "A" section of the SOAP note; in the SOAP note, they provide the rationale for the necessity of the skilled physical therapy services, interpret the data, and give meaning to the data.

Atherosclerosis: Fatty or cholesterol-lipid calcium deposited in the walls of arteries, veins, and the lymphatic system.

Autonomy: The ability to act independently of others.

Bloodborne pathogens: Pathogenic microorganisms that are present in human blood and that can infect and cause disease in persons who are exposed to blood containing these pathogens; examples of bloodborne pathogens are hepatitis B and HIV.

Bloodborne pathogens standards (BPS): A group of rules that provide information for preventing occupational infections in employees that have a reasonable risk of coming in contact with bloodborne infections such as HIV or hepatitis.

Closed question: A question that requires a "yes" or "no" answer.

Commission on Accreditation in Physical Therapy Education (CAPTE): The Commission on Accreditation in Physical Therapy Education (CAPTE) is an accrediting agency that grants accreditation to qualified entry-level education programs for physical therapists and physical therapist assistants.

Communication: The use of words, sounds, signs, or behaviors to impart information to someone else.

Competence: The ability to complete a task well and to a certain professional standard.

Congestive heart failure: The inability of the heart to pump enough blood to maintain adequate circulation of the blood to meet the body's metabolic needs.

Cryotherapy: Therapeutic application of cold such as an ice or cold pack.

Cultural competence: Cultural competence is a group of skills, behaviors, and attitudes that individuals acquire that allow them to provide effective clinical care to patients from a variety of cultural differences, such as ethnicity, racial, age, or gender.

Dementia: A progressive, irreversible decline in mental function.

Direct personal supervision: The physical therapist is physically present and immediately available to direct and supervise tasks performed by the physical therapist assistant.

Disability: The inability to engage in age-specific, gender-related, and sex-specific roles in a particular social context and physical environment; it is also any restriction or lack of ability (resulting from an injury) to perform an activity in a manner or within the range considered normal for a human being.

Domestic violence: A pattern of abusive behavior that keeps one partner in a position of power over the other partner through the use of fear, intimidation, and control.

Duration: The length of time that something lasts. In exercise, it could be the length of time spent doing a cardiovascular exercise.

Dyspnea: Inability to breathe or difficulty breathing (shortness of breath).

Dystonia: Impaired tone due to prolonged muscular contractions causing twisting of body parts.

Economic abuse: Attempting to or making a person financially dependent such as maintaining total control over financial resources, withholding access to money, or forbidding attendance at school or employment.

Edema: Accumulation of large amounts of fluid in the tissues of the body; swelling.

Electrotherapy: The use of electrical stimulation modalities in physical therapy treatment.

Emotional abuse: Undermining a person's sense of self-worth by doing things such as criticizing constantly, calling names, belittling one's abilities, or damaging a partner's relationship with the children.

Empathy: The feeling that you understand and share another person's experiences and emotions.

Ethics: Rules of behavior based on ideas about what is morally good or bad.

Ethnocentrism: The universal tendency of human beings to think that their ways of thinking, acting, and believing are the only right, proper, and natural ways; universal phenomenon in that most people tend to believe that their ways of living, believing, and acting are right, proper, and morally correct.

Evaluation: The use of information to make a judgment about a patient's condition.

Examination: The use of tests and measures to gather information about a patient's condition.

Experimental research: A scientific study of a hypothesis that includes a control group and a test group.

Flaccidity: A state of tone in the muscle that produces weak and floppy limbs.

Flexibility exercises: Activities that causes a lengthening of soft tissues.

Frequency: The number of times that an exercise is repeated daily, weekly, or monthly.

Functional limitation: Restriction of the ability to perform a physical action, activity, or task in an efficient, typically expected, or competent manner.

Functional outcome report (FOR): A measurement of a patient's function at examination and evaluation that is required by Medicare for payment. The FOR will also include a goal outcome and will periodically be updated to provide Medicare with information about a patient's progress toward the discharge functional outcome goal.

General supervision: The physical therapist is available by telecommunications to supervise interventions provided by the physical therapist assistant.

Health Insurance Portability and Accountability Act (HIPAA): The Health Insurance Portability and Accountability Act of 1996, among other things, provides rules that govern to whom, in what format, and when information about a patient can be released to others.

Health maintenance organization (HMO): An organization that provides health care to people who make payments to it and who agree to use the doctors, hospitals, etc., that belong to the organization.

Hydrotherapy: Physical therapy intervention using water.

Hypertonia: Increased muscular tension above normal resting level.

Hypotonia: Decreased muscular tension below normal resting level.

Informed consent: An agreement by a patient that grants permission for an intervention after having been provided information about the risks, benefits, etc.

Initiative: A personal characteristic that demonstrates the willingness and awareness to perform tasks without being directed to do so by someone else.

Interdisciplinary team: A group of health care individuals of different specialties that work together for a specific goal or purpose.

Intradisciplinary team: A group of health care professionals from the same specialty that work together for a specific goal or purpose.

Kinesthesia: A sensation that provides information about position and movement.

Kinesthetic sense: The ability to sense the direction of movement.

Learning: The process of assimilating, understanding, and utilizing information that is being taught.

Medicaid: A government program that provides money for health care services when patients cannot pay for themselves.

Medical diagnosis: Physician's identification of the cause of the patient's illness or discomfort.

Medicare: A medical program that provide money for medical care of older adults.

Morals: Concerning what is right and wrong in human behavior.

Multidisciplinary team: A multidisciplinary team (MDT) is composed of different health care professions that make treatment recommendations that facilitate quality patient care, but do not necessarily have common goals.

Networking: A cultivation of relationships with professionals within a field of study.

Nonexperimental research: Nonexperimental research is a study which does not control the variables but allows for collection of data which is interpreted to create a conclusion.

Numerical Rating System (NRS): A system created to provide a quantitative rating of a patient's pain.

Objective data: Data included in the "O" section of the SOAP note; they include information gathered by the health care provider through examination or assessment (or reassessment) of the patient; in the SOAP note are information that can be observed, measured, or reproduced by another health care provider with the same training as the initial provider.

Occupational Safety and Health Administration (OSHA): A government agency that provides policies, training, and education to assure safe and healthful working conditions for employees.

Open question: A question that requires an answer that expands beyond "yes" or "no."

Orthosis: A device added to a person's body to support, position, or immobilize a part to correct deformities, assist weak muscles, and restore function.

Physical abuse: Abuse by grabbing, pinching, shoving, slapping, hitting, hair pulling, or biting; also abuse by denying medical care or forcing alcohol and/or drug use.

Physical therapist assistant (PTA): A PTA is an educated health care professional that aides work under the direction and supervision of physical therapists.

Physical therapy diagnosis: The use of data obtained by physical therapy examination and other relevant information to determine the cause and nature of a patient's impairments, functional limitations, and disabilities.

Plan of care (POC): A plan of care is a list of goals and interventions developed by the physical therapist after evaluating the needs of a patient.

Policy: A plan of action chosen from all options to address a particular situation and allow consistency in response to the situation.

Preferred provider organization (PPO): A health care plan that allows members to choose any provider, within or outside of the network of professionals. Care provided within the network will be provided at a discounted price and care outside of the network may require an increased cost incurred by the patient.

Problem-oriented medical record (POMR): A medical record that is organized by the patient's impairment and treatment interventions.

Procedure: A series of actions performed in a particular order.

Proprioception: The awareness of posture, movement, and changes in equilibrium and the knowledge of position, weight, and resistance of objects in relation to the body; includes awareness of the joints at rest and with movement.

Prosthesis: An artificial appliance that replaces a limb that has been amputated.

Protected health information (PHI): Protected health information is any information about a patient's health, any health care interventions or health care payments that can be linked to a specific patient.

Psychological abuse: Abuse causing fear by intimidation; threatening physical harm to self, partner, or children; destruction of pets and property; mind games or forcing isolation from friends, family, school, and/or work.

Renal dialysis: The process of diffusing blood across a semipermeable membrane to remove toxic materials and to maintain fluid, electrolyte, and acid–base balance in cases of impaired kidney function or absence of the kidneys.

Research: A study performed to find new information about a particular topic.

Rigidity: Hypertonicity of muscles offering a constant, uniform resistance to passive movement; the affected muscles are unable to relax and are in a state of contraction even at rest.

Self-awareness: The understanding of your own personality and character.

Sexual abuse: Abuse by coercing or attempting to coerce any sexual contact without consent, abuse by marital rape, forcing sex after physical beating, attacks on sexual parts of the body, or treating another in a sexually demeaning manner.

Sign: A recognizable indication observed in a patient that demonstrates an illness, disease, or impairment.

SOAP format: A system of documentation that organizes information into subjective, objective, assessment, and plan.

Source-oriented medical record: A system of recording health care information that is organized by the provider that administers the care.

Spasticity: Increase in muscle tone and stretch reflex of a muscle resulting in increased resistance to passive stretch of the muscle and high response to sensory stimulation.

SQ3R: Survey, Question, Read, Recite, and Review (SQ3R) is a system for studying and learning information.

Subjective data: Data included in the "S" section of the SOAP note; they include information gathered through an interview of the patient or a representative of the patient; all information gathered by the health care provider.

Symptom: A complaint from a patient describing an illness, disease, or impairment.

Teaching: The act of imparting information to another person that they were not aware of or did not previously understand.

Therapeutic exercises: Therapeutic exercises are physical activities that restore and maintain strength, endurance, flexibility, stability, and balance.

Therapeutic relationship: A relationship that is developed between a patient and a caregiver.

Thermotherapy: Intervention through the application of heat.

Treatment plan: The projected series and sequence of treatment procedures based on an individualized evaluation of what is needed to restore or improve the health and function of a patient in physical therapy; the treatment plan gives direction to the medical care and provides an approach to measure the effectiveness of treatment.

Visual Analog Scale (VAS): A visual analog scale is a form of quantifying information, such as pain, by using a standardized line that a patient marks.

Index

budgets
   for physical therapy services, 65
   types of, 65. *See also* specific types
Buerger, Leo, 6
burns
   examination of, 83
   physical therapy for, 94

C

CAD. *See* coronary artery disease (CAD)
calendars, as learning resource, 198
capital expense budget, 65
capitation, 177–178
CAPTE. *See* Commission on Accreditation in Physical Therapy Education (CAPTE)
cardiac rehabilitation, 92
   phases of, 92–93
cardiopulmonary physical therapy, 78, 86
   interventions for, 92–93
caring, as professionalism core value, 117–118
Centers for Medicare and Medicaid Services (CMS), 179, 180
certified athletic trainer (ATC), 48
Certified occupational therapy assistant (COTA), 41
CHF. *See* congestive heart failure (CHF)
children
   examination of, 80
   as pawns, 128
   with special needs, physical therapy services for, 124–125
Children Act of 1989, 101
China, ancient, 4
chronic care facilities, 59
chronological resume, 61
CI. *See* clinical instructor (CI)
civil court, 133
client management
   in clinical practice, 51–52
   elements, in *Guide to Physical Therapist Practice,* 53
clinical instructional activities, 172–174
clinical instructor (CI), 48
Clinical Practice Guidelines (CPGs), 183
clinical settings
   acute care facilities, 58
   chronic care facilities, 59
   departmental meetings in, 64–65
   home health care, 59–60
   hospice care facility, 59
   outpatient care facilities, 59
   physical therapist's responsibilities in, 34–35
   policy in, 63–64
   primary care facilities, 58
   private practice physical therapy, 60
   procedure manual in, 63–64
   quality assurance in, 66–67
   rehabilitation hospitals, 59
   risk management in, 67
   role of PTAs in, 26, 34
   school system physical therapy, 60
   skilled nursing facility, 58–59
   subacute care facilities, 58–59
clinical trends, in physical therapy, 67–68
Clinton, Bill, 16
closed postures, body language, 151
closed questions, 149
CMS. *See* Centers for Medicare and Medicaid Services (CMS)
Code of Ethics for the Physical Therapist, 213–215
Codman, Ernest A., 7
cognition, examination of, 75
cognitive stage, of empathy, 143
coming back to own feelings stage, of empathy, 143
Commission on Accreditation in Physical Therapy Education (CAPTE), 22, 25, 125
commitment, as attribute of success, 204

common laws, 122
communication, 141–154
   defined, 141
   with family, 147
   methods, for teaching/learning, 171–174
   nonverbal, 141–142, 146
   for patient education, 174
   therapeutic, 142–143
   verbal, 141–142, 146–149
   written, 152–154
communication skills, in interview, 62
compassion, 117–118
competence
   as attribute of success, 204
   and PTA career development, 206
computer-based documentation, 169
concurrent peer reviews, 66
confidentiality, 101–102
   HIPAA and, 102–107
congestive heart failure (CHF), 78, 86
constitutional laws, 122
continuing competence, 118
continuous passive motion (CPM), 88
copayment, 178
coronary artery disease (CAD), 86
costs
   for physical therapy services, 65–66
   types of, 65–66. *See also* specific types
COTA. *See* Certified occupational therapy assistant (COTA)
courteous listening, 149
courts of law, 132–133
cover letter, and physical therapy employment, 60
CPGs. *See* Clinical Practice Guidelines (CPGs)
CPM. *See* continuous passive motion (CPM)
cranial nerves, examination of, 75
criminal court, 132–133
crossing over stage, of empathy, 143
cryotherapy, 90
cultural bias, identification of, 112
cultural competence
   application of, 113
   defined, 108
   ethics and, 109–110
   in health care, 110–112
   law and, 109–110
   in physical therapy, 112–113
   understanding of, 108–109
cultural differences, 112–113
Current Procedural Terminology 2014, 178
cyanotic skin, 78
Cybex I Dynamometer, 7

D

deductibles, 178
defensible documentation, 168
DeLorme, Thomas, 7
departmental meetings, in clinical settings, 64–65
dependent variable, 183
dermatomes, 75
diagnosis
   in *Guide to Physical Therapist Practice,* 54
   physical therapy *vs.* medical, 55
diagnosis related groups (DRGs), 179
diaphoresis, 78
diathermy, 6
direct access, to physical therapist's services, 18, 19
direct costs, 65
direct personal supervision, 26
directed listening, 149
disability, 7
   description of, 122
   in *Guide to Physical Therapist Practice,* 54–55

L

laws
- administrative/regulatory, 122
- common, 122
- constitutional, 122
- and cultural competence, 109–110
- documentation for, 156, 166–167
- for domestic violence, 131–133
- ethics *vs.*, 99–100
- licensure, 125–126
- malpractice, 133–134
- and physical therapy practice, 122–125
- sources of, 122
- statutory, 122

leadership, and PTA career development, 207

learning
- barriers to, 174–175
- communication methods for, 171–174
- defined, 171
- principles, 193–194
- resources, 197–198. *See also* specific resources
- strategies, 199
- styles, 194–196. *See also* specific styles
- test-taking skills, 199–200

Leithauser, Daniel J., 7

library, as learning resource, 197

Libro del Exercicio (Mendez), 5

licensure
- laws for, 125–126
- for PTs/PTAs, 125–126

linear learning style, 196

Ling, Per Henrik, 5

listening
- effective in verbal communication, 149
- ineffective habits, 150–151
- kinds of, 149. *See also* specific types
- methods of effective, 150
- purposes of effective, 150

Lovett, Robert, 6

M

malpractice laws, 133–134
- in physical therapy, 135

managed care, 178

manipulation, as manual intervention technique, 91

manual muscle testing (MMT) examination, 76

manual passive stretching, 90

manual techniques, interventions, 91

manual therapy techniques, 57

marketing
- medical records/documentation for, 156
- of PHI, 106–107

massage, 91
- history of, 5
- Swedish, 5

Massage and Therapeutic Exercise (McMillan), 10

mastery years (1970-1996), of physical therapy, 14–16

McMillan, Mary, 8–10

measurement scales, 185–186

mechanotherapy room, 8

Medicaid, 14, 180–181

medical diagnosis, physical therapy diagnosis *vs.*, 54, 161

medical ethics *vs.* medical law, 99–100

medical law, medical ethics *vs.*, 99–100

medical records/documentation, 155
- for assurance of quality care, 156
- computer-based, 169
- for continuity of care, 156
- defensible, 168
- for legal reasons, 156, 166–167
- for marketing, 156
- for reimbursement, 156
- reports. *See* documentation reports, physical therapy
- types of, 157–158

medical social workers, 47

Medicare, 14, 179–180

Mendez, Christobal, 5

mental health social workers, 47

mental preparation, for interviews, 62–63

Mental Status Questionnaire (MSQ), 82

methods section, of research articles, 187–188

Mezger, Johan Georg, 5

MMT examination. *See* manual muscle testing (MMT) examination

mobilization, as manual intervention technique, 91

morals, 100

motor control, 91

motor function training, 57

motor learning, 91

movement therapy in hemiplegia, 92

MSQ. *See* Mental Status Questionnaire (MSQ)

multidisciplinary health care team, 37

Muscle Function (Wright), 6

muscular tone, examination of, 76

N

National Committee for Quality Assurance (NCQA), 110

National Foundation for Infantile Paralysis, 12

National Physical Therapy Examination (NPTE), 23, 39

NCQA. *See* National Committee for Quality Assurance (NCQA)

NDT. *See* neurodevelopmental treatment (NDT)

Neer Test, 77–78

negligence, 134–135

networking
- and physical therapy employment, 60
- and PTA career development, 205

neurodevelopmental treatment (NDT), 92

neurologic physical therapy, 86
- examination of, 78

neurologists, 44

neurophysiologic approaches, types of, 92. *See also* specific types

newborns, examination of, 79–80

non-maleficence, 100–101

non-weight bearing (NWB), 91

nonexperimental research, 183, 184

nonverbal communication, 141–142
- body language as, 151–152
- defined, 146, 151

Normative Model of Physical Therapist Assistant Education, 17

notice of privacy, 103

NPTE. *See* National Physical Therapy Examination (NPTE)

NRS. *See* Numerical Rating System (NRS)

Numerical Rating System (NRS), 75

nurses. *See* registered nurse (RN)

NWB. *See* non-weight bearing (NWB)

O

OASIS. *See* Outcome and Assessment Information Set (OASIS)

objective data, in SOAP notes, 162–164

occupational health nurses, 46

Occupational Safety and Health Administration (OSHA), 15, 126
- bloodborne pathogens standards, 126
- and infection controls, 126–127
- and universal precautions, 127

occupational therapists (OTs)
- areas of expertise, 40
- employment of, 40–41

occupational therapy assistants, 41

older adults, examination of, 81–82

open postures, body language, 151

open questions, 149

operating expense budget, 65

optimism, as attribute of success, 203

orientation, examination of, 75

orthopedic physical therapy, 86
- examination of, 77–78

orthopedic surgeons, 44

orthotics, 91